Vanished in Hiawatha

THE STORY OF THE CANTON ASYLUM FOR INSANE INDIANS

CARLA JOINSON

University of Nebraska Press
LINCOLN & LONDON

Publication of this volume was assisted by
the Virginia Faulkner Fund, established in
memory of Virginia Faulkner, editor in
chief of the University of Nebraska Press.

Library of Congress Cataloging-in-Publication Data
Names: Joinson, Carla, author.
Title: Vanished in Hiawatha: the story of the Canton
Asylum for insane Indians / Carla Joinson.
Description: Lincoln: University of Nebraska Press,
[2016] | Includes bibliographical references and index.
Identifiers: LCCN 2015033012
ISBN 9780803280984 (hardback: alk. paper)
ISBN 9780803288249 (epub)
ISBN 9780803288256 (mobi)
ISBN 9780803288263 (pdf)
Subjects: LCSH: Canton Asylum for Insane Indians.
Psychiatric hospitals—South Dakota—History. | Indi-
ans of North America—Mental health services—South
Dakota. | Indians, Treatment of—North America.
BISAC: SOCIAL SCIENCE / Ethnic Studies / Native
American Studies. | HISTORY / United States / State &
Local / Midwest (IA, IL, IN, KS, MI, MN, MO, ND, NE,
OH, SD, WI). | MEDICAL / History.
Classification: LCC RC445.S8 J65 2016
DDC 362.2/109783—dc23
LC record available at http://lccn.loc.gov/2015033012

Set in Minion Pro by L. Auten.

This book is dedicated to my husband, Ray. Thank you for supporting me both practically and emotionally during many long years of research, and for helping me remember that I have a life outside an archive.

CONTENTS

List of Illustrations . . viii

Introduction . . 1
1. Where Will All the Insane Indians Go? . . 9
2. Life in an Asylum . . 27
3. The Bad Start Begins . . 41
4. Helpless . . 59
5. A Superintendent in Trouble . . 73
6. Which Way to Canton? . . 89
7. The Reign of Harry Reid Hummer Begins . . 101
8. Reforms and Canton Asylum . . 119
9. Let the Investigations Begin . . 137
10. Life among the Indians . . 151
11. Another Sort of Prison . . 161
12. The World Outside . . 173
13. Hummer Can't Keep Up . . 195
14. Ripples in the Waters . . 211
15. The Winds of Change . . 227
16. The Gale Blows . . 249
Epilogue . . 269
Afterthoughts . . 273

Acknowledgments . . 287
Appendix A: Patients Treated at Canton
    Asylum . . 289
Appendix B: Patients Interred in Canton
    Asylum Cemetery . . 335
Appendix C: Patients Transferred to
    St. Elizabeths . . 345
Notes . . 349
Bibliography . . 381
Index . . 391

ILLUSTRATIONS

Following page 136

1. The Canton Asylum for Insane Indians
2. Cold wash day
3. Oscar S. Gifford
4. Atkins Hall at St. Elizabeths
5. Attendant's room at St. Elizabeths
6. Q Building dining room, St. Elizabeths
7. A code of conduct
8. Hydrotherapy at St. Elizabeths
9. Hydrotherapy pack treatment at St. Elizabeths
10. Common room, St. Elizabeths
11. St. Elizabeths staff, ca. 1919 or 1920
12. Tourist plate
13. Patient craft
14. Patient Susan Wishecoby, 1922
15. Susan Wishecoby with friends, 1922
16. Group of female patients, 1925
17. Female patients, 1925
18. Group of male patients, 1925
19. Dolls made by patients
20. Trephining kit

Vanished
in Hiawatha

Introduction

Institutions filled with discontented people will always have problems. So it was at the Canton Asylum for Insane Indians. No patient wanted to be there, its employees were overworked and underpaid, and its superintendent, Dr. Harry R. Hummer, had a reputation for combining arrogance and petty self-interest with an exacting nature and an explosive temper. It had taken two decades to ratchet up the tension to near flash point, but now the bickering and accusations of mismanagement demanded that an outsider come in and see once and for all what was going on. Dr. Samuel Silk, a senior medical officer at the federal government's psychiatric hospital in Washington DC, was that outsider.

Silk expected to find some problems when he arrived at the small federal facility for insane Indians on March 20, 1929. However, he had *not* expected to see an epileptic girl shackled to a water pipe. He had not expected to see a ten-year-old boy in a straitjacket, in a padlocked room. Nor had he expected to see a bedridden, helpless man with a brain tumor also padlocked in a room. With growing revulsion, Silk discovered that patients were sometimes restrained for months in metal wristlets—so long, in fact, that attendants occasionally lost the keys and had to saw through the links to free their captives. Urinals didn't flush, the air inside the wards reeked of excreta from overflowing chamber pots, and the corridors and rooms were dark and unforgivably squalid. In Silk's words, the Canton Asylum was a place of padlocks and chamber pots. He found one elderly female attendant charged with caring for all the female patients on two stories in the main building as well as those in the separate hospital; the same overstretched situation applied to the male wards. Though that day's extreme shorthandedness had been created by the abrupt departure of three employees, the situation spoke volumes. The Canton Asylum for Insane Indians had bigger problems than anyone had realized.

Nothing could be further from the stereotyped Victorian image of a madhouse than this peculiar facility, its superintendents, its patients, and most of all, its setting in the remote West of the dawning twentieth century. When I first read about the institution, I almost believed it was fictional—except that too many documents supported its existence. I had never considered writing anything involving the Bureau of Indian Affairs or Native Americans, but I couldn't get the asylum out of my mind. I saw immediately that something called the Silk Report held crucial information. I submitted a request for it through the state archives at the South Dakota State Historical Society and took the first step in following the threads of information that would result in this book.

Fortunately, I did not have to start entirely from scratch. Two documents (besides the Silk Report) were particularly helpful to me as I gained my bearings on this topic: the first was a graduate thesis by Kelli Sweet, and the second a doctoral dissertation by Todd Leahy. Both were informative and well researched, and they gave me an excellent overview of the asylum, its staff, its problems, and its failures.

Of course, no two researchers will come away with the same book or will focus on exactly the same points. Sweet's thesis gave an informative snapshot of the asylum that included its history, patient population, and chronological high points from creation to closure. Leahy offered a broader picture of the institution as a means of social control and devoted substantial attention to the history of U.S. Indian policy and other governmental methods of coercion and control.

My own book is different from either of these works. I have not focused so much on the racism and institutionalized coercion within the Bureau of Indian Affairs as on an explanation of the asylum within the broader context of American society. I have tried to delve into why an institution like this asylum could exist for so many years, and what made it tick as a viable part of the Interior Department. I have been able to explore at least some of the patients' stories, though much of their lives can be seen only through fragmented documents and a few of their own words. Above all, I have tried to capture a time and place that was as real as the broken hearts of the ill-served people who spent so many hopeless years at the Canton Asylum for Insane Indians.

When Canton Asylum came into existence, the mental health field was very much a growth industry. In 1860, just before the Civil War, there were 27.1 patients in hospitals and asylums per 100,000 of the population. In the next decade, that number jumped to 46 per 100,000. By 1890 the number of patients had risen to 117.6. From 1870 to 1936, the total number of patients in U.S. institutions jumped from 45,000 to 566,000.[1] How did this happen?

Mid-nineteenth-century mental health specialists with new philosophies brought hope to what had been previously considered an incurable condition. This confident new breed of doctors convinced the public that institutional care was vastly superior to home care. Though commitment often remained emotional and a last resort, families clearly found asylums a resource of great help. Increasingly, they brought their most difficult, burdensome family members to institutions, which in turn began to lose their original focus on comprehensive, personalized treatment. Far too quickly, insane asylums started to become warehouses full of long-term, chronically ill patients who had little chance of recovery. As doctors felt the pressure to admit more and more patients to relieve family distress, their institutions became overcrowded, rundown, and poorly staffed.

Underfunding—always an issue—completed the disaster. Underfunding didn't curtail admissions so much as it undercut an institution's ability to provide decent care. Inevitably, staff became stretched too thin. Repairs weren't made. Patient care became patient neglect. In Tennessee's Eastern State Hospital, rats and roaches were so prevalent that one employee claimed to have seen roaches crawling out from under a bandage on a patient's wounds. Rats were such a problem that staff brought in three cats to control them . . . and the rats ate the cats. These incidents from modern times (1971) are not completely authenticated but are so substantially plausible that they are included in the Tennessee Department of Mental Health's own history of its mental handicap policy.[2]

Canton Asylum was by no means unique in its failure to provide adequate care for its patients. It was not unique in being overcrowded and underfunded. What was unique was its patient population. No other federal institution for a specific ethnic group existed, and questions then and now focus on why the U.S. government needed a separate facility for Indians. The Interior Department, also responsible for the health of native peoples in Alaska, did not create a separate insane asylum there. In that vast territory, a local facility might have actually made sense in terms of saving everyone involved the significant emotional, travel, and expense burdens involved in seeking treatment in one of the lower mainland states.

Instead, the Interior Department sent all mentally ill Alaskans to a state asylum in Washington, and then beginning in 1900, to asylums in Oregon.[3] Juries of six men tried and committed men, women, and children—usually without benefit of competent psychiatric exams—to an insane asylum and kept them in jail until the spring thaw if they were unfortunate enough to have been committed during winter. Patients were then sent to a climate and culture completely different from their own, to recover as best they could. Though there are striking similarities between the Alaskan and Native American experiences, mental health care in the former case was contracted into a mainstream facility that did not target native peoples exclusively.

Many researchers have rankled at the ease with which unfortunate native peoples could be banished to an asylum, particularly those who did not speak English well. Though English speakers certainly held a slight advantage, *anyone* accused of insanity stood on rather shaky ground in the early 1900s, when there were few laws to adequately protect their rights. Canton's patients seldom had any rights to protect, since for at least a part of the asylum's existence they were wards of the federal government—meaning they could not legally make their own decisions on many matters—rather than citizens. Cultural and language barriers further exacerbated their difficulties in disputing charges of insanity.

White citizens defending their reason did not often show to best advantage when dragged in front of an insanity board or to the doors of an asylum. Fear, anger, and other perfectly reasonable emotions only served to underscore their accusers' contention that these—by now horrified or terrified—victims had lost their reason and self-control. Indians brought before white staff at a reservation could almost be guaranteed to answer questions inaccurately or with truculence, fear, or anger. At the time of Canton Asylum's closing, only nine patients there had been committed through a court order. Most had had their fates decided by a reservation agent or superintendent, who likely based his decision on a doctor or family member's judgment, or on his own aggravation with the person's behavior. A potential patient might not have known what was going on at all or might have known all too well that he or she was being deprived of liberty unfairly.

In certain ways, Canton Asylum was a fairly mainstream institution. Though few of its patients were certified as insane by physicians actually capable of making that assessment, they were not necessarily all misdiagnosed. In an era when a condition like epilepsy was considered a form of insanity, epileptic Indians merely joined the ranks of white patients who had been similarly judged. Syphilitic patients often shared the same fate as epileptics, as did others—white and native—who did not conform to societal expectations. And just like other institutions, Canton Asylum could act as a safety net that provided food and shelter for those who were not being cared for well at home.

I have been pleased during my research to discover a great deal of interest in the Canton Asylum for Insane Indians. One of my goals has been to provide documented information about the facility and to shed light on some of the practices there. I have read that the asylum had no inspections until Dr. Silk arrived in 1929. The reality is that it was inspected on the same schedule as other operations within the Interior Department and in fact sustained several additional special inspections brought on by complaints concerning its superintendents. I have read that no patient left the asylum except through death, a statement unsupported by the many letters and reports listing patient discharges. Understandably, however, without the entire picture available it does seem as though the only way out of Canton Asylum was to die, or that inspectors couldn't possibly have missed the dreadful situation developing there.

That is part of the exploration—how and why did this institution thrive for so many years? Who and what allowed the asylum's mismanagement to reach the proportions it did? How could people on the spot have been indifferent to the misery before them? And what can we learn from the experience?

I was an independent scholar before I took formal training in history. As the former, I learned how to dig up facts. As a grad student, I learned what to do with them. To list information from documents is not enough for a historian; there must also be thoughtful analysis and fact-based interpretation of the subject matter, which allows the researcher and readers to come to an understanding or conclusion about the material presented. This interpretative process is often referred to as the writer's argument, or point.

In one particular class I took, a newly tenured and enthusiastic professor hammered into our student heads the importance of argument and methodology until it haunted our dreams. I remember discussing the difficulty of sometimes understanding—or even finding—an author's argument and the consequent frustration for all of us as graduate students tasked with discussing it in our inevitable papers. I vowed then and there that when I wrote a book, I would make my argument clear and concise for the (hopefully) many students who might have to turn in a book analysis. One friend laughingly vowed to do just the opposite—she promised a stream-of-consciousness introduction that would leave students even more baffled about her argument than we often were with our assigned authors.

As funny as her thought was, I intend to keep my vow. The argument I make in my book is this: the Canton Asylum for Insane Indians could only have existed in the particular time and policy period in which it did, *and* the very conditions that allowed its creation also doomed it to failure. What do I mean by this? At any earlier time, the federal government's policy of annihilation would not have sanctioned caring for helpless members of Indian society; any later, and reformers intent on returning cultural independence to Indians would have fought an institution that so clearly violated their societal norms. Instead, a peculiar vortex of compassion, paternalism, and belief in medical advances managed to combine with a federal assimilation policy (as well as a number of other factors) to create an environment that made the establishment of an Indian insane asylum sound like a good idea. By exploring these factors, I hope I can help my readers understand what made the asylum acceptable to the federal government as well as why these same elements ensured it could not carry out its mission.

Besides laying out the facts, I have tried to keep the narrative immersed in its own time period by using the era's contemporary language: *Indian, alienist, insane asylum, defective, Indian Office,* and so on. To keep the material manageable, I have been forced to merely touch on certain aspects of the complex Native American and mental health care histories surrounding the Canton Asylum situation; I take full responsibility for deciding what to emphasize or to condense. Hopefully, those who find my exploration of a certain topic inadequate will be led to other resources through my notes and bibliography. When able, I have turned letters, statements, testimony, and affidavits into dialogue to break up the narration, but I have never embellished or changed what was actually written in my sources. And finally, I consulted people I considered reasonable voices for the asylum on the matter of using photographs of patients. Our discussions left me comfortable making the decision to do so in a respectful way.

I hope you will commit some time to this unique story and come away with your own thoughts on it, as I realize my conclusions are not necessarily the only ones that can be drawn. Further information continues to come to light about the asylum and its patients, and the future may well see a second, more illuminating act concerning their painful history.

1. Where Will All the Insane Indians Go?

Patients Frank Bear, a Navajo, and William Abdulhena, a Shoshone, faced off in the narrow hallway. They were nearly alone, for their attendant had locked the ward so he could leave the building. Bear hadn't been out much lately. Until a few days earlier he had been weak and needed rest, and attendants had conveniently padlocked him in his room. The newly released Bear may have been excited or just in a bad temper, or perhaps he said something to offend Abdulhena. Perhaps it was the other way around.

It was the end of September and quite cold, but the rooms and hallway were stuffy as always. No one saw what happened next, but the two men fought until their noisy thrashing sent another patient scurrying outside to report the brawl. Frank Bear's taste of freedom ended badly—when attendant E. B. Colby returned to the locked ward, Bear's eyeball was lying on the floor. There is no record of an investigation, though the asylum's superintendent did report that both men were doing "as well as could be expected."[1]

While patients didn't routinely lose their eyeballs, the locked ward and lack of supervised care present a good snapshot of life at the Canton Asylum for Insane Indians. The asylum began as a simple pork barrel project that later took on a life of its own and ultimately died as an embarrassment to the U.S. government. Along the way, it highlighted the worst aspects of mental health care and the relationship between the U.S. government and Native American interests during the early part of the twentieth century.[2]

Though that relationship had become top-down and heavy-handed by the asylum's time, Native Americans and European settlers had a long history of engagement, conflict, cooperation, and misunderstanding behind them. Well before thirteen New World colonies banded together to found their own country, settlers understood that coexisting with the peoples already in place was of paramount importance. Colonists frequently found generosity and assistance in their first encounters with Indians, who in turn received useful gifts and trade items (beads, cloth, metal goods like axes and pots, and firearms) beyond their own capabilities to manufacture. Periods of goodwill existed between native peoples and newcomers, though they were also heavily sprinkled with clashes that worried both groups.

Much of the hostility and opposition between natives and newcomers originated with the very different worldviews they held. These differences prevailed on several fronts, primarily property, lifestyle, and religion. Europeans colonists were vested in the idea of private ownership of land and animals and could not understand the more respectful relationship Native Americans held with nature and the animal world. Colonists considered it a failing in either character or culture that native peoples did not own individual plots of land and had not domesticated animals to any great extent. Though some native groups *had* domesticated turkey and a few other animals, most found little need to invest their time and labor this way. Small game was abundant, and Native Americans found it easier to follow herds of deer or buffalo than to tame smaller animals with a lesser payoff in terms of protein and hides. Privately held land made little sense for peoples who typically worked as a group, shared assets, and domiciled intermittently over large ranges of territory.

When colonists began to stake out private claims to what had been Native Americans' publicly held land, property issues arose. Beyond curtailing the area in which native peoples could live—enough in itself to cause resentment—colonists created additional problems by letting their domesticated animals, particularly swine, roam free. (When swine went feral they could become both dangerous and destructive.) Colonists unreasonably demanded respect for their property rights and took quick offense when Indians killed ravaging hogs or other wandering livestock.

European misunderstandings about native spirituality only deepened the expanding rift. Native Americans believed some animals possessed spiritual power (*manit* or *manitou*) and that guardian spirits could take animal form.[3] Colonists confused these beliefs with animal worship, which reinforced other misconceptions about the supposed depravity of Indian culture. Though other factors were involved, Europeans found native peoples' apparent worship of animal deities—along with their failure to domesticate animals, own property, and subsist primarily through agriculture—sure signs that they were culturally inferior. It was only a short step, then, for colonists to feel that they had not only a right, but an obligation, to uplift Indians by imposing their superior European culture on them.

By the time the United States decided to establish an insane asylum especially for native peoples, an Indian Office with authority and tenure was firmly in place. Even before American independence, the Second Continental Congress had created the Northern, Middle, and Southern Departments of Indian Affairs. The commissioners were charged with preserving peace and friendship with the Indians in their jurisdictions and with preventing them from aiding the British. After independence, the Congress of the Confederation created an Indian Department composed of a Northern and a Southern District, each headed by a superintendent. These superintendents fell under the authority of the secretary of war.

Early leaders of the American nation realized how important Indians were to both its commerce and peace; they also realized how unfairly many Indians had been treated by traders. Entrepreneurs who were willing to live under frontier conditions had been quick to establish trade with Indians, in some cases forming firm and loyal ties with their trading partners. Others had merely taken advantage of their positions. For the price of a $1,000 bond, district superintendents issued licenses to trade with Indians, which sometimes turned into a license to steal. With the fur trade so lucrative for whites, traders too often gave in to the temptation to gouge their customers in unfair exchanges that left Indians with just a few goods to represent an entire hunting season.

To stop some of the abuses, George Washington suggested a system of trading houses, which would be run by government personnel as nonprofit entities.[4] These establishments were not popular with nongovernment traders, who saw their influence and profits slowly eroding. Their vehement opposition to the government's efforts eventually led to the closure of the trading houses in 1820.

Early on, Washington had hoped to bring Indians into a peaceful relationship with the United States by helping them become familiar with the new country's people and ways. The idea that whites should live among Indians to gain their trust and persuade them to accept these different ways was attractive. Treaties often called for government agents to live among the relevant tribes, and these men became the face of the federal government for most Indians.

Treaty obligations created moral and financial pressures for the new government, which embraced treaties almost recklessly. These documents often used sweeping and generous language concerning the welfare of tribes who signed them. The September 29, 1817, treaty with the Wyandots, Senecas, Delawares, Shawnees, Pattawatamies, Ottawas, and Chippewas, for instance, promised to pay the Wyandot tribe "*annually, forever*, the sum of $4,000"; the Seneca tribe, "*annually, forever*, the sum of $500"; and so on. Some treaties promised even more: a treaty made at Fort Bridger, Utah Territory, in 1863 said, "It is declared that *a firm and perpetual peace* shall be henceforth maintained between the Shoshones nation and the United States."[5]

As the frontier expanded westward, treaty obligations required more agents, goods, and services. Expenses for the Indian Department in 1792 fell slightly below $40,000. By 1822 its expenses were a little over $120,000 and included pay for agents and subagents, as well as a hefty expenditure for "presents to Indians." In the previous two years, the department had added at least eighty new personnel, including superintendents, interpreters, and blacksmiths.[6]

The department by this time supported ninety-five treaties, with associated costs of nearly half a million dollars. This was still a nominal expense for truly staggering amounts of Native American land: in 1804 Indiana territorial governor William Henry Harrison negotiated a shadowy Sauk and Meskwaki (Sac and Fox) treaty that ceded fifty million acres of land in what is now Wisconsin, Illinois, and Missouri.[7] Between 1800 and 1812, Harrison pushed through fifteen treaties that added millions of acres to U.S. territory at a cost of not more than one cent an acre.[8] Treaty by relentless treaty, colonists pushed Indians out of their way and overwhelmed them like a rolling tide.

Actual payment of the goods and services that had been offered through treaties became an enormous problem for the War Department in the early eighteenth century. Its accountant had to process every claim the department generated, including all the payments to vendors for supplies, equipment, and whatever else it needed to perform its duties. The secretary of war also had to process claims from white settlers who suffered losses from Indian attacks or thefts, acting as a de facto examiner and judge on matters that had occurred hundreds of miles away. By law, the secretary could not delegate these responsibilities, and eventually the paperwork overwhelmed him. A committee looking into the problem revealed that "the accounts of the Indian Department, without a solitary exception, had remained unsettled from 1798 to the date of their report in 1816."[9]

Clearly, something had to be done. By 1824, Secretary of War John C. Calhoun decided he had the authority to create a Bureau of Indian Affairs within the War Department. He offered the position of head of the bureau to former superintendent of Indian trade Thomas L. McKenney. This delegation of authority was not legal, and McKenney could not actually act for the secretary and relieve him of his onerous paperwork load.

In 1832, after much prodding by Calhoun, McKenney, and the Senate Committee on Indian Affairs, Congress finally created the position of commissioner of Indian affairs, at a salary of $3,000 a year.[10] Oddly, the department was seldom called the Bureau of Indian Affairs by anyone other than Calhoun. Instead, personnel referred to their organization as the Indian Office, the Indian Bureau, the Indian Department, or the Indian Service until the Bureau of Indian Affairs officially adopted its current name in 1947.

This structure and agency necessary to establish jurisdiction over native peoples emerged just as white settlers headed south after the Revolutionary War. They quickly encountered the Cherokee, Creek, Choctaw, Chickasaw, and Seminole nations, which stood in the way of white expansion. In 1814 and 1818, Andrew Jackson (later president) acquired millions of acres of land for the United States by defeating Creeks and Seminoles in a number of battles. Some Indians migrated west at this point, but the government pursued them with a powerful new policy: in 1823 the Supreme Court ruled that, though Indians could occupy land, they could not hold title to it.[11] This set the stage for wholesale exploitation.

As president, Jackson introduced the Indian Removal Act (1830), which exchanged Indian land in the east for land in the west. (One well-known result of this act was the Cherokees' forced migration known as the Trail of Tears.) An unorganized Indian Territory in the West at first delineated separate spaces where whites and Indians could settle. Whites continued to encroach on native lands, however, and the federal government accommodated them. By the mid-1850s, a reservation system encased Indian populations within lands they had once occupied completely but that whites were now determined to settle. Calhoun's agency expanded to meet this new need and began to supervise Indian affairs on reservations through its agent system.[12]

By the time Indian Agent Peter Couchman of the Cheyenne River Agency wrote to the Indian Service in 1897 about the unpleasant conditions insane Indians faced on reservations, a large and organized entity existed to process his findings.[13] His words were not merely an observation or idle complaint, either; Couchman premised his letter and its appeal on an understanding that the government had an obligation to help Indians suffering from health problems—which rightfully included mental afflictions.

Health care had often been referenced in treaties as part of the government's payment for ceded land, and an 1832 Supreme Court decision had underscored the implied obligations within the Indian and federal relationship. Chief Justice John Marshall wrote that Indian tribes were merely "domestic dependent nations . . . their relation to the United States resembles that of a ward to his guardian."[14] Furthermore, documents like the 1855 Yakama Treaty and the 1868 Fort Laramie Treaty held specific promises that the U.S. government would supply physicians and medicine to native peoples or would educate them to provide these services themselves. Clearly, the federal government owed its wards basic amenities like food, clothing, and medical care.

Just like most treaty provisions and other federal promises, these requirements were honored only fitfully. The War Department initially held responsibility for providing medical care, but its services were sporadic. (Fueled by a desire to prevent epidemics close to military posts, for instance, army doctors sometimes gave Indians vaccinations.)[15] Little improvement followed after the Bureau of Indian Affairs was transferred to the Department of the Interior in 1849. It took more than two decades for that agency to establish a medical and educational division—which was typically underfunded and lasted briefly, from 1873 to 1877. By 1880 there were only seventy-seven physicians serving the entire Native American population (306,543 people) in the United States and its territories.[16]

Obviously, an Indian Office that could not provide adequate medical care could not provide specialized facilities or programs to help the insane, and these afflicted men and women often wound up in their local guardhouses. Agent Couchman told his superiors that most state institutions for the insane didn't like to accept Indians, who were wards of the federal government. Even when they did, they charged what the agent considered exorbitant fees for their care. Couchman then made a relatively simple suggestion that started the whole ball rolling: might it be a good idea to simply create a separate facility for insane Indians?

That suggestion was all Richard F. Pettigrew, a senator from South Dakota and chairman of the Senate Committee on Indian Affairs, needed to see when he first got hold of Couchman's letter. He thought a special asylum for Indians would be a dandy project for his home state and promptly sank his teeth into justifying it.[17]

Though a federal asylum for a specific ethnic group was without precedent, there were racial theories that supported the idea that such an institution might soon be needed. A prevailing line of thought considered white civilization superior to any other and included a belief that introducing civilization to a "savage" race like native Indians would cause many of its members to become insane.

The fact that the theory wasn't backed up by extraordinary numbers of insane Indians didn't seem to matter. Nor did the theory even accord with other outlandish theories within the medical field. In the Notes and Comment section of the January 1906 issue of the *American Journal of Insanity*, editors drew attention to the findings on complexion in an article by Major Charles E. Woodruff, U.S. Army Medical Corps, which had appeared in the *New York Medical Journal*. Woodruff believed that "the man with dark hair, brown eyes, and olive or brown skin has a tremendous advantage . . . and can evidently stand mental and nervous strains which blonds cannot endure except in cloudy places like Scotland or Norway."

However, like many elected officials, Pettigrew, a somewhat dour-looking figure with sleek hair and a full beard and mustache, mixed his idealism with practicality and an eye toward gain for his constituents. An attorney with only briefly successful forays into politics, Pettigrew was a tough legislator who was prepared to wrangle for the westerners he represented. He was as unfazed by a lack of substantiated data to support his projects as he was by snipes about his character or the occasional screaming match in the Senate.[18]

One particular clash in early 1900 speaks both of Pettigrew's mixed vision and of his character. He had been arguing about the "Philippine Question" resulting from the Spanish-American War and stated that he wanted to withdraw troops from the Philippines and declare the territory neutral. In support of his position, Pettigrew said that "to hold the Philipinos [sic] without their consent gives the lie to every Fourth of July oration ever delivered in this country."

After some hot debate, a fellow senator rose and gave an eloquent harangue against Pettigrew that ended with:

> It is but a step from individual hatred to national hatred. It is but a step . . . to hatred of the flag and the government that nourishes and protects them. It is fitting that such people should be represented here, and I know of nobody in the whole United States so fitted to speak for them as the Senator from South Dakota [Pettigrew] who during all the years which I have served with him in this body—and I speak only of his public utterances—has never had a kind or friendly word to say of any person or of a single cause.

Pettigrew could and did survive such onslaughts and wasn't without his own unreasonable pontifications. Juxtaposed with his enlightened sentiment about the "Philippine Question" was the remark he had made moments earlier. Pettigrew had just told the Senate that it was "an historical fact that the Aryan race could not live in the tropics. He could no more live there than a polar bear."[19]

Certainly the senator was just as capable of making racial inferences about Native Americans, and in 1897 Pettigrew introduced a bill to purchase land in South Dakota and build an asylum there. He argued that "the peculiar mental afflictions of the Indians" would make it impractical to treat them in connection with white patients. "Association with their ancient enemy has," he continued, "a harrowing effect upon them."[20]

Though Pettigrew's motivations may not have been pure, his contention that insane Indians needed help wasn't necessarily wrong. At the turn of the twentieth century, Native Americans were traumatized peoples who had faced genocide and been displaced numerous times due to the encroachment of white settlers on tribal lands. In the course of their displacement they had lost much of their cultural independence, as whites increasingly insisted they assimilate into the dominant Anglo culture. Their traditional foods, medicine, language, and religion had been dismissed as barbaric and unnecessary. And, as they lost almost everything of value—both physical and spiritual—Native Americans also fell into extreme poverty. Life on reservations meant poor-quality flour and beef instead of wild game and an abundance of roots, berries, and other traditional foods.[21] Vast landholdings within rich forests and on arable land dwindled to small allotments on reservations that could not support the population.[22] Loss was a new way of life.

Researchers studying the issue have seen strong links between poverty, social inequality, and mental health problems. Poverty was rampant on reservations, with land so poor that residents could not survive without supplemental federal rations. Simultaneously, native people were told that they belonged to a substandard race and culture. Their condition at the time would have been ripe for the development of problems like depression, excessive worry and anxiety, paranoia, and neuroses. That so very few Native Americans succumbed to these afflictions is a testament to their inner strength and resiliency.

Additionally, native peoples did not conceptualize insanity as Europeans did. Native Americans embraced the idea of balance; this concept made room for many deviations in behavior among the members of a community. A deaf woman could be a great healer, or a mentally impaired man might be a good hunter; both could still contribute to the well-being of the tribe and remain valuable members of it. Mind, body, and spirit were entwined in such a way that mental ability (or disability) did not receive special emphasis. Native Americans did not recognize mental conditions as a separate issue from the balance that all sought. Because they made little distinction between the physical and spiritual/mental, each tribe very likely treated a mentally afflicted person in the same way it treated a physically afflicted one.

Still, they and many other non-Western cultures held a concept that some people could not control their minds and therefore acted inappropriately, whether the cause was supernatural malevolence, a broken taboo, or an offended spirit. Despite some (white) experts' contention that there weren't any insane Indians at all, Native Americans had long recognized mental problems such as hysteria and depression in their people. They called these alienated states "soul loss" or "being lost to oneself."

Native Americans typically used herbal medicines, rituals, chants, drumming, and purification ceremonies to care for the sick and wounded; these were rendered through specialized professionals whose roles can be roughly translated as medicine men or women.[23] Most of these healers' efforts were directed at restoring stability, balance, harmony, and purity to the person or situation experiencing the problem. These learned practitioners also helped those who were considered "out of mind" or whom Westerners would label "insane."

Few practices were universal among the hundreds of Native American tribes living in North America, and that diversity included treatments for the insane. Most of the earliest accounts of Native American therapy necessarily come from European observers and show a variety of responses to mental illness. Some accounts cite the same indifference and violence toward the insane that Europeans had demonstrated for centuries, which included confinement, abandonment, or even execution.

Cases of acute, violent mania were supposed to indicate a cannibal (windigo) spirit that possessed the body of an insane person, and sufferers were killed so they could not become a menace to others. In a memoir, John R. Jewitt described an Indian driven insane by the ghosts of two men he had killed. When asked how to deal with the man's hallucinations and distraught behavior, Jewitt suggested a common remedy of the time: a beating. The beating was delivered with a will but did no good, and the man was allowed to simply remain mad.[24] Though other accounts also note a superstitious shunning of the afflicted, instances of stigmatization and violence are rare. The preponderance of written observations show clearly that most tribes considered insanity just another type of illness.

Healers tried to determine why a person was insane, often using dreams and divination. Many tribes believed that invisible spirits could interfere with the living by bewitching or possessing them. "There are very few madmen or idiots among the Indians," wrote Colonel Richard Dodge in 1882. "They are never confined or maltreated, but, being looked upon as directly under the malevolent influence of the Bad God, are rather avoided."[25]

If healers thought the supernatural was at fault, they tried using special rituals to counteract the evil power involved. Native Americans also believed that an enemy could obtain a charm or poison from a medicine man in order to inflict insanity on someone and that a counter-remedy or charm by a stronger healer would cure the afflicted.

The Creeks thought that a man who killed another could be haunted by the dead man's spirit and become insane, or "troubled in spirit," unless he was purified. To do so, a medicine man selected and placed four white pebbles in a cup of clear water. After performing ceremonies and singing specific songs, "the medicine man took some of the water into his mouth and spurted it violently upon the head of the insane man, also causing him to drink from the cup four times. It was believed that this performance gave the medicine man power over the insane person who thereafter was compelled to do his bidding and was treated in various ways until finally cured."[26]

The Pimas, who had always been bitter enemies of the Apaches, felt that even a drop of Apache blood could cause them sickness. Though it was laudable for a Pima to kill one or more Apaches, "it was believed that some of the progeny of that man would become insane or otherwise injuriously affected." To prevent or treat this disaster, a tuft of Apache hair could be tied "with a chicken hawk feather and an owl feather and burned in a certain way with greasewood, [and] would cure any sickness induced by the contact with the Apache."[27]

The Navajos believed that some mental afflictions were caused by breaking taboos or moral codes. For example, sibling incest was thought to cause generalized seizures. The Navajos called these seizures "moth sickness" because an afflicted person's twisting and convulsing movements resembled moths flittering around flames. These troubled patients could go through a curing ceremony (the Moth Way) for cleansing and atonement. A person who touched or brushed against a corpse might go mad, lose fertility, or die and needed a ceremony like the Enemy Way to release the dead person's ghost (which had come back to harm the living). Curing rites, like the Night Chant, called upon the spirits of sacred mountains to act on a sufferer's behalf.[28]

Native American cures surely didn't work all the time, but traditional methods did treat the mentally afflicted within their own cultural norms.[29] Pettigrew's proposal, however, would wrench them away from both their families and familiar surroundings. Almost all white patients' published accounts of their time in an insane asylum underscored their bewilderment and distress at entering such an unfamiliar world. At least these patients knew in a general way where they were and what was going on and could understand what they were being told to do.

Many of the patients targeted for treatment at the Canton Asylum for Insane Indians couldn't speak or understand English. This drawback would serve first to magnify the terror that accompanied commitment and then to interfere with effective treatment. The inability to communicate may not have been seen as an especial problem to lawmakers, if they even thought about it, but it was a fundamental reason the asylum could not fulfill its mission. However, the deeper problem with an asylum in Canton was its very existence: did the U.S. government really need the facility at all?

Then as now, congressional pork projects weren't always founded on truth or necessity. South Dakota boosters had unsuccessfully tried to make a case for moving the U.S. capital from Washington DC to South Dakota, citing the latter's balmy weather and gentle Chinook winds as healthier than Washington's humid atmosphere.[30] Anyone who believed them would have frozen to death after stepping off the train into a howling fifty-mile-an-hour wind in a South Dakota blizzard, but few Washington lawmakers believed every word coming from their compatriots. They declined to consider the proposition.

At the turn of the twentieth century, South Dakota did indeed present a different and much harsher type of life than that of the settled East. In the northern plains, a person could ride for days and see only a wolf or a rippling stream. The grassy land spread out so wide and empty that people could get lost in broad daylight if they didn't have a landmark to guide by.

This condition was amply demonstrated by Indiana governor Winfield Durban on a camping trip out west in 1904. He broke away from his friends to take an ill-advised solo horseback ride—providentially with two sandwiches—across the South Dakota plains. After deciding he'd ridden far enough, Durbin discovered that he couldn't see his friends, his campsite, or any landmarks.

He slept in the open that night, while his companions recruited several Indians to hunt for their missing pal, who was found two days later. The Indians quickly discovered him by following a trail that "had baffled his friends," according to the *Washington Post*. Durban was "nearly starved," the paper also noted, as the sandwiches he had taken had been small.[31]

South Dakota's endeavor to establish an asylum within its borders did not meet with any great degree of enthusiasm. Pettigrew tried hard to justify the need for such a separate asylum for Indians and sent his bill to the secretary of the interior, asking for a report "as to the practicability and utility of such an institution."[32]

He did have the support of the principals in the Indian Service, notably the acting commissioner of Indian affairs, Thomas P. Smith. Smith sent a letter to the secretary of the interior, saying that "the establishment of a government asylum, for insane Indians only, would, in my opinion, materially advance the interests of the Indian Service."[33] A week later, Smith informed the secretary that there were currently seven insane Indians being cared for in asylums around the country.

In September, after sounding out Indian agents and reservation superintendents, Commissioner of Indian Affairs W. A. Jones reported to the secretary of the interior with new numbers on possible candidates for an Indian insane asylum. The Pottawatomie Agency, Kansas, had two Indians, "partly idiotic," but not troublesome, while the Quapaw Agency, Indian Territory, had "six harmless idiots."

Rather than being a cruel or careless label, idiocy was an actual classification of mental deficiency, along with *imbecile, moron, borderline*, and *dull normal*. The term *idiot* generally meant a person with profound mental retardation and a mental age below three years. A *moron*, on the other hand, had a mental age of between seven and twelve. None of these intelligence-measuring terms implied insanity.

Jones continued his report, stating that Mission Agency, California, had seven insane Indians who should be cared for in an asylum. White Earth Agency, Minnesota, had eight who needed care; Crow Agency, Montana, had a few Indians who were slightly insane, but not requiring restraint in an asylum; and the Uintah and Ouray Agency, Utah, had "two harmless insane Indians." However, the reservation agent thought the two would "do better if allowed to remain on the reservation than to be confined in an asylum."

After investigation, the Committee on Indian Affairs found "fifty-five insane Indians and from fifteen to twenty idiotic Indians." The commissioner of Indian affairs, who had conducted his own inquiries, found "fifty-eight insane Indians, one doubtful, six idiotic, and two partly idiotic."

These figures were meant to justify an establishment like an asylum, if one could just ignore the preponderance of answers that showed how few among the Indian population needed such services. W. H. Clapp's reply to Pettigrew's inquiry is typical:

> There were 6,481 Indians belonging to this reservation at the last census. I have no knowledge of any insane person among them, nor have I learned of there being any such for several years, except in the case of one woman who had been mildly insane for some time, and who was transferred last summer to the Government Hospital for the Insane at Washington, where she now is.
>
> I do not think insanity nearly so common among these Indians as among whites.[34]

The secretary of the interior had forwarded Pettigrew's proposal to Dr. W. W. Godding, the superintendent of St. Elizabeths in Washington DC, the only existing federal institution for the insane. Godding pointed out that five of the seven insane Indians currently in asylums were already being treated at St. Elizabeths.[35]

Formally known as the Government Hospital for the Insane, St. Elizabeths had been created through the Civil and Diplomatic Appropriation Act of 1852 and received its first patient in 1855. Championed by mental health reformer Dorothea Dix, the facility's initial 250 beds were offered "to provide the most humane care and enlightened curative treatment of the insane of the Army, Navy, and the District of Columbia."

The hospital opened its doors to wounded soldiers during the Civil War. Patients hated to write home that they were staying in an insane asylum, so they began referring to the place as "St. Elizabeths," the name for the colonial land where the hospital stood. The hospital's name wasn't officially changed until 1916, but its nickname was firmly established by the time the existence of Canton Asylum became a question.[36]

Cycles of overcrowding and new construction occurred at St. Elizabeths as the government's needs grew, and in 1897 the hospital was overcrowded. However, Godding pointed out that $75,000 had been recently appropriated by Congress to ease overcrowding and that there could be no justification for a separate facility for Indian treatment. If any special provision were needed anywhere, he said, it should be for the much larger number of "African citizens" who needed help.

Congress ignored the objections and passed Pettigrew's bill, appropriating $45,000 for the asylum under the Indian Appropriation Act of 1899 (for fiscal year 1900). Oscar S. Gifford, the ex-mayor of Canton, South Dakota, and a former South Dakota congressional representative, supported Pettigrew's plan wholeheartedly. He was also convinced that his own city of residence, Canton, South Dakota, would be the best place to site the facility.[37]

Gifford, a popular, handsome man with a statesman's visage and a well-trimmed beard, could speak easily after years of practicing law. He argued that South Dakota was a particularly ideal spot for an asylum since it was close to reservations in all the western states. He added, "The value of favorable surroundings recognized in the treatment of insane whites has been entirely ignored in the case of the Redskin, with their insane growing more neglected, violent, and unmanageable."[38]

With South Dakota nominally established as an ideal general site for the insane asylum, Gifford pushed to show that Canton was ideal as the specific site for it. The bustling community had been an established town and the site of the (Lincoln) county courthouse years before South Dakota became the nation's fortieth state in 1889. Its small huddle of sod homes had survived grasshopper plagues, Indian hostilities, and harsh winters during its early territorial years. With its hotels, college, and railroad depot, Canton had been considered the gateway city to Dakota Territory and, afterward, to the state of South Dakota. By 1903, housing in Canton was so scarce that the new county treasurer couldn't move his family until he had built a dwelling from scratch.

Canton had a population of two thousand forward-looking people, including the influential Gifford. He and Pettigrew could make a good case for their project, at least on paper to congressmen in the east. They were eventually successful in landing the asylum, and Gifford handled the legal work to obtain one hundred acres near the Big Sioux River for thirty dollars an acre. Canton residents were thrilled, for the asylum meant a steady stream of work and trade, as well as a chance for the town to become famous through the asylum's unique patient population.

Speculation in the local papers ran high as to who would be the institution's first superintendent, the favorite being Canton's own Gifford. Architect John Charles, who had experience building asylums, designed the facility, and the lowest bidder for construction, H. S. Pelton and Company, began work on it in 1900. With only a few glitches here and there (a fire in the paint storage area halted construction for a short time), the facility went up as fast as weather conditions would permit.

When completed, the building was impressive, positioned as it was on an otherwise empty landscape two miles from town. The asylum overlooked the Big Sioux River, which was visually appealing to visitors but undoubtedly a cruel sight for homesick eyes that could follow the line of its flowing water. Even though the grounds were set on plenty of acreage under a soaring South Dakota sky, the layers of brick and stone spoke of nothing but lost freedom and compulsion. A woven steel fence seven feet high surrounded the grounds.

Designed to resemble a Maltese cross, which looks like four arrowheads pointing toward the center of a circle, the two-story building, with its jasper granite foundations, looked as solid as the authority that had placed it there. The four wards (two in the east for males and two in the west for females) were 52 by 64 feet each, with hard maple floors and lofty, eleven-foot ceilings that gave them a spacious feeling.

A cement-floored basement ran under the entire seventy-five-room building, a solid 184 feet in length and 114 feet wide in the center. Ward doors led into a cheerful dining room, just north of the kitchen.

The building had all the modern amenities, too, a marvel for patients and probably most staff. Electric light, supplied by the Canton General Electric Light Company, fed 120 lamps that shone like trapped stars on a moonless night. Steam radiators kept the rooms comfortable, water was supplied by a convenient well, and range toilets negated the need to dash to outhouses in inclement weather.[39] A sewer system siphoned waste from the building into a septic tank in the approved, hygienic manner.[40]

Funds allowed for a staff consisting of a superintendent and assistant superintendent, a financial clerk, an attendant, three laborers, and a night watch, for a total personnel expenditure of $7,180 per annum. The asylum was completed on October 1, 1901, and Gifford was indeed selected as the asylum's first superintendent. He accepted the position November 6, and then he and his wife traveled to Washington DC to complete plans for furnishing the asylum.

On December 31, 1902, the entire asylum staff turned out in below-freezing weather to meet their first patient, a thirty-three-year-old Sioux man named Edward Hedges, at the train station.[41] Heading the facility was Canton's favorite son, Oscar S. Gifford, an attorney without any experience whatsoever in medicine, mental illness, or hospital management. The asylum was thus launched with a grand bad start that set up a pattern of mismanagement until the day it shut its doors.

2. Life in an Asylum

If there is a wailing and gnashing of teeth by those condemned to hell, it might sound like the anguished lamentation of patients first entering the Canton Asylum for Insane Indians. Torn from their homes, family, and friends, they arrived at Canton in varying states of confusion and fear. To deal with their anxiety and upheaval, these Native American patients often resorted to cultural practices that still offered comfort and couldn't be ripped away. Some fell back on silence and observation, while others gave vent to their feelings through heartbreaking chants and singing. Clara Christopher, a longtime asylum employee, said she had to "hold my ears so I couldn't hear 'em."[1]

Indian patients' decidedly negative introduction to asylum life was not so different from that of non-Indians. Almost no one went to an insane asylum voluntarily and many white patients wrote about the trickery or force used to get them into one. However, the Indian experience included a feature that undoubtedly made everything else worse: they were far from home. State institutions across the country were just that: asylums servicing patients within a relatively small geographic area. And, in recognition of the difficulties long distances imposed on both families and patients, many states built more than one insane asylum so they could provide services regionally. Despite their dismay at confinement, state asylum patients at least knew that if need be, family or friends could get to the institution in a timely manner.

Unlike state facilities, Canton Asylum took patients from across the nation. Canton, South Dakota, might have been centrally located for most Indian populations, but it was still hundreds—sometimes more than a thousand—miles away from its patients' homes. Their families might never be able to afford a trip there, even if they could negotiate the intricacies of long-distance travel. And, since many families had not sought the commitment in the first place, they were left nearly as forlorn and helpless as the relative they might never see again.

Whether or not psychiatric help was necessary, a long-distance trip to a lonely, foreign setting would not have been therapeutic for most Indian patients. Wrenched abruptly from kin and community, their isolation and loneliness would have exacerbated any underlying problem and added to their misery. The enormous disservice of sending Native American patients to a facility so remote from their own cultural experience and language cannot be overemphasized.

Nothing about the typical top-down, question-dotted Anglo medical exam would have been comfortable for a new patient. In modern times, Dr. Lori Arviso Alvord, the first female surgeon in the Navajo tribe, describes her own initial patient consultation with another Navajo doctor as akin to "drawing verbal circles around each other." In a typically nondirect Navajo style, their conversation lasted at least a half an hour before they began to discuss Alvord's problem; they first needed to get comfortable with each other by exploring their respective clan relationships until they could discover where their lives intersected. The two doctors spoke English, but Alvord noted that the Navajo language is nuanced with tones and inflections that would simply escape the notice of a nonspeaker. An encounter between white doctors and Native Americans at the turn of the twentieth century would have been marked by both discomfort and miscommunication under the best of circumstances.

Federal assimilation policy did not offer the best of circumstances, nor did it concern itself with any nuances of Indian language or culture. Assimilation—admittedly more humane than annihilation—was still cruel. While the government had abandoned its attempts to kill all Indians physically, its leaders still wanted to kill them culturally. Captain Richard H. Pratt's famous remark at an 1892 convention embodied the new attitude best: "A great general has said that the only good Indian is a dead one, and that high sanction of his destruction has been an enormous factor in promoting Indian massacres. In a sense, I agree with the sentiment, but only in this: that all the Indian there is in the race should be dead. Kill the Indian in him, and save the man."

Pratt had earlier (1879) founded the Carlisle Indian School at Carlisle Barracks, Pennsylvania, and most of the government's nearly 150 Indian boarding schools were modeled after it. In the boarding schools' quasi-military setting, Pratt and other administrators systematically "assimilated" Indian children by stripping them of every aspect of their tribal culture—including their names. Once in school, they were expected to adopt the hair, clothing, education, food production—and medical practices—prevailing in the larger Anglo culture.

Unfortunately for Indians, whites had become quite comfortable with both "scientific" medicine and insane asylums in the decades just prior to and following the Civil War. With all these years of experience to draw on, doctors rooted in European thinking firmly believed that the help they offered would be far superior to anything "savages" could have devised over thousands of years. Indeed, asylums provided a necessary service for the feebler members of even white society, since the rate of insanity was rising in that population. Alienists (an early term for doctors trained in mental health) attributed the increase in mental distress to the rapid social changes of the nineteenth-century. They assumed that "uncivilized" Indians suffered from this shock of progress even more than whites.

Despite their unintended trauma to Native Americans, asylums presented a breakthrough in both the nation's attitude toward and its treatment of mental illness. Though the condition still held a stigma, most people saw sufferers as "unfortunates" who needed help and kindly care—best given in a centrally located "mind hospital" like an asylum. This had not always been so.

Since before the country was founded, mental health care had been a family affair, with members doling out whatever treatments their ignorance or enlightenment suggested. The extreme stereotype of a disheveled madman in chains was birthed in reality; families might restrain mentally ill members for convenience or safety for days, weeks, or months at a time or beat, maltreat, ignore, and starve them with few curbs on their decisions.[2]

When colonial settlements grew large enough that the indigent insane became a problem, town fathers usually resolved the issue by farming out their care to the lowest bidder. Churches and charities also stepped in, but eventually, most mentally ill people wound up in jails, poorhouses, and hospitals, where care was indifferent if not down-right cruel. Reverend Louis Dwight, an agent for the American Bible Society in the early 1800s, wrote of an insane man housed in jail who had left his unheated room "but twice in eight years."[3]

Institutions like jails and poorhouses could not address the problems of the insane, and housing them there only created hardships for the sane cohabitants. Over time, hospitals began to set aside areas for insane patients, until in Virginia, the Public Hospital for Persons of Insane and Disordered Minds (established in 1770 and opened in 1773) became the first state hospital in America built exclusively for the insane. The country's oldest hospital (Pennsylvania Hospital, 1751) was founded much earlier and did treat the insane, but not exclusively.

Despite their recognition that the insane had special problems that did not warrant incarceration or punishment, community leaders did not often extend them much beyond the barest of custodial care. Relief came from influences overseas, primarily France, where work by Dr. Philippe Pinel did much to stop the practice of incarcerating the insane in dismal conditions for life. Pinel had a novel idea for the time: that the insane were sick and could actually get well if they were properly treated. Defying tradition, Pinel spent time with insane patients, talked to them and discovered their histories, and treated them with kindness and consideration for their feelings.

Pinel eventually extended his radical break in tradition even further—he decided to discard restraints. To everyone's surprise Pinel wasn't attacked and murdered by his unloosed patients but instead enjoyed an amazing cure rate. With that success, he opened the door for a new kind of thinking about insanity—that patients could be cured, that kindness was preferable to brutality, and that insanity need not be a life sentence. Pinel's new method was known as "moral treatment," appealing as it did to patients' own discipline and moral sensibilities to aid in their recovery rather than physical restraint and force imposed from the outside.

Pinel's work began in the late 1700s, as did William Tuke's similar work in England, and by the early 1830s their philosophy began to influence America.[4] When early psychiatrists (alienists) adopted these gentler, individualized approaches, they *did* cure patients in astonishing numbers compared to anything that had gone before. To alienists, it began to make sense to build centralized hospitals for treating the insane in a stabilized, systematic fashion.

The idea was a hard sell to legislators and the general public, who didn't always understand the return on their investment. However, in one of life's incongruous juxtapositions, a frail spinster accomplished what medical men could not force. In 1841 Dorothea Lynde Dix taught a Sunday School class for female prisoners in the East Cambridge House of Corrections. She was dismayed to discover that insane people in the same jail were housed in bitterly cold rooms because they supposedly did not feel the cold. Without political clout or even the right to vote, she launched an attack on the Massachusetts legislature amid both approval and stormy protest. The result was the enlargement of Massachusetts's overcrowded lunatic asylum in Worcester, which had opened in 1833. Combining whirlwind energy and pit bull stubbornness, Dix campaigned for the relief of the insane for the rest of her life. Besides helping to establish the Government Hospital for the Insane in Washington DC, Dix was instrumental in establishing or enlarging thirty-two other mental hospitals.[5]

Though earlier institutions at times were clean and cheerful and provided kindly care, some had been little more than mediocre poorhouses. Pragmatic Americans, fired up by Dix and the idealism of the era, eventually embraced the idea of asylums, especially when their masters—insane asylum superintendents—revealed astonishing treatments and astounding cure rates. Hope had finally entered the field.

Burgeoning interest in mental disease during the 1830s and later brought some of the most dedicated and eager men of the era into practice, and they gradually imposed a certain degree of standardization and cohesiveness to the treatment of mental illness. In particular, they considered the facility itself—the very building—to be an important contributor to patient wellness. They urged state legislators to establish asylums in peaceful, lovely settings and to make the structures magnificent. Consequently, palatial asylums became almost the norm, and their grand architecture, imposing grounds, and beautiful interiors impressed vacillating relatives who might be reluctant to release a family member to a doctor and institution away from home.[6]

The Canton Asylum for Insane Indians, though small in comparison to the country's grander asylums and to St. Elizabeths in Washington DC, was nonetheless a handsome building with cutting-edge amenities that were considerably admired by visitors. Indian patients and their families, however, never had the opportunity to visit before a commitment, and this impressive domicile and treatment center would not have held much emotional comfort to anyone outside the white culture that had built it. Instead, it would be the same old story for Indian patients: discard every traditional way of managing stress and illness and submit to the white way of doing it.

Native Americans on reservations did have limited experience with white doctors and their medical practices, but their own medicine was (and is) far richer in ritual and community. At home, something like a Navajo "sing" or chantway was a communal affair that could take several days or nights and involve dozens of memorized songs. At home, healing ceremonies and chants were attended by dozens of people who knew the afflicted person. At home, patients could understand the language spoken around them despite their fear, pain, or confusion. Healers usually knew both the patient and his or her community well and could take the sufferer's dreams, possible encounters with evil forces, and imbalances in psychic harmony into account as they unhurriedly assessed the problem and gained the patient's trust.[7]

Part of the healing was undoubtedly due to faith and the comfort of known ritual—or superstition, as most medical men saw it. Alienists sought to substitute their scientific approach for native methods and beliefs, no matter how jarring or incomprehensible the attempt might be. Even whites of the time who might have believed implicitly in the power of prayer and the comfort of hymns could not transfer their experiences with the prevailing Christian culture to see the similarities in Native American experience. The result was that nothing of value to Native Americans' mental health was incorporated into any treatment they received in an asylum.

For the most part, the Indian patient's introduction to the white way via Canton Asylum would begin in the most distressing manner possible. A good many patients had spent their precommitment time in a reservation guardhouse or a town jail before the Indian agent and Superintendent Gifford could make arrangements for their trip to Canton. Indians arriving at Canton Asylum from outside the immediate area were stressed and fatigued from a long train trip. Many would be frightened or confused and desperately unwilling to stay.

If typical Indian Service procedure is anything to go by, new patients could expect little empathy from the Canton Asylum staff, though the callousness and indifference some showed later might have been tempered initially by excitement and a considerable effort to make the institution a success. Few documents that describe Canton Asylum's patient routine remain, but the Indian Service's attitude toward its charges consistently reflected the same sense of white superiority and high-handedness that other groups displayed toward Native Americans.

When Indian day schools were first established on reservations (usually by religious societies), new students faced a similar type of displacement as Canton Asylum's patients, along with a typically authoritarian introduction to their new way of life. "Our first work was to wash and clothe them. . . . We had a tub of water for ablutions; then Mr. P. armed with stout shears, soon reduced their hair to our notions of taste and comfort," wrote one former staff member about the Fort Coffee Academy.[8]

A similar disregard for culture took place when new patients arrived at the Canton Asylum. They were first searched by attendants, who were to "take charge of all valuables and weapons" by turning them over to the superintendent. Attendants then examined and inventoried the patient's possessions and issued new clothes if necessary. Attendants gave the newcomer a bath, during which they examined him or her for obvious cuts or sores and deloused him if necessary. It is not too much of a leap to believe they would have cut patients' hair if they felt the need—a traumatic enough event for a school-aged youth in Indian culture, and a nearly debilitating one to an adult who believed long hair had a spiritual dimension. Much of this in-processing would have been done without explanation if there were language barriers. The bottom line: patients were intimately examined by strangers, stripped and washed, their valuables taken away, and possibly humiliated or psychologically traumatized by a change to European-style "citizen clothing" or a haircut.

At some point in the process, attendants would introduce new patients to their roommate(s), show them how to use the sink, tub, and toilet, and if they were ambulatory, show them over the ward and grounds. Almost everything about the asylum was guaranteed to be strange and uncomfortable, from the bathroom facilities to rooming with strangers. As one patient put it, "They call this an Indian Asylum and then why don't the Indians have it more like their home?"

As in most asylums, the day was regimented and task-oriented, and it began *early*. Patients got up shortly after attendants arose and then dressed and ate.[9] Patients assisted with chores if they were at all able and the weather reasonably clement. Men worked in the garden or on the farm (typically hoeing weeds and picking and preparing vegetables for cooking) or helped one of the laborers in his duties. If skilled enough, female patients might sew a little, but they were often put to a more energetic use in scrubbing floors and working in the laundry, dining room, or kitchen. Patients also helped tend to their fellow patients, usually by dressing them, taking them to the toilet, or wheeling them to the dining room.[10] It might be noted that these latter activities were strictly against Indian Office rules.

At least at first, patient rooms were scrubbed down once a week, and the asylum hallway and stairways twice a week—an ambitious undertaking for the few attendants to manage amid all their other duties. They were fortunate indeed to be able to draw upon the unpaid labor of their charges. The original, therapeutic intent of this labor was both to occupy patients' minds and time and to instill routine and discipline into their days. Labor was designed to be light and of short duration, but complaints in patients' letters from later in the asylum's existence suggest that the original intent was lost. Their resentment is apparent in such phrases as "all I do is work," and "we got to do it all."

Some patients appreciated that chores helped the time pass more quickly, but one who wrote about scrubbing the floors of her ward and then varnishing them (with the help of an attendant), as well as cleaning the walls, clearly did more than light, therapeutic labor.[11] After what could certainly be a long, wearing day, patients were taken to their wards at eight o'clock and locked in by nine o'clock.[12]

How did life at Canton Asylum around the turn of the century compare to that of other asylums? Getting beyond the very foreign nature of the Native American experience, it probably did not differ that much. Like most other new facilities, Canton Asylum was well sited, clean, and modern. And unlike many other asylums, it did not face immediate overcrowding. New state asylums were often built because existing ones were bursting at the seams; a rush of backlogged patients quickly filled the new one and left it little better than its older counterpart. Canton Asylum took several years to fill to capacity, a bit of breathing space that ought to have given the staff time to implement best practices and iron out any glitches. There was never enough money, of course, but the same was true of other asylums. One exception might have been Massachusetts's McLean Asylum, which catered to the very wealthy and could afford the best of amenities, both scientific and domestic.

Though built much earlier, by 1908 McLean Asylum offered all that Massachusetts's blue bloods could want for their unfortunate sons and daughters. Its gutters were copper; every patient's room had a fireplace, closet, and toilet; rooms were soundproofed; and the food ran toward lobster and lamb rather than the endless beans and beef of more bare-bones establishments. Four- and five-bedroom "cottages" with servants' quarters, living room, dining room, and sunroom (as well as kitchen, pantry, and the like) housed *one* patient and support staff. (There were only four of these cottages, but their presence suggests the lavishness the rest of the patients enjoyed.) The asylum had tennis courts, a golf course, an art room, a recreation room, and by 1904, a forty-four-hundred-volume library. Among its building were houses for "excited" men and women, two gymnasiums, a chapel, and stables.[13]

Despite being able to offer such luxury, McLean still relied at heart on the age's standard treatment for insanity: exercise and healthy habits, agreeable busywork, hydrotherapy, and hypnotics and other medicines that alleviated patients' worst symptoms. Though its residents were considered too refined for manual labor to provide any benefit, the asylum offered lessons in woodcarving, drawing, painting, and fancy work. One innovation that would have served Canton Asylum's patients well was McLean's incorporation of special nursing care during a patient's first few hours, to "lessen the shock of admission."

Admission to an asylum could indeed be a shock for Indian patients. One night a man might find himself in a jail cell after a bit of trouble, and the next day he would be waiting for a room at the Canton Asylum. Though the commissioner of Indian affairs was the only one with authority to commit an Indian to the asylum and the asylum superintendent the only one who could say whether there was room for another patient, it was the Indian agent who ordinarily requested that an Indian be admitted to the facility. It was at this local level that any abuse of the commitment process was likely to start.

Outside Washington DC, Indian agents were second in hierarchy after field superintendents. They usually handled the day-to-day details of running Indian affairs and were the primary government representative most Indians encountered. Agents distributed annuities, licensed traders, enforced alcohol bans, supervised Indian education, and acted as the final government authority in resolving most problems on reservations. They had little supervision and great power; men of integrity could do a great deal of good, and men without it could behave almost any way they wanted.

It was to this agent that families who wanted help dealing with a difficult family member, doctors who noticed deteriorating patients, and even law enforcement officials tired of coping with problem Indians turned when the issue of insanity arose. The agent (a man with no medical background) assessed and validated the psychiatric need, then requested permission from the commissioner of Indian affairs to send the person to Canton Asylum. The commissioner, in turn, ascertained whether the asylum had room and was willing to accept the patient. If so, permission was given and one of the asylum's staff would usually go to the patient's reservation to escort him or her back to Canton. Few patients were certified insane through any court or board hearing, but legal or medical certification wasn't a prerequisite for commitment. The commissioner of Indian affairs and Gifford alike simply accepted the agent's word that the patient required the asylum's services.

This relaxed commitment procedure, coupled with the lack of psychiatric training available on reservations, certainly led to unfair commitments. Some were undoubtedly made in good faith, but others stemmed from exasperation, spite, or convenience. On November 19, 1907, an Indian agent requested that William L. Greenfeather (Cherokee) be admitted to Canton Asylum. He and another man were considered too dangerous to be at large and were being held in jail awaiting commitment. On December 4, 1907, the agent told Gifford that Greenfeather had recovered. It was an insane episode of remarkably short duration.[14]

Peter Thompson Good Boy represents another example of an Indian railroaded into an insanity diagnosis for the convenience of law enforcement and perhaps his Indian agent. Good Boy was accused of stealing two horses, a crime he had been similarly convicted of (and received a pardon for) years earlier. This time he was considered to have developed a "mania" for horse theft. Good Boy acted somewhat oddly in jail, and his defense counsel requested a sanity hearing. The county insanity commission agreed that Good Boy was insane, and for some obscure reason he was sent to St. Elizabeths in Washington DC in 1913.

Good Boy was a model patient at the institution. He displayed no mental symptoms or hallucinations (the supposed cause of his commitment) and passed his time either beading or helping the hospital staff. Good Boy's only mental aberration was a belief that he had been sent to St. Elizabeths because he had pled not guilty to horse theft and because he had some damning information concerning one of the men who had accused him of it. Friends apparently agitated for his release strongly enough that two congressmen looked into the matter.

A St. Elizabeths staff member wrote a synopsis of the case, saying that Good Boy's "past conduct here has been exemplary, and aside from his ideas concerning Whipple [the man accusing him of horse theft], he has manifested no signs of psychosis." He suggested Good Boy be sent to a facility closer to home until the conflicting stories surrounding his situation could be cleared up.

Good Boy arrived at the Canton Asylum for Insane Indians on May 3, 1916, where he was diagnosed with "constitutional inferiority" (obsessions and compulsions), delusions of persecution, and litigiousness—all related to his (presumably false) allegations. As the asylum superintendent had time and opportunity to observe the patient, he found that Good Boy was a leader among the patients, preferred his fellow Lakota (Sioux) patients, teased other patients, could be profane, and was occasionally depressed. Good Boy remained at Canton Asylum until 1918.

Unfortunately, few records exist about Good Boy's time there, his experiences, or even why he was suddenly released. Though no one at St. Elizabeths believed Good Boy was sent to their facility because of the reasons he stated, it seems extremely odd that his reservation agent or the county insanity commission would choose to send a Sioux Indian from a South Dakota reservation (Rosebud) to a Washington DC institution nearly 1,500 miles away rather than to a facility around 250 miles away.[15]

These troublesome cases reflect the same types of abuses that had occurred—and continued to occur—in white society whenever vulnerability met loose commitment laws. Elizabeth Parsons Ware married a minister named Theophilus Packard in 1839 and bore him six children. As time went on, Mrs. Packard became interested in Universalism and phrenology, and eventually her husband decided she had gone insane. He brought two doctors from his congregation (and the sheriff) to his home. The doctors took Mrs. Packard's pulse, declared her insane, and sent her to the Jacksonville asylum in Illinois.

Mrs. Packard was eventually released (as incurable) to the care of her husband three years later. Locked in her room, she managed to communicate with a friend who secured an attorney for her. In 1864, Packard embroiled her husband in a very public legal dispute during which a jury—after deliberating seven minutes—pronounced her sane.

Thereafter she used her fame as a platform to campaign against unfair commitment laws as well as for the protection of married women's earnings. Mrs. Packard detailed her experience in a book, *Modern Persecution; or, Insane Asylums Unveiled*. Her services on behalf of the insane resulted in reform of commitment laws—particularly bringing more people into the process—and patient safeguards; these reforms are generally referred to as Packard Laws.

Though Packard's case was a cause célèbre, not much had changed by 1910, when New York resident Alice Stanton Smith was arrested for carrying a small revolver for protection. She was sent to Bellevue Hospital, stripped, forced into a chair, and injected with morphine. Later she was examined by doctors and released as sane. Adorned with diamonds and other gems, Smith appeared the following week in the Harlem Police Court—not nearly so much to defend herself against the crime of carrying a revolver as to plead with the court not to send her back to Bellevue.

The court magistrate called the psychopathic ward at Bellevue to talk to the examining physicians there, who told him that Smith "was only a little nervous and eccentric." Her brother, however, had sent his agent to court, saying that Smith had been doing "crazy acts" for twenty years. When pressed for an example, the agent said that Smith had once slapped the faces of guests at a dinner party.

Smith told the court that her relatives had tried to have her declared insane a number of times, adding, "It is only through publicity that I can be freed from these attacks my relatives are making on me." The court magistrate, stressing that he had the latitude to do so, sent the heiress back to Bellevue. Smith, evidently the owner of a large home on Long Island and worth $100,000 in her own right, did not appear deranged to the reporters in the court.[16] Plainly, even wealth and social connections could not protect persons against commitment if a more powerful adversary pushed for it. Indian patients at Canton Asylum had neither and were particularly vulnerable to abuse from men in authority.

The Canton Asylum for Insane Indians differed radically from other mental institutions in some respects. A physician offered medical care to asylum patients, but a matron rather than a nurse supervised his attendant staff. This arrangement mimicked Indian boarding schools, but unlike the schools, Canton Asylum did not have the interpreters who could have made life so much better for everyone involved. The asylum also had no laboratory, on-site hospital, or staff training program, nor a regional body to provide oversight (such as a board of trustees, board of state charities, board of visitors, etc.) as other mental institutions did. Instead, Canton Asylum depended on the time and expertise of its lay commissioner of Indian affairs more than a thousand miles away.

Consequently, the asylum reflected federal Indian policy and societal attitudes more than the possibilities of advanced psychiatric care. As the century marched on and the asylum dealt with the pressures of a changing era, observers close to it found much to praise and to criticize. Their voices created a record of arrogance, insight, obliviousness, concern, and callousness as they imposed their views and values on a vulnerable population.

The only voices that would not be heard were those of patients.

3. The Bad Start Begins

Though some of its mythic elements were fading, the West was not quite settled at the beginning of the twentieth century. Calamity Jane died the year Canton Asylum opened, and plenty of people were alive who had actually known Jesse James, Billy the Kid, Sitting Bull, and Crazy Horse. Towns like Deadwood, South Dakota, and Tombstone, Arizona, had barely wiped the shine off their history of gold and silver mines, gunfights, and gambling. And Pancho Villa's attacks on the United States and his escape to Mexico would take place more than a decade in the future.

The end of the nineteenth century had teemed with invention and breakthroughs. Thomas Edison's incandescent lightbulb brightened the world in 1879, while Guglielmo Marconi's 1895 invention of the wireless radio—along with Alexander Graham Bell's 1876 invention, the telephone—connected its people. Felix Hoffman synthesized aspirin in 1897, and three years later surgeons began to use rubber gloves. Wilhelm Rontgen took the first X-ray in 1895.

The mental health field, however, had not seen the same breakthroughs. Though decried by many, wrist and ankle restraints, handcuffs, camisoles (straitjackets), rope, and chains were still commonplace in many American insane asylums and were sanctioned methods of control. Alienists from Europe who visited these asylums often criticized their free use of restraints. American alienists simply replied that the spirit of freedom instilled in the American psyche made their patients harder to handle than European ones.

When the idea for Canton Asylum first arose, medical science could offer only a few hypnotic medicines, like chloral, sulfanol, hyoscine, and bromides to relieve the suffering of patients in asylums. Sigmund Freud had coined the term *psychoanalysis* only a few years earlier (1896), but his time-intensive, personal approach to probing the psyche did not become popular in the United States for many years. Asylums with hundreds or thousands of patients didn't have the luxury of using the method and instead kept patients calm and occupied with old stand-bys like occupational and water therapies.

The study of insanity itself was in a relatively freewheeling state at the turn of the century, just as it had been for many years. The premier issue of the *American Journal of Insanity* in 1844 described a spontane-ous attack of insanity (apparently brought on by a robust prescription of bleeding, purging, and blistering for dyspepsia) and the fortunate man's subsequent instantaneous recovery. By 1900 most alienists felt that spontaneous recovery from madness was highly unlikely, but they could only theorize about insanity's actual cause and cure. Certain condi-tions like alcoholism or syphilis could bring on symptoms of madness, but not every alcoholic or syphilitic became insane. War could drive men mad or create heroes, and though some women became deranged enough after childbirth to harm their infants, the vast majority of moth-ers cared for their children tenderly. What, then, created insanity?

Insanity was attributed to many nebulous causes, like excessive men-tal stimulation, a disordered stomach, domestic difficulties, sunstroke, jealousy, kidney disease, gout, faulty education, and sudden frights or shocks. Professor W. H. Walling, MD, in his interesting book *Sex-ology* (1904), related the case of a child who contracted the masturba-tion habit "spontaneously at the age of five years, who, in spite of all that could be done, died at sixteen, having lost his reason at eleven." Doctors warned parents about the "dangers of puberty" and railed against marriages that could pass on hereditary insanity from epilepsy.

In fact, alienists were still floundering with the problem of describ-ing and diagnosing their patients. These learned men bundled most mental conditions under the all-encompassing term *dementia*, which essentially meant "weakening or deterioration of the mental faculties" as opposed to problems present at birth. After that essential tag, how-ever, alienists could have a field day slapping on whatever descriptive term best suited the symptoms: *senile* dementia, *epileptic, organic, par-alytic, hysteric, acute, chronic,* and so on. The term *mental defective* or simply *defective* could mean almost anything the physician chose it to mean, while the public's kindlier label of *feeblemindedness* also encompassed a world of conditions.[1]

Frustrations arose because symptoms of insanity varied so much from patient to patient and had nebulous criteria. Physicians dealing strictly with physical problems could easily diagnose a broken leg or a fever, but when did an idea stop being an interest or passion and develop into an obsession or monomania? How long could a man or woman remain in a blue mood before one decided such melancholy required professional help to overcome? At what point did a frightening temper or frenzied reaction to a situation cross over into a manic disturbance? What one family could tolerate might nearly destroy another, just as some portions of society had a wider tolerance for erratic or odd behavior than others. The American Psychiatric Association even today readily admits that there are few reliable laboratory tests or biomarkers for mental illness—which leaves enormous flexibility in deciding what is or is not "normal." In the end, insanity tends to be a subjective diagnosis (typically) arrived at by people other than the suspected victim.

Normative behavior has changed over time, making it difficult to nail down a definition of true mental illness. A mystic who would have been readily accepted as the mouthpiece of God five hundred years ago might need to accompany his message with a miracle to be credible today. A rambunctious child labeled as "all boy" in the 1800s might be on medication for attention deficit disorder in the modern classroom. With a few exceptions such as incest and murder, almost no behaviors have been universally described as aberrant. Even the definition of murder has been fluid, considering that human sacrifice was once acceptable in some cultures and self-defense continues as a legitimate reason to kill someone.

Modern critics are wary of the medicalization of mental disorders, as well as their proliferation. The point is valid: the American Psychiatric Association's "bible" of mental disease, the *Diagnostic and Statistical Manual of Mental Disorders* (currently DSM-5) has gone from a volume of 130 pages listing 106 disorders in DSM-1's 1952 edition to 991 pages describing over 300 disorders today. Some people hesitate to swallow all its data. Is a first-class case of coffee jitters really a "caffeine-induced sleep disorder"? Do children have "intermittent explosive disorders" rather than temper tantrums? Just as important—are all the named conditions actually types of mental illness rather than individual deviations from the average?[2]

The history of psychiatry as a defined field is relatively short. And like most new fields, psychiatry presented a somewhat murky picture as new practitioners began to sort out fact from conjecture, the absurd from the practical, and to create and evaluate theories about the origins of mental illness. Though groundbreakers, alienists coupled their real lack of understanding about the causes of insanity with an inability to treat it effectively. This led to much experimentation within asylums as alienists applied treatments based on their own worldviews, experiences, and backgrounds toward resolving the problems they saw in their patients.

One enthusiastically touted treatment was static electricity, administered to patients through a battery. Dr. H. R. Niles's 1897 article in the *American Journal of Insanity* described its advantages over the galvanization method, which required stripping the patient almost completely and then rubbing a wet electrode over his or her skin for ten or twenty minutes. With the preferred *static* electricity treatment, however, the patient could sit comfortably in a chair next to revolving glass plates.

"No accurate and satisfactory means of measuring the dose has yet been discovered," Dr. Niles acknowledged. However, he added in the next sentence, "To augment the dose, we make a direct metallic connection between the machine and the patient by placing his foot upon the connecting rod or chain."

The treatment presents a surreal picture at best, as do some of the medically sanctioned water treatments—hydrotherapy—of the early 1900s, which were sometimes carried on for days. Attendants might take an excited or violent patient and forcibly plunge him headfirst into a cold bath while restraining his limbs. Sometimes attendants wrapped a patient snugly in a wet sheet for several hours or days. They often wrapped a blanket around the sheet, and if the patient resisted, added another wet sheet to the layers and tied it to the bed. Restrained like mummies, the patients were often violently frantic until they finally quieted down from exhaustion.[3]

Dr. Emmet C. Dent, writing in 1902, gave a case study of a woman identified as "R.B., age 30; married," with a diagnosis of "mania acuta with delirium." The woman received a number of baths, accompanied by ice packs on her head, and according to Dent, "she was removed from the bath, given a stimulant and placed in a number of warm woolen blankets in order to continue the perspiration. She remained in the dry pack for about two hours, after which she became quiet and slept soundly for several hours; the bowels and kidneys acted freely."

After describing a number of patients who underwent some rather extraordinary baths, wraps, and packs, Dr. Dent added, "Of course we meet with more or less opposition on the part of the patient to these baths."

Oscar S. Gifford joined this unrestrained and largely self-regulated group as the newly minted superintendent of an insane asylum. When he visited Washington to see about furnishing his new asylum, he undoubtedly visited St. Elizabeths and picked up as much practical advice as possible. Otherwise, he had no training or experience and probably couldn't have deciphered much of practical use from an article in the *American Journal of Insanity* if he had wished to educate himself. As superintendent, however, he likely felt that his role was to manage and that a trained physician would look after the technicalities of caring for his insane patients. Meanwhile, he could continue to reside at his comfortable home, unlike most superintendents, who lived at the facilities they supervised, and continue to stay involved with business and social affairs.

This third year of the new century was looking like a good one for Gifford. Besides his new job, he had just pulled off a coup for the city by getting the new insane asylum placed there: that victory gave him the approval and applause of his fellow businessmen and civic boosters. He—and any merchant with a little business savvy—knew that government money would roll into the town's coffers via wages, supplies, and services to the (hopefully) expanding facility. For Canton to become famous through this unique institution was a hoped-for bonus.

On the home front, things were also sweet. Though he had married the Ohio native Phoebe Fuller in 1874 and had a son, Oscar Bailey, who would graduate from college that June, Gifford had been a widower for several years before remarrying in 1899. His civic efforts had now certainly secured his bride, the former Jenny Rudolph, a place as one of Canton's preeminent hostesses.

Small though it was, Canton had a bustling social scene that included church outings and festivities, lectures, plays, numerous civic clubs, and at-home entertaining. As a newlywed, Jenny Gifford had given a "delightful talk" on recent literature at the Teacher's Institute in Lincoln County. As an established matron with a prominent husband, she now filled her parlor with lilies and hosted friends using fine china and silver, or more casually with bouquets of chrysanthemums, card games, and midnight repasts. As the wife of a unique government facility's administrator, her opportunities for social advancement may have looked boundless.

Gifford was already successful as a businessman and attorney, and this new venture must have looked like an especially tasty piece of metaphoric cake to savor. His new position involved a heartening mix of uncomplicated assets and responsibilities: Gifford had seven employees, one patient, and a brand-new facility. No one could have foreseen that he would take a little less than five years to bungle matters irretrievably.

It was an astonishing turn of events when it happened, because Gifford was Canton's favorite son for a reason. The town was a bustling little metropolis-in-waiting in 1903, with big ideas as well as modern telephone service, fine churches, a number of impressive brick buildings, and the first real schoolhouse in Lincoln County.[4] Gifford had been Canton's mayor before Dakota Territory even became a state and could be counted on to throw his energy behind any forward-thinking initiative. He was the kind of go-getter that every up-and-coming community needed: smart, energetic, friendly, and loyal.

Like many white men in the old West of that era, Gifford came from the East. Born in New York in 1842, he moved with his parents to Wisconsin and then Illinois, where he served in the state's Elgin Battery as a private from 1863 to 1865. He studied law in Belvidere, Illinois, and was admitted to the bar in 1870. Gifford moved to South Dakota's Lincoln County in 1871 and from that time forward maintained a reciprocally loyal relationship with South Dakota that would continue until he died.

Gifford stood out from many of Canton's residents simply because he was so well-educated, well-traveled, and politically connected. Many of the town's residents had been homesteaders or came from that stock, typically from a Norwegian background. Early schools in the region had often taught children—and sometimes their parents—English. And even at the turn of the century, many schools still kept to a farming schedule that required only three months of school during the winter and one in spring. Eighth-grade graduation was an achievement.

Socially, Gifford could dance circles around any competitor. He was a Mason and the organization's former grand master of the Territory of Dakota (1882–84), as well as a member of several other social organizations. He had a knack for making friends and forming relationships that helped him get elected to a number of influential positions, including territorial delegate to the Forty-Ninth and Fiftieth Congresses.

Gifford was generally credited as the legislative force that helped create the state of South Dakota. During his term as a territorial delegate, he pushed what was known as the omnibus bill, a measure that split the huge Dakota Territory into North and South Dakota and also allowed Montana and Washington to become states. Gifford later helped establish industrial schools for Indians at Flandreau and Pierre (South Dakota) and many day schools on reservations.[5] Any project he couldn't get behind and make a success of didn't seem worth doing, and yet . . .

It was dark and lonely inside the asylum when Gifford's first patient died. One unsupervised night watchman, making rounds in whatever manner he chose, flashed a lantern occasionally amid the dark walls of the nearly empty building. Since only eight people (counting Gifford) were employed at the facility, the probability is good that only a couple of them were on duty that night.

Robert Brings Plenty, a twenty-one-year-old Sioux from South Dakota's Pine Ridge Reservation, had been diagnosed with chronic epileptic dementia, denoting the era's judgment that epilepsy and insanity were intertwined. His seizure that night began with a cry—the involuntary scream or moan caused by spasms in the larynx. He fell, convulsed, rolled his eyes, and thrashed in violent spasms. Blood-specked foam dribbled from his mouth as he gasped for breath, lost control of his bowel and bladder, and died alone in his room about an hour after he had gone to bed.[6]

In most of Canton Asylum's reports, few words were wasted on people when the facilities could be praised. Brings Plenty's death warranted only a quarter of a sentence in Gifford's annual report to the secretary of the interior for 1903, though the assistant superintendent, Dr. John Turner, managed to give the incident a whole sentence in his portion. What neither man mentioned was Brings Plenty's lone grave, disturbing the bucolic grounds at Canton Asylum like a grim wound. Gifford had just run into what was to become a surprisingly common occurrence: no one would claim the body.

Whether the young man's seizure could have been prevented is anyone's guess; treatment for epilepsy at the time consisted primarily of dosing the patient with bromides and sedatives.[7] Gifford made it clear (as did later inspectors) that Dr. Turner very properly administered these kinds of preventatives, along with sedating hot baths. The real question is not about Brings Plenty's medical care, but why he died the way he did. Even if medical treatment couldn't have prevented his death, did he have to die alone?

Perhaps that was inevitable. Though there were only sixteen patients—ten males and six females—staying at Canton Asylum on May 20, 1903, surely anyone with a modicum of scheduling expertise could have anticipated trouble. Only eight people were available to run a twenty-four-hour caretaking facility, and three of them had nothing to do with patient care.[8] The remaining five personnel had to somehow split shifts and provide coverage to the separated male and female quarters while allowing each other a little time off.

To make matters worse, the only female employee was a laborer who likely did laundry and cooking in addition to a few attendant duties. The two male laborers cared for the building and its grounds, though they were also likely to be conscripted at times for attendant duties. That really left only a male attendant and Dr. Turner specifically designated to provide twenty-four-hour care and attention to sixteen patients. It simply couldn't be done.

Though the number of personnel increased as the asylum added patients, the workload continued to stretch staff to the limit. Attendant Mary J. Smith gave an inspector a taste of her responsibilities in 1907: in the morning she dressed six patients—two paralytics, one with spastic diplegia (a form of cerebral palsy characterized by severe stiffness in the legs), and "three that are so crazy they do not know enough to put their clothes on." After that, she waited table in the dining room, gave medicine to patients and took them to the toilet, and then made eleven beds. Wednesday mornings she scrubbed five small rooms, one large room, one large hall, three short halls, and a pair of steps. She then dusted and changed bandages on her patients if they needed it. All the while, she undoubtedly found herself called to do other things as patients' needs arose, and sometimes she battled physically with them. Smith bitterly told about a patient who threw a cuspidor at her and bit her, and she mentioned other instances of patient violence against herself and others. The attendant finally got her patients to bed around nine o'clock, and at six the next morning she rose and started it all over again. It was a wearing life, particularly since attendants had their rooms on the wards and could never really get away from the pressure and the atmosphere. Even twenty years later when the asylum employed more staff, attendants' days lasted from 6:00 a.m. to 6:00 p.m. (and until 8:00 p.m. every third day), with one half day off each week and a couple of Sundays off a month.[9]

The situation at Canton certainly merited a smug "I told you so" from St. Elizabeths' former superintendent, Dr. Godding, who had flatly advised that a separate Indian asylum wasn't necessary. Canton Asylum's small scale made it impossible to run with the same efficiencies of manpower and supplies as the larger institution, which had by now received nearly a million dollars for new buildings. Though Canton's sixteen patients could still have been easily absorbed into St. Elizabeths, such a course of action wasn't even considered.

These first patients' experiences might have been worse. Many asylums in 1903 did use restraints and experimental courses of treatment, while others centered their programs around rest, hydrotherapy of some sort, and manual labor. As a layperson, Gifford probably found the latter approach quite acceptable and apparently tried to implement it. As presented in his reports, his facility offered an almost enlightened approach to patient care: cleanliness, light manual labor, amusements, and tonics, sedatives, or antispasmodics as needed. His female patients were being taught "calisthenics, numbers and object lessons" as well as how to clean their rooms and help in the dining room and kitchen.

The heart of his patients' troubles lay in their identity. It was a given, of course, that "normal" behavior mirrored that of white society. When confused or frightened Indians entered Canton Asylum, they could easily have reacted with violence or disorientation that further "proved" their insanity. Sadly, Pettigrew and Gifford hadn't been lying when they argued that care for insane Indians often suffered when they were thrown in with whites; they had just been too blind to see that bringing them to an institution *run* by whites would simply add its own painful twist.

For their parts, both Gifford and his assistant superintendent, Dr. John F. Turner, saw their asylum as far more palatable for their patients than the reservation. "The agencies or school officers have no proper means to care for them, and the miserably wretched condition of many of these patients when received can scarcely be exaggerated," Gifford told the Indian commissioner in 1905.[10]

His reports spoke of patients who came in, filthy and wretched, from their home reservations to a place where they could receive medical care, food, shelter, and compassionate treatment. Gifford claimed, "The establishment of the asylum was certainly a humane and proper thing to do. . . . Previous to opening the asylum this unfortunate class of Indians were without proper care or attention. None of them were wanted anywhere, nor by anybody."[11]

Young James Hathorn was one of the wretches from that "unfortunate class" that made their way to Canton. His mother had endured a difficult delivery due to a narrow pelvis and likely an unskilled midwife. Hathorn's brain had been compressed at some point during birth, causing a hemorrhage that led to motor problems. His muscles clenched in involuntary spasms that traveled down his flesh without warning, while his hands and feet writhed in slow, snakelike movements that kept his body in constant motion. Though bright, the Navajo child couldn't speak. It was a hopeless situation for an Indian boy.

Canton staff hung the eight-year-old Hathorn by the shoulders from an oaken frame with a horizontal beam, his arms imprisoned in a tightly laced jacket. He dangled for an hour three times a day, suspended by spiral springs. He was also given antispasmodics and tonics. In an article appearing in the *New Albany Medical Herald*, Dr. Turner said the child was greatly helped by the treatment, which was given in an attempt to straighten Hathorn's limbs from almost permanent contraction.

Turner gave no indication whether this treatment was private or took place in a room accessible to other patients, but the facility never had a separate place for the children sent there. At best, the boy would have been placed with the quietest of the twenty-three male patients confined to the facility when he arrived, or in one of two single-bed rooms in the north wing, which unfortunately didn't receive daylight.

Little James Hathorn was eight years old when he came to Canton. After living thirteen years in the insane asylum—most of his life—he died there at the age of twenty-one.[12] The fact that a child was in an asylum at all says less about the reservation that gave him up and the facility that took him in than it does about the government agency that would allow a child that age to be placed in such a situation.

Within the Indian Office as a whole, sensitivity toward Indians and their needs was actively discouraged, and its assimilation program clearly reflected that attitude. Indian children were sent to boarding schools for the express purpose of breaking their family and tribal bonds, and they were sternly reminded not to start speaking their native languages again upon their return to the reservation. Indian agents often gave adults jobs and allotments of food and supplies based on their ability to adopt the white man's ways.[13]

In 1887 another far-reaching piece of legislation, the Dawes Act, had worked to devastate traditional Indian life and culture. Senator Henry Dawes of Massachusetts, who introduced the act, believed that holding land in common as tribes did was inefficient and not in the best interest of either Indians or whites. His act proposed to allot Indians a certain amount of land (which they would own outright after twenty-five years) within the vast western acreage set aside for them and then open up unallotted land for white settlement.[14]

Some people believed that this system would help Indians assimilate into the white population more easily. By owning private land, Indians could farm—a new and disdained occupation for many tribes—and become self-sufficient. Adopting the superior white way of making a living would make reservation Indians less "Indian" and also end their dependence on government assistance and oversight.

What the act actually did was to strip Indians of vast landholdings and force them to farm on mostly arid, poor land that couldn't sustain them. Their populations became riddled with disease. The government began distributing food and supplies to reservations, partly to keep people alive and partly as a tool to coerce impoverished Native Americans to do as they were told.

The government's policies played out in a number of ways, but they were consistently biased. In his 1902 annual report, Commissioner of Indian Affairs W. A. Jones wrote to his superiors about the furor that a "short-hair" order had caused. The text of this order would be comical if it were satire instead of reality:

> This office desires to call your attention to a few customs among the Indians which it is believed should be modified or discontinued.
>
> The wearing of long hair by the male population of your agency is not in keeping with the advancement they are making, or will soon be expected to make, in civilization.
>
> . . . On many of the reservations the Indians of both sexes paint, claiming that it keeps the skin warm in winter and cool in summer, but instead this paint melts when the Indian perspires and runs down into the eyes. The use of this paint leads to many diseases of the eyes among those Indians who paint. . . . You are therefore directed to induce your male Indians to cut their hair, and both sexes to stop painting.

Jones explained to the secretary of the interior that for some inexplicable reason this order had caused an uproar in the press. He wrote, "To my surprise this letter [the order] created considerable excitement . . . and the impression seemed to prevail that the Government intended to accomplish its desires by main strength and awkwardness." Jones added that "from beginning to end there is not a single suggestion of force as applied to the untutored Indian, but, on the contrary, patience, tact, perseverance."

What Jones seemed to miss in the order (which he quoted in its entirety to the secretary) were these words: "With your Indian employees and those Indians who draw rations and supplies, this will be an easy matter, as noncompliance with this order may be made a reason for discharging (the employee) or withholding rations and supplies. . . . Employment, supplies, etc., should be withheld until they do comply. If they become obstreperous about the matter a short confinement in the guardhouse at hard labor with shorn locks, should furnish a cure."[15]

The attitude behind this order was part of the problem with the Indian Office's leadership. It gave tacit permission to ride roughshod over Native American culture, and perhaps it is the reason that Gifford thought nothing of arranging an Episcopal burial service for the dead epileptic Robert Brings Plenty.

At least Gifford hadn't adopted the Indian Office's apparent attitude that Brings Plenty's death didn't matter at all. When the superintendent informed the young man's reservation agent of his passing and asked for instructions about the body, he received no answer. Gifford then took it upon himself to find a pretty area on the grounds to start a cemetery, draw a map that showed where the body was buried, and arrange for a service. When he asked the Indian Office for money to erect a marker, the agency did give him some attention—it replied that the expense was unwarranted.

Perhaps Gifford did the best he could in this and many other unanticipated situations. As a merchant, attorney, and politician, Gifford couldn't have enjoyed the mundane details involved in caring for people with ailments he didn't have the training to understand. He may have seen his position as one of management and delegation, contentedly passing on the real work to the people under him. By the end of fiscal year 1903, Gifford's patients represented nine different tribes that embraced languages and customs he and his staff couldn't understand—a mixture that would have brewed up trouble for even the savviest of administrators.

One stark deficiency at the asylum was that no staff members except Dr. Turner, who had graduated from Baltimore Medical College in 1893, were actually trained for the positions they held. From Gifford on down, the basis for presumed competence came solely from any practical knowledge employees may have picked up during their lives. The civil service exam for candidates who wanted to register for positions at the asylum consisted of three subjects: age (twenty points), physical condition (twenty points), and experience (sixty points).[16]

Though experience held more weight than the other two qualifications, few people in the small town of Canton could be expected to have the relevant experience needed. Yet what qualified individuals wanted to uproot themselves from a city to live in the still rough-edged town of Canton, where they would earn at most forty dollars a month?

Schoolteachers anywhere could earn forty-five dollars a month, and they were at a premium on the frontier. In March 1903 the *New York Sun* reported a "teacher famine" in South Dakota. Tacked to the local schoolhouse in Hye County was this sign: "TEACHER WANTED—If single, must be old and unattractive, as two wealthy bachelors threaten to marry the next teacher of this school."

Noncompetitive salaries aside, the unskilled employees at the asylum didn't even really know what they were supposed to do. Excepting Dr. Turner and the night watchman (who could be presumed to understand that he was supposed to walk around the building at night), employees at Canton Asylum had little idea what their positions required.

Even Turner had never worked in an insane asylum before. Gifford certainly hadn't, and neither had the clothing merchant—now the facility's financial clerk—Charles Seely. Seely's wife became matron of the establishment, while Anna Turner became its seamstress. As housewives, both women presumably knew a bit about feeding, clothing, and managing dependents, but neither had any actual experience in their new positions. Though well-defined instructions existed for employees (nine for the superintendent and forty-three for the others) Gifford didn't distribute them. Consequently, staff treated patients just about the way they felt would be best.[17]

Some of Gifford's problem also lay in his choice of staff: the ex-mayor deliberately favored Canton residents over other job seekers. At least one inspector would explain that delinquency with the admission that the asylum didn't pay a wage that made its jobs attractive to anyone coming from a distance. Regardless, Gifford dipped only into a pool of workers with the backgrounds, prejudices, and skill levels likely to be found in a remote western area.

Despite his own and his staff's deficiencies, Gifford *could* keep up the pep talk and boosterism that defined his political personality. Gifford's 1903 report to the commissioner of Indian affairs presented a lovely façade that, for a while at least, hid the fact that Canton Asylum had been built on a foundation of problems.

The facility itself probably looked as good as an insane asylum could. Two steel arched gates embraced the entrance, and the words "Hiawatha Asylum" had been placed upon the archway. Though the archways were erected with the consent of the commissioner of Indian affairs, there seems to be no record that speaks to the reason behind this embellishment. Locally, however, the asylum was nearly always referred to as "Hiawatha."

The grounds included the main building, a pump and power house, sewer and receiving tank, horse barn and cow barn, and grazing meadows. Gifford mentioned that twelve hundred trees had been planted, including evergreens, elm, maple, and mountain ash, along with many ornamental shrubs. A grass lawn surrounded the building, and cows grazed in adjoining meadows. It was a pleasant place in the summer, when Gifford wrote and submitted his report, and it was a pleasant picture that he painted.

However, Gifford had lived in Canton for over twenty-five years and knew the idyllic scene he presented couldn't last. The windswept land in his adopted state turned brittle in the searing heat of summer and iron-hard during winter, when temperatures plunged below zero, often into the negative double digits. On May 1, 1903, a relentless sleet storm encased the hands of the courthouse clock in ice so thick that they stopped turning. Two years later—again in May—a late snowstorm caused a heavy loss of livestock when it dumped a foot of snow on the tender, green prairie grass.

Almost always the wind blew: steady onslaughts that could chill a man to the bone in winter or suck him dry in summer. In March 1902 a blizzard sent three feet of snow and a line of zero temperatures along the eastern part of the state. A month after the blizzard, papers reported temperatures in the nineties. What were his patients going to do outside, when the elements decided to act this way?

Their comfort inside the building wasn't guaranteed, either. Besides the surface water that collected around the boiler pit, the region's hard water itself had begun to present a problem. Gifford observed in his second annual report (August 1904) that "the capacity of the soft-water system is insufficient to store enough soft water for the entire year."

The system he referred to may have simply been a holding tank, but he made it clear that the insufficiency caused a problem. In the same sentence he wrote that "the well water is not suitable for drinking and bathing purposes."

Though the well water was hard, the heating coal was soft and therefore created a dirty burn that left a light black film on every surface.[18] Mentally ill patients were often physically ill as well, and the contaminated air would have exacerbated the tubercular patients' symptoms. Between the extra filth supplied by the coal and the inability of the hard water to make good suds, the institution rapidly lost its shine. No amount of washing could get the grungy sheets and clothing really clean, and subsequent investigations showed that the staff at Canton didn't always put their backs into their jobs, anyway.

Like many a political animal before and after, however, Gifford could ignore unpleasant realities and spin a situation to present its best side. That spin began almost immediately, though his first report in 1903 (with a new building and freshly hired staff) didn't need much help from him. Gifford wrote proudly, "The asylum is so equipped and managed that the patients are provided with well cooked, wholesome food; frequent bathing is required; absolute cleanliness is enforced; regular and proper exercise is practiced."

Dr. Turner added in his portion of the report, "Our large gardens are a source of great benefit to the patients. On every suitable day during the summer season each male patient who is able and competent is required to spend a part of his time at some light work in the gardens. . . . Since the middle of May the patients have been bountifully supplied with fresh vegetables from the gardens, and they have benefited by them."

However, not every patient was as pleased to be at Canton as Gifford and Turner were to have them, and some acted on their discontent by leaving. A few slipped away while strolling the grounds or fishing; deaf-mute Sam Black Buffalo took advantage of a rainstorm to hop a freight train going west.[19] Escaped patients often hightailed it to their reservations, making it relatively easy to recapture them, though one Mesa Grande Indian named Moxey made it all the way to Virginia. He remained at large for two years before he ran afoul of the law there and was returned to the asylum.

A dangerous patient referred to as "Lo" escaped from his locked room on June 30, 1905, by somehow breaking out of the handcuffs attendants had placed on him as an additional precaution against his leaving. Lo made it out a window, unclothed, and anyone who could be spared from the asylum staff began searching for him after he was discovered missing. Gifford received a telephone call saying that the patient had been seen near Newton Hill and took off after him.

Ten hours later, financial clerk Charles Seely, armed with a shotgun, and a companion armed with a revolver found Lo in an oat field a mile west of the city. Lo, by now clothed in strips of gunny sacks, gave up and raised his hands. He was carted back to the asylum in a wagon, where he could trust that restraints would be more vigorously applied in the future.[20]

Despite the superintendent's inability to deal with truly violent or determined cases, Gifford's lack of knowledge about insanity probably worked to the benefit of his patients: he felt none of the typical alienist's urge to try out pet theories in order to advance his career in the field.[21] Turner did study to improve his knowledge of insanity, but the specialty never became his primary interest. Within a couple of years, he had released patients like John LaDeaux (melancholia) and Moses Kenote (hysteric angina pectoris) as cured.[22] Despite his lack of psychiatric credentials, Turner was undoubtedly correct in his summation of such cases: a change of scenery or the patients' removal from problematic local situations to a sheltered space had probably effected a real cure.

Turner provided medical care that certainly made a difference to some patients. Alice Short, a Bannock woman with syphilitic dementia, came to the asylum raving uncontrollably and stinking from unhealed ulcers. According to Turner, within a year, her ulcers were healed, she had gained nineteen pounds, and she had become rational enough to work in the ward. Many of his patients suffering epileptic seizures were helped by the bromides he administered, and those suffering from poor diets were given more nutritious food than they had received on the reservation. Some patients undoubtedly had been neglected, shunned, or abused by family and found a safe haven at Canton Asylum.

And for the first few months of 1903, Canton Asylum perhaps did fulfill its promise. The gardens and grounds *did* look lush and beautiful, a far cry from the intimidating bull-yards of other asylums; patient-to-staff ratios *were* low; programs for stimulating, teaching, and perhaps even curing patients *were* both promising and possible.[23] The place was so small, so new, so gloried and gloated over that it was insulated from trouble.

Unfortunately, the shine was wearing off and the charade was wearing thin. Canton Asylum was far from the triumphant piece of cake Gifford thought he had sliced in 1903. Its sweet taste would soon turn bitter as he saw his great accomplishment transform into a heavy liability.

4. Helpless

Any lurking misgivings an outsider might have had about the welfare of Canton Asylum's patients would have been allayed by a quick visit there. Whether in person or via a newspaper, concerned citizens could easily see that Indians were better off in Canton's special facility than anywhere on a reservation. Certainly in the summer of 1905, most visitors or inspectors focused on the pleasantness of Canton Asylum rather than the contentment of its patients.

Neatly dressed men and women walked or milled about on grassy lawns, enjoying a breeze that played across the shrubs and flower beds. On the front porch a ninety-year-old Sioux medicine man contentedly smoked a pipe, while in the men's ward an old Umatilla chief named Peo sat and watched attendants come and go, smiling occasionally at his favorites.

Forty-one patients lived in the facility by then, but in reality they did not all stroll leisurely about the grounds or sit in repose after a difficult life. Bob Tom, a Paiute from Nevada, ate his meals in the dining room while cuffed and shackled.[1] A younger man raved in his room, clothed in a one-piece garment fastened with snaps in the back. Joseph Langer, a strong young man who had escaped three times, caused such mischief on his home reservation that he was kept in shackles upon his return to the asylum. Sturdy mittens covered his hands, which were tied behind his back so he couldn't get them loose. For all its bucolic setting, the asylum was an exceedingly disagreeable place for many of its inmates.

Of course, it wasn't only Native Americans who didn't go willingly to a madhouse (or stay); unsuspecting white patients often had to be duped into entering an asylum or appearing before an insanity board. These boards were often hit-or-miss as professional bodies; they were composed of medical men and perhaps a few prominent citizens without a medical—let alone a psychiatric—background. Sometimes merely unsophisticated, on occasion they could be overtly hostile to the purported lunatic.

The tragedy was that even under the best of circumstances, insanity boards looked primarily at *current* behavior to make a determination about a person's mental state. The more patients struggled and protested, the more they became agitated, defensive, and angry, the more they made the case against themselves that they were uncontrollable, confused, potentially violent, or liable to harm themselves or others. Native Americans were at an exceptional disadvantage under these circumstances, as their behaviors would often appear incomprehensible, and certainly abnormal, to most white board members.

An additional turn of the screw came from alienists themselves. Early on, they had studied, defined, and treated insanity, and asylum superintendents had become the elite managers of care in institutional settings. As a rule, asylum superintendents did not take kindly to interference from public committees or government boards or other forms of regulation. Thomas Kirkbride, an authority on asylum construction and the highly regarded superintendent of the Pennsylvania Hospital for the Insane from 1841 to 1884, summed up their attitude in his "one man, one rule" mandate. That is, *one man* needed to be in charge of an asylum, and that man's rules needed to take precedence over outsiders' opinions, advice, or feelings.

This high-handedness had not died by the twentieth century. In the 1916 landmark book *The Institutional Care of the Insane in the United States and Canada*, the authors (presumably speaking through lead editor Dr. Henry Hurd) state that "the movement toward the prompt treatment of curable cases *without the formality of legal commitment . . .* gives every hope that at an early day cases of recent attack may be received everywhere promptly, and that greatly increased numbers can be cured" (italics in original).

Completely convinced that they knew better than the public, alienists were not apt to listen to the voice of mere laymen speaking up on behalf of a patient. Unfortunately, U.S. commitment practices of the period often fell right into place with the alienists' sense of authority to work against the accused instead of protecting them. All it took in many states was a certificate from one or two doctors and a letter from a family member to have someone committed to an insane asylum. It becomes nearly impossible to believe that relatives didn't sometimes commit unwanted family members to asylums for convenience, out of spite, or as punishment.

Some critics have maintained that an "insanity" label has always been society's way of controlling behavior. Whether it banishes targeted persons to the countryside or takes them to asylums, society has typically used the tools at hand to rid itself of misfits who put a strain on the majority. At times, these tools could be applied very easily. In 1885 the District of Columbia required jury trials for commitment, but Congress overruled the requirement in 1899. By 1904 any member of the Washington DC metropolitan police could apprehend and detain—without warrant—any insane person or person of unsound mind found in a public place.[2]

The Washington DC metropolitan police superintendent could also order the arrest and detention of an insane person, again without warrant, whenever *two or more respectable residents* of the District of Columbia filed an affidavit saying they believed someone to be of unsound mind. Undoubtedly many disgruntled relatives enjoyed the privileges afforded them under so loose a provision. If homeless and friendless, committed persons were often taken to the government insane asylum, St. Elizabeths.

Some patients gamely fought back, but typically the brick wall they ran into was not the solid reality of an asylum's outside structure. Instead, it was the nearly insurmountable bias of its superintendent. In 1905 a former soldier named Daniel O'Keefe hired attorney Charles Poe to get him released from St. Elizabeths. Poe took the case and first attempted to see the facility's superintendent, Dr. William A. White, as a courtesy before committing to any court action. White happened to be out at the moment Poe arrived, so the attorney walked over to his client's ward.

"You can't see the patient," said Dr. Harry Hummer, a young doctor who served as a senior assistant physician under White. He turned away, evidently thinking he had dismissed Poe.

Poe wasn't afraid to butt heads with a mere doctor, though, and stood his ground. "I've prepared a petition for a writ of habeas corpus for the man," he told Hummer.

"O'Keefe can't sign it," Hummer snapped.

That didn't sit well with Poe, who snapped right back, "You're a little ignorant on that subject!"

Dr. Hummer wasn't used to being opposed, but Poe wasn't used to seeing the law challenged, and the two men walked back to Dr. White's office to argue the matter further. By then, they fortunately found Dr. White on hand. White, who hadn't seen O'Keefe's record, reviewed it and also declined to allow O'Keefe to sign the petition for a writ of habeas corpus.

Poe wasn't having it. "You'd better read the Code of the District," he told White, who countered that he'd rather communicate with the district attorney.

"Then you'd better do it by telephone," Poe rejoined. "It's a pretty serious thing to refuse to allow a man to sign a petition for a writ of habeas corpus."

White did call the district attorney's office and after a short conversation told Poe that O'Keefe could sign the petition. Later Poe argued O'Keefe's case in front of the district supreme court. Dr. White and Dr. Hummer testified that O'Keefe was insane. O'Keefe took the stand, however, and acquitted himself well, resulting in a hung jury. In a later trial, O'Keefe was adjudged sane by a jury and released from St. Elizabeths.

Dr. Hummer was not gracious in defeat, refusing to give O'Keefe any lunch that day until he was coerced into it by Poe. The only possession Hummer gave O'Keefe on his release was a razor, and to add insult to injury, he and White refused to enter on the hospital record that O'Keefe had been found sane by a jury. Alienists—whether young or well-established, in government or private employ—clearly did not like to be challenged, questioned, or proven wrong.[3]

Doctors on insanity boards didn't like to be challenged, either. Realistically, patients had little chance against the forces of authority who declared them insane, unless they were championed by someone who had money, clout, or the law to wield. For presumed insane Indians in the West, such champions seldom existed.

The lack of patient safeguards went hand in hand with the amazingly loose criteria for insanity as applied to Indians. One reservation superintendent wrote to the asylum concerning the admittance of James Black Bull, saying, "I can safely say that he is insane as it is plain for anyone to see by just looking at him that he is not sane."[4]

His statement isn't as extraordinary as it sounds. At a murder trial in 1846, Dr. Amariah Brigham, superintendent of the Utica Asylum for the Insane and the founder of the *American Journal of Insanity* in 1844, sat in a court of law and told the New York state attorney general that he could diagnose insanity by sight. Asked if he relied on the nose, the chin, the mouth, and so on to make his diagnosis, Brigham replied that he relied upon all features, with special emphasis on the eyes and mouth.

Nothing shook his confidence, and after the "nervous tension of the entire mass of people had become painful," Brigham demonstrated his skill by scrutinizing the audience one by one and finally pointing out an insane man. The man thus pinpointed jumped up, gesticulated wildly, "shouted a volley of oaths against any one who would call him insane," and then rushed to the bar. He was dragged out by officers of the court, with Brigham's outrageous diagnosis apparently confirmed by his behavior.[5]

Though this incident had occurred many years before, it was related in a paper read before the fifty-ninth annual meeting of the American Medico-Psychological Association in 1903. Its audience received the information enthusiastically. Based on the discussion comments concerning the paper, alienists more than fifty years after the incident didn't seem to doubt Brigham's accuracy nor consider that the targeted man might have been highly insulted rather than insane. Instead, they seemed to believe that Brigham's action showed brilliance rather than an extraordinary degree of presumption and arrogance.

Almost any unusual action could raise the antennae of a spirited alienist, and these specialists were more than willing to offer their insight to Indian agents who might consult them. The Native American Helen Groth fainted one day from overwork and fatigue, then became hysterical after being poked and prodded by strangers who were called in to see what was wrong with her. The doctor in attendance asked her if she'd heard evil spirits during previous nights. He took it upon himself to call the doctor on the board of Canton's insanity commission, who declared Groth "dangerous and insane" and told her he'd have to take her to the hospital for treatment. After that, matters took a decided turn for the worse.

The doctor had also called the police, who dragged Groth—protesting all the way—to the station. She stayed there for two days in December, cold and miserable, without an examination or any questioning by the board. She was isolated from friends and family and, to her dismay, had only two prostitutes for company.

"After being slapped in the face three different times by the jailer, I was taken to the courtroom where I was promptly informed by the doctor on the board that I was insane," said Groth. "It was, as you might know, somewhat of a surprise to me."

Another doctor urged some further deliberation, and Groth was put back in jail until her mother could come from Missouri to take charge of her. A judge set her free, but one of the doctors on the board decided to pursue the insanity diagnosis. Nearly paralyzed with fright by this time, Groth refused to go to Canton Asylum for an examination and instead opted for the Yankton State Hospital (in South Dakota), where she was declared sane and released after a short stay.[6]

Groth's relatively prompt release was due in large part to her vigorous insistence on the rules of law pertaining to her case and to her fighting spirit. Not every patient had her advantages, and no matter what incident instigated a commitment, treatment that began with yanking a frightened and confused individual from his community and culture did not bode well. Unfortunately, it represented a typical exchange between the Indian Office and Native Americans.

The *Washington Post* reported on May 24, 1904, that "braves" from the Black Hills of South Dakota had called upon the "White Father" at the White House and received the sage advice to "sell your ponies and buy cattle." The article went on to say that the Indian visitors complained of broken treaties and their need for more provisions and that the president "endeavored to impress upon them the delights and advantages of agriculture." The encounter pretty well summed up the federal government's relationship with its wards.

In the case of Canton Asylum, the White Father's wishes for his Indian wards fell in happily with the era's generally accepted therapy for the mentally ill: keep them busy, especially at practical work that helped defray the expenses of the institution where they resided. Of course, Canton was no worse than any other institution of the time. Here, as elsewhere, physically able patients hoed, weeded, and gathered vegetables in the gardens. They grew and ate corn, oats, potatoes, and a variety of vegetables and tended hay for the livestock. Amenable patients were guided in cleaning their rooms and learning domestic skills.

During the first couple of years—at least during the summer—life at Canton Asylum was relatively pleasant given the circumstances. The day began with a cooked meal and included leisure amusements and quiet time. Many Indian patients wanted to be outdoors if they were able, and it was good that they could get out. Though the weather could be harsh in winter, summer days were hot enough indoors to soften and bend candle tapers, and one patient noted in a letter that "it won't be long before we can't stay in the house for it will be too hot."[7]

Gifford encouraged fishing, ball games, and quoits (a game similar to pitching horseshoes), as well as strolls and light calisthenics. Patients enjoyed an occasional picnic and sometimes went to town. Besides working in established gardens, patients picked wild berries and other fruit. During the winter, patients played cards, sang, and danced. Few demands were made upon the weak and elderly.

By the time Gifford made his fifth report to the secretary of the interior in 1907, Canton Asylum had sixty-three patients under treatment for conditions ranging from alcoholism, syphilis, toxic insanity, and imbecility to epilepsy. Of these patients, thirty-six were male and twenty-seven female; they ranged in age from ninety-eight-year-old Kay-zhe-ah-bow, who had arrived the same week that Edward Hedges died, to young Hathorn, admitted at the age of seven or eight.[8]

There is little reason to believe that Gifford had any personal agenda against either Indians or the insane. He and Dr. Turner—though patronizing and paternalistic to be sure—were enthusiastic, proud of their asylum and its mission, and likely doing the best they could with what they had. They admitted patients who appeared to be needy of attention, allowed most of them what laxity they could, and shackled the runaways and the violent when they couldn't control them any other way.

Given that the facility didn't have a working hospital or any equipment to speak of, Turner didn't lean toward anything cutting edge in the way of treatment. Instead, patients like the deaf-mute runaway Sam Black Buffalo, admitted at age eighteen and discharged two years later as "trustworthy and alert," probably received basic medical care for conditions that Turner was well able to recognize. These and other releases were beginning to buck a trend in psychiatry, in which superintendents of large institutions found they were dealing mainly with "incurables."

During the reformist movement of the 1830s, alienists believed that nearly all insane persons could be cured—one reason to build large asylums where they could go for treatment. By 1887, when Dr. Pliny Earle published *The Curability of Insanity*, they weren't so sure anymore. Besides the fact that overcrowding and understaffing kept madhouses from being "asylums" in any sense of the word, alienists also began to think that genetics and heredity played a major role in insanity and that cures might not be possible.[9]

Official attitudes toward patients seemed to change as well, with referencing language about the insane transforming from *unfortunates* to *defectives*. At the fifty-ninth annual meeting of the American Medico-Psychological Association (May 12–15, 1903) in Washington DC, Dr. A. B. Richardson, superintendent of St. Elizabeths, remarked that the attendees must appreciate the extent of the problem . . . to curtail the evil of insanity. By caring for patients so well, he said, "The general result is that the survival of the unfit is extended. . . . They are nursed, protected, housed, brought to a procreative age and then turned loose on the community in large numbers, and as a result we have a constantly increasing class of defectives."[10]

Gifford was pretty far away from this rhetoric as a layman out West. For all the incompetency he later displayed, Gifford didn't really seem to view his charges as defectives. His policies at the asylum were fairly relaxed toward his patients' cultural expression, and to their credit, Gifford and Dr. Turner approved of crafts like beadwork and basketmaking. Gifford and his wife took two patients to Canton's Congregational Church when a guest from the Santee reservation spoke and sang in their native language there. The city's weekly paper merely noted their presence at the church, as it noted any special events and their attendees, and seemed to find nothing special in the situation.

In an interview with the *Chicago Daily* on January 3, 1904, Gifford said, "Our treatment is simple. We allow the Indians to follow their own likes and dislikes, so far as can safely be done." This was a startling departure from the attitude of most government officials associated with Indian affairs.

Veering even more sharply from the typical government mindset, Gifford continued, "We even allow them [patients] to indulge in native dances, if they are not dangerously exciting, as we think the normal habits of the Indian are most apt to bring him back to a possession of his faculties."

Unfortunately, Gifford did reflect other attitudes in vogue, which often made Canton Asylum a destination for curiosity seekers as much as an institution for mental health care. Throughout the country, many officials, doctors, board members, or town fathers involved in operating institutions for the insane had few qualms about opening up "their" asylums for viewing by visiting physicians or the public. In this they were following a practice that began with London's first lunatic asylum, where gawkers could pay a penny to see lunatics, as well as grab the opportunity for entertainment by poking sleeping lunatics with a stick to stir them up.[11]

Though Canton Asylum didn't go that far, it was certainly a public place, and anyone with even an inkling of social stature could expect a pleasant tour of the facility. Visitors generally returned the favor by talking up the asylum in glowing terms. The editor of the *Hudson (SD) Hudsonite* dropped by the institution on August 4, 1905, a day when visitors weren't expected (Wednesday). He received a tour from the financial clerk, Charles Seely.

"Everything fairly shone throughout the place, from the basement throughout the wards, in the kitchen and dining rooms, everything was bright and cheery," the editor wrote. He went on to describe the contented patients (except for the shackled ones) and commented on the comfortable iron bedsteads with their white sheets and spreads. He finished with a round of applause for the management, the facility, and the government's sagacity for building the place.

His admiration was echoed by the people of Canton, none of whom seemed to be either put off by the idea of going inside the asylum or squeamish about the idea of staff living in one. Seely's son, Merritt, bicycled to school from the asylum and children from town came up to play with the children of staff members. Staff spouses like Mrs. Seely and Mrs. Turner hosted gatherings as they would in any ordinary home, once jointly entertaining forty guests at a party where the four-player card game Five Hundred and refreshments were the highlights.[12] For its white inhabitants, the asylum was truly a home.

The town's lack of dismay concerning the asylum may have been simple tolerance or a case of swallowing the bad with the good in accepting the institution's economic impact on the area. Additionally, by the turn of the century, laypeople had begun to entertain new ideas concerning the mind. One of these new notions was the concept of mental hygiene (also called *psychophylaxis*), which focused on the development of healthy mental and emotional habits, attitudes, and behavior and the prevention of mental illness. Though the concept was developed in the late 1800s, it began to thrive as a specific area of study in the early 1900s, helping to divorce insanity somewhat from the mystery and fear that had previously surrounded it.

The nation's population seemed open to change of all kinds, embracing novel ideas and behaviors as the old century gave way to the optimism and excitement of the new. Comedians Fatty Arbuckle and Harry Bulgar were the first entertainers to give cigarette testimonials in advertisements, Einstein postulated the theory of relativity, and toasters and vacuum cleaners began to make housework just a little easier.[13] Teddy Roosevelt, who had visited Canton during his 1900 campaign, had been reelected president in 1904 and by 1905 had established a number of national parks, as well as the National Park Service.

It was an exciting era, with both opportunity and convenience delightfully close at hand. The good housewives of Canton could buy ten pounds of rice for thirty-nine cents at Chraft & Hanson's or get a copper-bottomed teakettle for $1.25 at The Enterprise. In ladies' fashions, leg-of-mutton sleeves were very popular for summer wear, and within just another few years, waist sizes on shop mannequins would go from eighteen to twenty-four inches. Buggies and wagons remained the most common mode of travel for Cantonites, but asylum staff could reach Superintendent Gifford at home by telephone if an emergency arose while he was absent.

Proud as they were of their modernity, Cantonites—and South

Dakotans more generally—could scarcely pretend that their amenities were on par with those of the East. The *Washington Post* actively refuted the notion that the West was settled or occupied to any large degree, as some of its readers apparently believed. Its January 3, 1905, article "Still Room for the Settlers" described the splendid opportunities for newcomers to the West and pointed out that South Dakota farms averaged 362 acres while farms in states like Missouri and Iowa averaged 119 and 151 acres respectively. Readers were urged to consider rolling up their sleeves to give the West a try.

The notion of settling out West was undoubtedly attractive to the vast numbers of immigrants coming to the country. The sweatshops in Manhattan's Garment District were thriving, and garment workers (often young girls), fortified by a breakfast of a cup of coffee and roll and soup with a slice of bread at lunch, typically worked from 7:00 a.m. until 6:00 p.m. The idea of life on a farm—growing plenty of food—was undoubtedly appealing.

There was a darker side to the West, of course. In 1904 there had been a violent clash between cattlemen and sheepmen in Butte, Montana when a band of cowboys raided a sheep camp and killed hundreds of animals. The reason: their range around Granite Hill Valley had been invaded. That same year, fourteen miners were killed by a bomb in Cripple Creek, Colorado, during an acrimonious labor dispute, and the Wild Bunch's Kid Curry met death at his own hand rather than surrender to a posse.

Canton Asylum had a dark side as well, and it was beginning to show. Never mind its burgeoning sanitation problems—compared to most American homes of the era, Canton Asylum was a pretty decent place to be. A good number of people in the western states still lived in sod houses and dugouts, and two- or three-room shacks meant home for many families in the southern and eastern states. A major achievement in Washington DC legislation was regulation that "no person shall expectorate or spit in or upon any paved sidewalk . . . on any part of any street-railway car . . . or in or upon any part of any public building."[14] Outhouses and wells prevailed throughout the country, though urban dwellers at a certain economic level were now attaining the comforts of indoor plumbing and electricity. In many rural areas, however, electricity wouldn't show up until Franklin Roosevelt's New Deal provided it through the Tennessee Valley Authority (TVA) in the 1930s.

White coal miners breathed in methane and carbonic acid and died of black lung from inhaled coal dust, while "breaker boys" sorted slag and lost their fingers and their lives in the coal chutes beneath them. Children peeled shrimp that oozed acid so strong it ate holes in their shoes, or they developed chronic lung diseases working in cotton mills. Sweatshops and piecework in the garment industry ruined the health of whole families as it kept them in helpless poverty.[15]

It is little wonder, then, that in the first decade of the century, most visitors looking at Canton's physical aspects—the focus of most tours— would have found little to complain about. The facility was almost luxurious with its electric lights, plumbing, coal heat, and indoor range toilets. Since most of these visitors weren't competent to judge the mental health care patients received, they took their host's word that it was excellent.

Though improvements were regularly made (forty new storm windows, two storm houses, five thousand square feet of cement walk, and a cistern were added within a couple of years of the asylum's opening), anything to do with patient care was woefully underfunded. Men and women were housed in separate wards—a moral rather than mental health consideration—but the old and young, the violent and peaceful, the contagious and healthy were not separated. Tuberculosis plagued the patient population, as it did the Indian population as a whole, but Canton Asylum never established a sanitarium or even a separate building or ward for these chronically ill cases.

Gifford and his successor alike recognized these problems and repeatedly requested funds for separate cottages to house the types of patients they wished to segregate (in Gifford's case, the violent from the nonviolent). Asylums are noisy and sometimes chaotic, and many institutions rewarded obedient patients with a move to a "quiet ward" where they could live with others who were well-behaved. There, patients could actually rest at night, undisturbed by groans and screams from their more disturbed comrades and free from the countless aggravations inherent in living with people who had only a fragile grasp on reality. In quiet wards, it was easier for staff to interact with patients and to spend more time with them, and the changed atmosphere undoubtedly helped many mildly disturbed patients to get well.

Though a hospital was finally erected on the grounds, Washington never shook loose the finances for other physical assets at Canton Asylum that would have brought badly needed comfort or aid to patient care. Instead, the tractable and violent, the delusional and merely melancholy, children and adults, were housed together; only extreme cases of illness or violence were ever isolated. To make their experience worse, many patients could not communicate with each other or with staff because of language barriers. Confused, medicated, and overwhelmed by the strangeness of it all, far too few of these displaced people could get their bearings enough to recover.

Of course, less than perfect facilities weren't the real problem—the real problem lay in almost everything else associated with the asylum. Gifford was an intelligent, energetic man who probably had the best of intentions when Canton Asylum was a pie-in-the-sky prize. He just didn't have what it took to run an asylum. He was used to dealing with businessmen, congressmen, and other committed and educated people who typically labored for a common cause. His asylum staff, however, were largely uneducated and unmotivated. (Dr. Turner had to show attendant Mary Smith how to use a thermometer so he could be absent a few days.) In a 1904 advertisement, the positions of attendant (both male and female), cook, assistant cook, dining room girl, laundress, and night watchman were advertised. No position required an educational test.[16]

Gifford apparently didn't know how to light a fire under his employees to get all the work done, stop their feuding and complaining, or get rid of the staff who didn't work out. He also might have found it hard to face his friends in town if he had disciplined anyone on staff too severely. As an administrator, he wasn't proactive enough to use his available manpower effectively or to see beyond the needs of the moment.

In February 1905 the *Sioux Valley News* reported on a particularly hectic week at the asylum. On Monday, Dr. Turner and another employee had just returned from Idaho, where they had picked up two Shoshone patients, and on Wednesday, financial clerk Seely had brought back an Apache brave. During his time away from the asylum, Seely had visited Pasadena, Los Angeles, and Catalina Island. That Friday, Dr. Turner was to start for Indian Territory to get someone from Union Agency, and Gifford himself was to leave shortly to go to Minnesota to pick up a patient.

From July 1, 1905, to July 1, 1907, Gifford was absent from the asylum on official business (mainly bringing in new patients) for 77 days, Seely for 27, and Turner for 124, for a total of 228 lost man-days in only a couple of years. It seems almost inevitable that Gifford and such staff as he had could do little more than control the chaos. On his watch, a large barn burned to the ground, destroying farm equipment as well as hay and grain and killing several horses.[17] After the first flush of confidence, Gifford seems to have settled for whatever got him through the day. One bright spot was the marriage of his son, Oscar Bailey, to Alice Cedarbloom of Minneapolis in October 1906. Oscar Bailey had graduated from the state college in Minnesota after taking a course in pharmacy and held a position at one of Minneapolis's leading drugstores.

It was Dr. Turner who felt the brunt of the staffing issues. Because Seely and Gifford had business interests in town, it fell to Turner to go after patients much of the time. He often recruited other Canton doctors to care for his patients while he was gone; usually they filled in free of charge, but sometimes Turner paid for their services out of his own pocket. To add to his frustration, staff members often didn't obey his orders, or Gifford himself overstepped them. Unfortunately for Gifford, Dr. Turner was not a loyal Cantonite who could be depended upon to let the superintendent do as he wanted.

The situation was deteriorating, fast, and when Gifford crossed a line that Turner couldn't live with, the doctor put his foot down. When he picked it back up, Gifford didn't have a job.

5. A Superintendent in Trouble

Star-sprinkled South Dakota nights may have seemed endless, fleeting, filled with bewildering shapes, or simply voids that gave rest to the weary patients at Canton Asylum. That they were filled with dark horrors to some is undeniable, given the mental conditions and circumstances they endured. In some cases, however, Gifford's carelessness allowed an extra dollop of suffering.

Lizzie Vipont, a thirty-year-old Paiute woman from Churz, Nevada, entered the asylum in 1905 as an epileptic with delusions, auditory hallucinations, and occasional violent spells that required restraint. She could speak only a few words of English, and no one at the asylum knew her language. Vipont had a husband and young daughter, but the distance between Canton and Churz was too great to allow visits. She was completely at the mercy of the institution.

Frank Shanahan, a Chippewa with delusional melancholia, was prone to bouts of sleeplessness that left him anxious for activity at all hours of the night. He was also young and strong, and Gifford saw no harm in allowing him to leave his ward to help in the boiler room or with other chores the engineer might have for him. Dr. Turner considered Shanahan far too treacherous for this kind of freedom and ordered him locked in his room at night. Turner was away from the asylum during most of February and March 1906, making trips to pick up patients. While he was gone, Gifford overrode his lockup order, declaring that Shanahan was "all right."

Whether he committed rape once or many times, entered a consensual relationship, or did what he wanted with someone too delusional to care is not known, but Frank Shanahan found a key to the women's ward, slipped past the night watchman, and had sex with Lizzie Vipont and perhaps her roommate as well. Shanahan may have been more attracted to Vipont or found her an easier target, because he later admitted to having sex with her more than once—even during daylight hours. He additionally claimed to have had intercourse with Vipont behind a bush out on the grounds, close to the female ward.

When Turner returned from his trip, he was furious at finding Shanahan roaming freely and immediately ordered him locked in at night. The damage was done, however—Lizzie Vipont was pregnant. Turner's records were meticulous enough that he kept a menstrual chart for the women patients; Vipont's last cycle had occurred between February 15 and 18, pinpointing the impregnation as having occurred sometime during his absence.[1] He delivered Vipont's "full-term, bastard, imbecile child" November 6, 1906.[2] This blotch on his record of care and upon the institution did not sit well with Turner, and he put the blame for the situation squarely on Gifford. This was not the first time that Gifford had stepped on Turner's toes. The two occasionally differed on what was in the best interest of a patient, and Gifford didn't seem to back Turner's orders to the attendants.

Another thing had reached a boiling point with Turner: all these exhausting trips. He got stuck with most of the patient fetching, "excepting when they [Gifford or Seely] wish to make a visit to a section of the country they have not seen."[3] His duties in this regard were so onerous that when he was in Pennsylvania visiting his terminally ill father, Turner had to retrieve the escaped patient Moxie, who had made it all the way to Virginia. The elder Turner accompanied his disgruntled son and the prisoner back to Canton Asylum.[4]

However, the straw that broke the camel's back came when Gifford ordered Turner not to tell Vipont's husband about her pregnancy. Rather than lie on an official report, Turner stopped making them. He was sure that Vipont's husband or the superintendent at her agency would begin to make inquiries, and he wanted help in deflecting the blame he was sure he would get.[5] He wrote in December to Charles Dickson, supervisor of Indian schools in Washington DC, whom he had met in New Mexico. Turner detailed his exasperating situation at Canton, ending his letter bitterly: "I acknowledge that I was unfortunate enough not to be born at Canton but I still insist that I could not help it and that it is really no disgrace to be in the civil service."

Dickson relayed Turner's information to the assistant commissioner of Indian affairs, Charles F. Larrabee, and the Indian Office managed to launch an investigation by the end of July 1907. Reuben Perry, supervisor at Fort Peck Agency in Poplar, Montana, visited Canton Asylum in August and found a lot to write home about.

Plenty of things were wrong at the facility, though not all of them were Gifford's fault. For one thing, Gifford was supposed to reside at the asylum. That proved impractical because there wasn't enough room for two families (Gifford had a wife and infant daughter, Frederica, at the time). As the facility's only physician, Dr. Turner's on-site presence at the asylum was practically mandated, so he got the family accommodations. However, nine beds were available for staff members, and Gifford reserved one for himself so he could spend the night if needed. Otherwise, he continued to live in his home.

Gifford said he had the Indian Office's permission for the arrangement (and nothing indicates that he didn't). A supervisor named Wright had inspected the asylum in early 1903, and Gifford said he had particularly called his attention to the asylum's living arrangements. It seems reasonable to believe that over the subsequent four years something would have been done about Gifford's residence if the Indian Office had a real problem with it.

A more serious charge was that Gifford and Seely spent inordinate amounts of time away from the asylum on personal business. After sifting through depositions—most of them from employees loyal to Gifford and Seely (and from both Gifford and Seely, each avowing that the other scarcely left the premises)—Perry concluded that Seely really did spend too much time at his business in Canton. Gifford seemed to be at the asylum a reasonable amount of time, but in Perry's opinion, all three officers (Gifford, Seely, and Turner) were away far too often on trips to pick up patients.[6]

Gifford swore that he had never told the night watchman to let Frank Shanahan loose at night, but other deponents contradicted him. He also told Perry that he had heard about some suspicious circumstances concerning Vipont in July or August (of 1906) and had immediately suggested to Dr. Turner that he examine her. According to Gifford, Turner refused because Vipont was violent; he then informed the superintendent a month or so later that she was probably pregnant. That would have placed Turner's discovery of Vipont's pregnancy around September, two months before she gave birth—hard to believe if he had eyes in his head and was charting her menstrual cycle.[7]

Gifford had never given employees a copy of the rules governing the asylum or a list of their duties. He explained that each employee had to perform so many duties other than his or her own that it didn't make sense to give them a list of duties and then make continual exceptions to it. In this part of the deposition, it came out just what kind of facility the asylum had become in only five years.

"The Asylum has been and is a place for the treatment of the insane of all types, feeble minded, imbicile [sic] and idiots, infant injured in child birth, condition absolutely helpless and hopeless every way, incorrigible—and for juveniles who should be in reform school," said Gifford. He continued, "In fact it is a hospital for physical and mental deformities of almost every name and character; and all ages from five to seventy years of age."

In his subsequent report, Inspector Perry gave an interesting counterpoint to Gifford's words: "The officials and employees should always keep in mind that this institution was not established solely for the purpose of having a safe place for keeping this class of unfortunates, but that its ultimate object is the physical and mental improvement of its inmates, especially the latter."[8]

Perry did have a certain amount of sympathy for Gifford's problems. Though he faulted the superintendent for the fact that during the life of the asylum's operation, only three employees had come from anywhere other than Canton, he also pointed out that the calls for examinations were made properly and widely advertised. After March 1904, appointments had been made by the Indian Office, which further took hiring decisions out of Gifford's hands. However, the fact that favoritism had been and continued to be a factor in hiring was borne out by a sharp letter Gifford received from Acting Commissioner Larrabee a few months after Perry's inspection. In it Larrabee said, "It is observed that you nominated for this position Norman C. Rogers, subject to the approval of this office. After careful consideration . . . the Office is at a loss to understand why you should nominate Norman C. Rogers [a local] for the position in preference to Mr. Coleman. . . . It is observed that you have given both applicants a rating of 70 per cent in experience, while an examination of their papers shows that no comparison whatever exists." Larrabee then overruled Gifford to give Coleman the appointment.[9]

A larger issue lay in how employees were used. Laborers, who needed no examination, were frequently used as attendants, who did. Unqualified people could slip in this way if Gifford wanted them to, but it was just as likely a case of Gifford not being proactive enough to request the right categories of workers. Perry suggested that one female and one male laborer position be abolished and replaced by attendant positions. This change was instituted the following month.

In an undated letter to Supervisor Reuben Perry, the Canton physician John W. Corrigan declared that the institution's methods of operation were "lax in the extreme" and that something was "radically wrong" at the Indian asylum. He added that ward attendants often neglected patients, couldn't be found when needed, and didn't always try to control violent patients. Additionally, Perry discovered that Sarah Revel, a laborer who acted as an attendant, was said to be addicted to morphine. Perry told Gifford that her case needed to be investigated immediately. She instead turned in her resignation.

When Perry ended his investigation and prepared to leave Canton, several men approached him to offer statements regarding affairs at the asylum. Six prominent citizens made sworn statements, and a general statement was signed by six other citizens. Perry said that the gist of the statements was to the effect "that superintendent Gifford has given his undivided time and attention to the Asylum and probably more so than the physician." Perry took the statements with a grain of salt and merely noted that they showed the standing that Gifford had in the community.

Gifford didn't need to agonize unduly over the investigation. It showed that he was a little too lackadaisical in the way he hired and didn't discipline workers, let patients do what they wanted rather than institute regimens to enrich their mental health, and let attendants follow their own leads rather than Turner's rules. But, except for a sharp letter, he wasn't sanctioned in any particular way. Life pretty much went back to normal, though documents from around this period show Gifford's signature starting to slant downward rather than horizontally.[10]

The reality was that investigations were an inherent part of the job. Any community of workers, especially groups isolated the way staff at the Canton facility were, could breed considerable gossip, backbiting, and blame. Patients in asylums—angry, delusional, paranoid, or vindictive—often brought up accusations against their doctors and attendants. Canton's sister asylum, St. Elizabeths, had just come off its own investigation. The difference was that Canton Asylum got away with a fourteen-page report from a lone inspector, Reuben Perry. A special congressional probe produced over two thousand pages of testimony in an investigation conducted in 1906 over allegations of abuse at St. Elizabeths.

In February 1906 a group called the Medico-Legal Society made allegations of horrific abuses at St. Elizabeths. The society printed charges in the *Washington Times* on February 18, 1906, but declined to give St. Elizabeths' governing body the information from which the charges were derived. The *Washington Herald* wrote, "Society a Mystery," and both papers noted that the society was new to the district and that few names of its members were known.

Various societies interested in the legal questions arising from medical practice had formed during the 1800s, but the most influential was probably the Medico-Legal Society of New York, which oversaw the publication of a quarterly journal (the *Medico-Legal Journal*) from 1883 to 1915. The journal offered articles like "Is Criminal Anthropology a Science?" and "The Medico-Legal Relations of Abortion" and focused particularly on court cases where medico-legal questions arose.[11]

The society alleged in 1906 that patients at St. Elizabeths were beaten at will and restrained with contraptions like the saddle (a device upon which patients were placed in a reclining position, then fastened hand, foot, and neck so that no movement was possible). Additionally, feeding tubes were used for spite or punishment, and needle baths (a full-body shower spray) were given indiscriminately.[12] The group also alleged that the hospital charged excessive per capita costs per patient and then rounded out their complaints by saying that the superintendent neglected his patients.[13]

Congress launched an investigation, and testimony covered nearly everything that could go wrong with a building, staff, and patients. A former employee complained of bad meat and a shortage of food, while a former waitress testified that the food was not clean and sometimes had cockroaches in it. She apparently had an otherwise high tolerance. When she commented on how good her patients were, she said that "the worst things they did at table was to break up the dishes and throw prunes at each other."

Personnel clashes, perhaps inevitable, were sometimes intense. One former employee testified that he and three other attendants had been supervising some patients who were cleaning bricks, when Dr. Harry Hummer (O'Keefe's former physician and attorney Poe's adversary) ordered the attendants to help. When the attendant replied that he wasn't hired to clean bricks and wouldn't do it, he was fired.

Dr. Hummer's name cropped up again in the testimony. Attorney Richard P. Evans, while attempting to interview several patients (his clients), had found Hummer extremely discourteous and interfering: "Dr. Hummer insisted upon being in the room with an attendant present. They [patients] wanted to see me, not relative to getting out, but relative to some other matters. I took their statements down and used a little of the hospital paper, a couple of sheets."

If Hummer had been petty after O'Keefe's jury trial, he now descended into an almost awe-inspiring level of spite. "After I was through with the interview," said Evans, "Doctor Hummer threatened to have me arrested for stealing hospital property and compelled me to leave my notes on the table."

Evans testified further concerning the ongoing issue of committing patients who weren't insane to St. Elizabeths. His experience showed a strong inclination on the part of the superintendent to resist discharging patients; however, the few who managed to get to court were usually discharged as sane. (Interestingly, Evans was the Medico-Legal Society's attorney.)

However, St. Elizabeths' records showed that it had a fairly typical rate of discharge (either as cured or nonrestored but given to the care of relatives) compared to other institutions.[14] Violent patients were restrained, but Superintendent William A. White had absolutely forbidden use of the saddle in a letter to hospital staff in 1904, shortly after his arrival. Patients were "toweled" by attendants, who would place a towel around a patient's neck and wring it until the patient was subdued, and they sometimes struck patients in self-defense. However, straitjackets didn't seem to be routinely used. More usually, suicidal or violent patients were confined to their beds by placing a sheet across their chest and tying it to the sides of the bed.

Facts were gathered by the investigating committee, down to the number of eggs fed to bedridden patients. Many of the charges seemed to be unsubstantiated or isolated in nature, though beatings and other violence against patients apparently had occurred as unsanctioned incidents. Family members of confined patients wrote supportive letters to White, and his reputation remained high. Another asylum, another investigation . . . though trying, they were one of the burdens of the job.[15]

At least White's problems had come from outside. Back in Canton, however, tensions between Gifford and Turner likely ran a little high after Perry's investigation; Gifford had to have known that the initiating complaint came from Turner. Whether to prove his authority or to tweak Turner's nose—or for some other reason entirely—Gifford overrode Turner once again in what turned out to be both a literal and figurative fatal error.

Gifford, as superintendent of Canton Asylum, had absolute control over its operation. He was supposed to direct its affairs, delegate all its tasks and duties, and make decisions about personnel and patient care. Elsewhere, asylum superintendents were doctors who had the knowledge required to make these latter decisions. Canton Asylum was run like an Indian boarding school, and no one had thought to substitute a physician for a lay superintendent. Consequently, even medical decisions were subject to Gifford's ultimate authority.

Gifford obviously had no medical background, but he seemed to feel (as in the case of Shanahan) that he was competent to determine a patient's mental or medical status. Additionally, attendants frequently disregarded Turner's instructions regarding patients, and Turner felt that a few had died as a result. Gifford apparently did little or nothing in the way of disciplining the attendants or backing Turner, either out of animosity toward Turner, friendliness toward the Canton employees, or a feeling that few things were as serious as Turner made them out to be.

With this background, the situation was ripe for a really serious incident. Gifford had once disagreed with Turner over an epileptic girl, sending her home over the doctor's objections. Now he prepared to overrule Turner again. In October 1907, Charles Brown, a sixty-three-year-old Winnebago Indian, fell ill with intestinal problems (biliary calculi).

Turner treated him but believed that the real problem was an obstruction. He told Gifford that surgery was the only answer. Turner brought in two doctors from town (Drs. Corrigan and Rogers) for a consultation, and they agreed that there appeared to be an obstruction in the common bile duct.

Turner couldn't operate without Gifford's permission, and it must have been galling to ask for it. He and Dr. Corrigan went to Gifford's office, but Gifford wouldn't entertain the notion of an operation and abruptly asked Corrigan into his private room.

"Are you really positive about the condition?" Gifford asked Corrigan once the door was shut.

"Everything points to it being an obstruction [of the bile duct], but of course, it's possible to be wrong," Corrigan replied. Then he added, "Whether that's wrong or right, it's a surgical condition—an operation is positively indicated."

Gifford hesitated. "He's too weak."

"Dr. Turner and I think he's in fair shape," said Corrigan. "I've operated on a number of such subjects."

"I'm afraid he might die from the operation," said Gifford. "And the revenue of this institution is in live Indians, not dead ones." Opposing the opinions of all three doctors, Gifford refused permission for the operation.

Turner took his consultants back to Canton. He knew money might be an issue for Gifford and asked Corrigan his fee.

"I'll do it for the love it," Corrigan replied.

"If I can get permission from the superintendent, I'll telephone you on Sunday, and we can operate Monday morning at 9:00," Turner said, evidently hoping he could prevail against whatever other objections Gifford might have.

He gamely went back to see Gifford, but the superintendent countered every suggestion.

"I don't know whether or not the Indian Office would allow a fee as they do for veterinary or dental services," he first told Turner.

"Dr. Corrigan won't charge a fee," Turner reassured him.

"I don't think Charles can stand the operation. He may die later even if he can get through it."

Gifford flatly refused to allow the operation, and three weeks later Charles Brown died. Turner incised the tumor in the presence of the night watchman and an attendant and removed a calculus, which he kept.

Somebody wrote to the Indian Office, whether promptly after this incident or after a period of reflection and growing concern, or about another matter entirely. That somebody had enough clout to raise real concerns, because the department responded by sending out special agent Edgar A. Allen, who arrived without fanfare on Tuesday, April 8, 1908, to check out the "rumors that had reached the Office" of his superiors. He set out to unobtrusively observe the comings and goings of Gifford, Seely, and Turner until Thursday, when he had to abandon his anonymity and get to the asylum before Seely departed to fetch a patient from Arizona.

Allen was not impressed with much of what he saw. He observed leaky cotton fire hoses that wouldn't put out a fire, and no chemical fire extinguishers. The institution's septic tank had been bypassed because it wasn't working properly. The sewer discharged into an open ditch about three hundred yards away from the building, emitting a stench foul enough that neighbors complained about it in the summer, when it could be counted upon to smell especially ripe. Employees were keeping poultry at government expense. Gifford later averred that everyone got their eggs, but the cook stated that patients rarely did; butter and other extras also went to the employees rather than patients. Allen did note that the patients received the same food as provided at a well-conducted Indian boarding school.

Though he discovered other minor problems (like the two horses kept at the asylum for personal use at government expense), Allen found most of the grounds and buildings in good shape.[16] He apparently had a particular mandate to look at a laborer named Berney Christopher and the financial clerk, Seely, though he made additional observations about the employees in general.

Christopher had been accused of immoral conduct, profanity, and various other infractions, and the investigation may well have been initiated by a communication from Dr. Corrigan. Corrigan gave an affidavit stating that Christopher had asked him to perform an abortion, which he would not do. Since Christopher's morals were of prominent interest to Special Agent Allen, this may have been the main reason for his visit. Corrigan got another grievance off his chest, though, since his affidavit also discussed Gifford's refusal to allow the operation on Charles Brown.

The investigation played out like most: accusations, counteraccusations, finger-pointing, and denial were the order of the day. Gifford stated that he had heard about Christopher's profanity only a few weeks earlier, from Dr. Turner, and had asked him to make the complaint in writing (which Turner wouldn't do). He then countercharged that the cook who made the complaint, Hannah Mickelson, was herself foul-mouthed and insolent and had even referred to Mrs. Seely (the financial clerk's wife and matron of the institution) in insulting terms. Christopher, he said, had always been a competent and satisfactory employee.

Gifford again averred that his clerk, Seely, had attended only to asylum business when in town and had never conducted personal business there on government time. The cook, Mickelson, mentioned that Seely took his son to and from school each day, unless the boy rode his bicycle (in good weather) or caught a ride with the asylum farmer.

Allen, however, noted that he had seen Seely in town working in his store, and his investigation confirmed Berney Christopher's unfitness for employment.[17] Allen was especially irate that Gifford had hidden behind the excuse that Turner hadn't put his complaint about Christopher in writing and then had attacked the cook, Mickelson, who had been at the asylum since it opened and had just received an "excellent" rating from Gifford himself. Allen noted that Gifford was prone to absence, took no meals at the asylum, and hadn't slept there for months.

After sorting through the mess, Allen concluded, "Dr. Turner is doing the work of one man and Superintendent Gifford and Mr. Seeley [sic], together, about the work of another."

If the air had been frosty at the asylum before (Allen noted that relations were very strained between Turner and Seely during a meal he had shared during his investigation), it had to be freezing afterward. Allen suggested that a doctor be appointed superintendent of the asylum, with another doctor to act as assistant superintendent and clerk combined. That would not only allow the asylum to have one physician always present, it would also eliminate the clerk's position.

Gifford's superiors digested Allen's report and reviewed Perry's previous one. Whether it was Gifford's lack of administrative ability, the pregnancy of a helpless patient, or the botched medical care given to Charles Brown, something finally snapped at the Indian Office. A few weeks after Allen filed his report, Larrabee asked Dr. William White, the superintendent at St. Elizabeths, to recommend a suitable person for the position of superintendent at Canton.

Meanwhile, Gifford had to perform what may have been his most difficult task to date at the asylum: fire his friend Seely. The Department of the Interior had agreed with Special Agent Allen that a financial clerk, at $1,100 annually, wasn't worth the government dollar and decided to abolish that position and substitute a mere clerk—and an inexpensive female one at that—at $600 a year. Allen's suggestion that they create a combined physician-clerk position hadn't gone over so well, the office probably recognizing that not many physicians would be interested.

Gifford, probably couching the termination in as palatable terms as possible, told Seely he would have to go. Gifford respectfully asked the commissioner of Indian affairs to let Seely stay on until July 1 so he could do the quarterly returns. Then he practically begged the commissioner not to send a female clerk to the asylum: "A female clerk can do nothing in the way of receiving, handling, weighing coal, freight and supplies generally for the Asylum and she would be utterly useless in taking care of violent male patients, (or female patients either for that matter) in case of emergency." Gifford foolishly cited the clerk's need to be on the road to pick up patients—one of the reasons the financial clerk's position had come under scrutiny—as another argument for appointing a male clerk.[18]

This letter was dated May 19, 1908, and on May 20 South Dakota's taciturn senator Alfred B. Kittredge sent an urgent telegram to Commissioner of Indian Affairs Francis Luepp, asking him to reconsider

Seely's dismissal. The commissioner told his staff to move forward. He also told Kittredge that he had talked the case over with the secretary of the interior, that the actions at Canton were "morally obligatory," and that he had decided to reorganize the asylum on "common-sense lines." The matter was settled.

As for Gifford's replacement, Dr. White's first choice, Dr. B. R. Logie, didn't want the position because it didn't pay enough.[19] Early in June, White sent Assistant Commissioner Larrabee two other names: Dr. George H. Schwinn and Dr. Harry R. Hummer—the same Hummer who had butted heads with attorneys Poe, in the O'Keefe case, and Evans, in the 1906 congressional investigation of abuse at St. Elizabeths. Hummer visited the Indian Office in June to meet with staff members, who weren't impressed by him. However, Luepp said Hummer would suit him if he could get White's endorsement—they needed to replace Gifford and Hummer had good credentials. Hummer submitted his application to Commissioner Luepp on June 28, 1908, along with White's endorsement.

Less than a month later, Gifford was invited to resign. Eben W. Martin, a congressional representative from Deadwood, South Dakota, immediately telegraphed an inquiry on Gifford's behalf to Larrabee. Larrabee politely told Martin that the secretary of the interior and Commissioner Luepp had decided on a change of management at the asylum. Gifford accepted the inevitable and on July 29, 1908, wrote a terse note of resignation.

Part of Luepp's "common-sense lines" included getting a medical man in charge of the asylum (his chief complaint with Gifford), but he was evidently alarmed by some of the incidental problems his investigators had mentioned concerning the asylum's facilities. In late May, he directed John Charles, his supervisor of construction, to go to Canton and look into the fire safety issues and sewage problems the inspectors had discovered. Ironically, in his subsequent report, Charles made some of the most cutting comments in a government document to date about the conditions of the patients.

Shackles, muffs, and camisoles (another version of the straitjacket) were nothing new at Canton and had been described in the *Hudsonite* quite matter-of-factly following the editor's visit to the asylum in 1905. What hadn't been mentioned much by either newspapers or government inspectors—and which Charles now documented—was the overcrowding and illness at the facility.

"A great deal of sickness exists among the patients who have been brot [sic] here," reported Charles.[20] He found that about a fifth of the patients admitted to the asylum since its opening had died and that typically a tenth of the patients were too ill to get out of bed.

The facility held sixty-one patients, at the time of Charles's visit, plus theoretically another three who were absent without leave, rather than the forty-eight for which it had been designed. A dozen or so additional patients may not have seemed like much, but considering that several required constant medical attention and that several others were dangerously violent, the attendants would have been stretched thin. Canton Asylum's small size always told against it—a few extra patients who might have been absorbed within a larger institution presented a significant drain on manpower when the entire staff consisted of eighteen people, of whom only four were actually attendants.

Charles recommended a separate hospital building that could accommodate at least a dozen patients. He speculated that a building costing about $30,000 could include a dispensary, operating room, kitchen and dining room, and quarters for nurses or attendants. As a layman, he likely did not realize how spreading the staff to another building would *decrease* their availability to patients, or he may have simply assumed that the Indian Office would authorize additional attendants.

Charles went on to discuss the conditions he had actually been sent to observe. He recommended chemical fire extinguishers to use for any small fires that might occur within the structure, instead of relying on the leaky cotton hoses. Then he tackled the situation that probably made life miserable for both the patients and the staff.

Charles probably smelled the problem before he saw it—raw sewage. The receiving tank for waste sat a few hundred yards away from the building. The tank automatically discharged when the sewage reached a certain level, and the discharge was supposed to disperse over sewage beds in a thin sheet, spreading over a liberal area.

The ground for the beds had never been leveled properly or prepared for receiving the waste, so the sewage pooled in a low-lying portion of the field and dribbled across the railroad track and onto the property of other people—who didn't like it one bit. The tank's siphon, which trapped air to hold the waste back until it could be released with sufficient pressure to allow distribution, had never worked properly and had been removed. Thus sewage in its crude state ran onto the ground in a constant stream. Charles suggested a septic tank and recommended that the range toilets be replaced by seat operating closets whenever a change in the plumbing was made.

This was the situation that Dr. Harry Reid Hummer walked into when he took over as superintendent of Canton Asylum on October 1, 1908. Although Gifford had offered his resignation at the end of July, he remained at the institution until the end of September—due to the "number of requests from prominent persons in South Dakota, asking for delay in acting on this case."[21] Whether Gifford actually wanted to remain as superintendent or simply felt a bit of stung pride, he allowed friends and associates (such as South Dakota's former secretary of state, a current member of the Republican National Committee) to raise a clamor on his behalf at the Indian Office.

Those same friends and associates, unsuccessful at keeping Gifford in place, had also clamored to make sure that Turner didn't get his job. There they found more success, though Turner apparently did not seriously consider putting in for Gifford's position. The Indian Office didn't consider him for it, either. Whether they felt he was too close to the problems there or wasn't qualified, or because they automatically turned to the East and St. Elizabeths once they perceived the need for a new superintendent, his name was never brought up for the superintendency. Hummer arrived in Canton with the knowledge that after Dr. Logie's refusal, he had been the Indian Office's only real contender.

Hummer was perfectly at ease taking charge of a situation. He immediately distanced himself from Gifford and made sure that Turner knew who was in control. From his first day, Hummer was the point person for anything to do with Canton Asylum. Confident in his medical abilities, up-to-date on treatments for the insane as well as theories about insanity's origins, Hummer was a young physician ready to make a name for himself. He was familiar with the government's civil service requirements and other regulations and understood the scrutiny that federal establishments came under. His confidence at a high, he set about resolving one deficiency Gifford had been unable to resolve:

To: The Honorable
The Commissioner of Indian Affairs
Subject: Inquiry concerning tombstones

Sir:

I would respectfully request to be informed as to whether or not there is any fund out of which headstones for the graves of deceased patients might be bought.

> Very respectfully,
> H. R. Hummer
> *Superintendent and Special*
> *Disbursing Agent*

Sir:

In answer to your question of the 29th ultimo, you are advised that the Office has no fund out of which the cost of headstones for the graves of deceased patients might be paid.

> Very respectfully,
> *Acting Commissioner* [22]

Gravestones were all well and good for a large facility like St. Elizabeths in the heart of Washington DC, but out in Canton, they were just a waste of money. Hummer may have been discouraged by the rebuff, but the Indian Office's indifference also sent Hummer a heartening message. Out here, without much oversight and treating patients that nobody cared about, he could do almost anything he wanted. And with very few checks in place, he did.

6. Which Way to Canton?

n 1902 Dr. Frank A. Jones of Memphis, Tennessee, addressed the fifty-third session of the American Medical Association, saying that a high school education and the knowledge of English grammar and rhetoric were sufficient qualifications to study medicine. Even though many states were licensing physicians by this time (usually requiring a diploma from a four-year medical school that held six months of courses each year), the academic credentials of any particular physician could be hit-or-miss. Proprietary schools, whose courses consisted of lectures delivered by physicians who owned the school and had no incentive to disenroll poorly performing students, were the norm.[1] Except for a few state-chartered schools, most medical colleges were chartered by the state to private corporations, which ran them without oversight of any kind.

Aspiring physicians could alternatively receive hands-on instruction as apprentices to a local practitioner, which may have given them more practical knowledge than going the typical academic route. The soundest medical training was a hybrid that embraced the best of both practices: attending a university that gave both lectures and clinical training. Hummer's training fell into the latter category.

Born in Washington DC in 1879, Hummer was bright and confident, graduating in 1896 from Eastern High School with a scholarship to Georgetown Medical School. Upon graduation in 1899 at the age of twenty, Hummer worked at Columbia Hospital, one of the district's oldest, leaving it three months later to begin an internship at St. Elizabeths. One month into his internship, he took a civil service exam for a junior assistant physician position, to which he was appointed.

In 1904 he was promoted to senior assistant physician. That earned him an assignment overseeing the detached building group at St. Elizabeths, with more than 650 patients under his care. Hardworking and ambitious, Hummer had a wife (he married Norena Guest in 1901) and two young sons by 1908. He was also a member of the District Medical Society and the Medical Association of the District and an associate member of the American Medico-Psychological Association.

Why on earth did this man want to be superintendent of the Canton Asylum for Insane Indians? Hummer was an easterner through and through, with an easterner's disdain for the unsophisticated culture of the West. More than that, he was rightly proud of having an education that was unequivocally superior to that of many of the country's practicing physicians. Canton Asylum held a tenth of the patients he was supervising at St. Elizabeths, and there is nothing to indicate that Hummer wasn't as ambitious as he was hard-working. So what about the job appealed to him?

Perhaps Hummer just didn't like working the night shift at St. Elizabeths, which undoubtedly affected the quality of his family life. He had sworn under oath during St. Elizabeths' investigation in 1906 that he had had only one month and three weeks of vacation in seven years and that he was at the hospital at all times, day and night. Such grueling work at the government hospital may have made the opportunity for more control over his time as superintendent at a smaller asylum quite attractive. Far more likely, however, was Hummer's need to get out from under the shadows of a couple of men who reminded him that he was not yet as successful as he wanted to be.

His wife's cousin, Edgar Guest, wrote a column in the *Detroit Free Press* that acted as a springboard for his immensely popular poetry. Sentimental and often folksy, Guest's verse had a huge following that eventually led to a collection of poems that sold over a million copies in 1916. Though he had not yet reached that accomplishment by 1908, he was probably the family member who consistently got the most attention and acclaim within Hummer's extended family. Hummer may have had a perfectly cordial relationship with Guest or even enjoyed his poetic skills. However, given the character and personality traits he displayed, Hummer very likely did not enjoy playing second fiddle, even socially, to an in-law.[2]

Of far more consequence was his relationship to the enormously respected Dr. William Alanson White. A professor of nervous and mental diseases at both Georgetown University and George Washington University in Washington DC, as well as a lecturer at the Army Medical School, White was already a well-established psychiatrist before President Theodore Roosevelt appointed him superintendent of St. Elizabeths in 1903. White authored *Outlines of Psychiatry* in 1907, a book that became the standard medical text on the topic for almost three decades. He frequently testified as an expert in court cases, including the famous Thaw murder trial, in which the multimillionaire Harry Thaw was prosecuted for murdering his wife's ex-lover, Stanford White, in Madison Square Garden's rooftop theater in 1906.

Only nine years older than Hummer, White had a career that was on an increasingly lofty trajectory. Hummer probably realized he could never catch up to his superior if he remained where he was, and he had not worked so hard for his own education and internship to merely orbit a man who had such a career head start on him. Heading his own institution rather than remaining an assistant physician in White's would have appealed to a man with ambition. At Canton Asylum, Hummer would enjoy both position and power—something he later proved he enjoyed immensely.[3]

More practically, as the superintendent of his own institution, Hummer would gain the kind of credibility and expertise he could never achieve otherwise. And, as Canton Asylum's superintendent, he would be particularly well placed to add his thoughts to the burgeoning theories concerning heredity and race in the development of insanity. No one had really done in-depth studies concerning insane Indians, and Canton was a unique facility full of them. Hummer might eventually be considered a bona fide expert in the field.

Whatever ultimately drove his decision, Hummer accepted the government's offer of $2,500 annually (with quarters, light, and fuel provided free of charge) and set off for Canton, South Dakota. A couple of weeks after his arrival, Hummer took the practical step of dropping in at the *Sioux Valley News* office to introduce himself to editor George Nash, who publicly encouraged the town to welcome the newcomer.

Nash had taken over the paper after the death of his father, Newman C. Nash, in 1905. The senior Nash had been a dedicated newspaperman with considerable clout—when he backed a political candidate, that candidate's worries were generally over. A fervent and vocal town booster, Nash threw himself and the power of his paper behind many important improvements and enterprises in Canton. George Nash continued in the same vein, openly encouraging civic projects and lending a strong voice to community affairs. It would not hurt anyone to earn his favor, particularly an easterner coming in under a cloud.

Canton's leading citizens wanted to keep the asylum open and flourishing, but they were not inclined to like Dr. Hummer. The only reason they gave was that he appeared young, but the fact was that Hummer was replacing a very popular citizen whom many felt had been treated unfairly. The new superintendent did not seem to appreciate this and apparently put forth little effort to ingratiate himself with the town's leaders.

Though it may be presumed that Hummer had a certain grace period in which Canton's leading citizens would have swallowed their indignation enough to extend him and his family invitations to the numerous social events enjoyed by the townspeople, there is no mention in the paper—for months—of any parties or functions where Hummer was a guest.[4] Whether he didn't get the invitations or chose not to accept them, Hummer still occupied a prominent position as superintendent of Canton's insane asylum. His absence from the roster of any reported town functions is striking.

Hummer and his wife might have fit into Canton society if they had chosen to enjoy the town's amenities. Though not to be compared to the nation's capital, Canton had a thriving downtown with plenty of businesses. There were several clothiers, among them Seely & Tank (the store to which the ousted financial clerk Charles Seely had devoted so much of his time), where ladies could purchase stylish wardrobes and men could find suits by manufacturers like Hart Schaffner & Marx. The town had doctors and lawyers, an optician, jewelry stores, drugstores, restaurants, a buggy shop, grocers, a hardware store, banks, hotels, a train depot, a college . . .[5]

There was plenty to do, as well. Each Friday the *Sioux Valley News* ran a serialized novel that ladies might then discuss at any of their various ladies clubs. Citizens could enjoy numerous concerts and plays, as well as lectures, like the one in which Mrs. Oscar Gifford and her friend, Mrs. DeLong, gave accounts of their childhood experiences during the Civil War at a twenty-fifth anniversary banquet of the Grand Army of the Republic Post No. 11. Canton had a baseball team, several fraternal organizations, and social clubs to suit anyone's tastes. Despite these enticements, the Hummers kept to themselves, probably the worst thing they could have done to make themselves welcome.

Gifford, comfortably ensconced in Canton, had stayed on at the asylum until Hummer could arrive, which gave the appearance of a deliberate transfer of power. The *Sioux Valley News* kindly reported that Gifford was retiring because the Indian Office had decided to combine the positions of superintendent and chief physician. In a paper that routinely published such minute details of Canton life as who had dropped by the office to renew a subscription, not one word of the investigation had hit print. It probably soothed Gifford's spirit when the friendly paper also reported on October 9, 1908, that an inspector named Harris from Flandreau, South Dakota, had come to check on the asylum during the transfer of leadership and "found it in exceptionally good order."

Some of the paper's silence was due to Canton's pervasive boosterism and Nash's cheerleading of it, but some of it was assuredly due to Gifford's standing in the community. Though prominent citizens were aware of the investigations, they didn't seem to hold it against their longtime friend and simply restored "Judge" to Gifford's name in place of his title of superintendent. Nash, of course, had no incentive to rake up a scandal in his beloved Canton.

Two weeks after Hummer took over Canton Asylum, the Giffords hosted a supper party—mentioned in the paper—for many current and former employees, including the dismissed Berney Christopher. Gifford's friend Seely continued to bring Indian patients to the asylum for the next several months, the Indian Office apparently sticking to its guns by insisting that officers of the asylum shouldn't leave for such a task. Within a year, Gifford was an important player in the Inter-State Land and Investment Company. Seely and his family stayed at the asylum until the end of September; their move to town made it into the paper the same day that Dr. Hummer's arrival was noted.[6]

For his part, Hummer threw himself into his work, reviewing records and bringing his own expertise to the front. Initially, at least, he was inclined to discharge patients whom he felt didn't belong in the asylum. A week after he assumed his position, Hummer asked the commissioner of Indian affairs to allow Ida Todd, a thirteen-year-old patient, to attend an Indian school in Flandreau, South Dakota.[7] He stated explicitly that "the surroundings [at the Canton Asylum] are not suitable to the development of this future woman." However, the letter he wrote was revealing in several ways.

Hummer, in very formal language, engaged in the farce that the commissioner might do something other than follow the asylum superintendent's recommendation when it came to patient treatment. He asked both permission and advice on the situation, perhaps testing Luepp's inclination to give either. Hummer also, even at this early stage, made it clear that he did not like to relinquish control of patients. He told Luepp that he was not recommending "an unconditional discharge, but a furlough with the understanding that she might be returned here at any time her condition would necessitate it."[8]

And what was her condition? In Hummer's own words, Todd was an epileptic with infrequent convulsions that weren't particularly severe. She was quiet and well-behaved and assisted with light work in the dining room. Hummer's main concern was that she was sometimes irritable, as though irritation ought to be surprising to find in a thirteen-year-old girl confined to an insane asylum. Whether irritability was permissible under any circumstances or not, Hummer's real concern seemed to be that because of the epilepsy, Todd probably had a mild degree of idiocy.

It is telling that Hummer, a trained psychiatrist, did not differentiate between idiocy and insanity, nor seem to find anything amiss in such a young person being at an institution with so many insane adults, nor feel reluctant to bring the patient back to an institution that he was telling the commissioner couldn't help her. Even at this early stage, he seemed loath to let patients slip through his fingers completely.

Many patients at Canton Asylum were diagnosed with senility, congenital imbecility, or idiocy. Hummer's failure to take a stand to clear the asylum of anyone who wasn't insane seems deliberate. Unlike Gifford (and for that matter, Turner), Hummer had the training to actually know who belonged in the asylum and who didn't. At this pivotal moment, Hummer set the direction that the Indian Office was bound to follow. Rather than establish professionally endorsed guidelines that limited patients to those who fit the criteria for an insane asylum, Hummer took anyone that reservation superintendents wanted to send him and irrevocably transformed Canton Asylum into a shameful holding tank for unwanted Indians—only some of whom were insane.

Hummer had been described as arrogant when he was a young physician at St. Elizabeths. Congressional testimony during the asylum's 1906 investigation showed that Hummer was not afraid to throw his medical expertise around or to challenge people who interfered with his agenda. Now, at Canton, Hummer's self-confidence was further bolstered—he knew that as both superintendent of the asylum and its primary physician, his medical decisions were not likely to be overturned by a layperson in the Interior Department. His trust was borne out; there are fewer than half a dozen instances on record in which the Indian Office challenged either Gifford or Hummer when it came to decisions concerning their patients.

That he didn't choose to clear the facility of all but the insane is obvious, though it is difficult to fathom how a person with Hummer's credentials could have tolerated the caretaking of such a gamut of "defectives" as Canton Asylum housed.[9] Perhaps Hummer simply didn't want to empty the asylum of a great many of its patients. Alternatively, he could have regarded all his patients as offering potential data to test theories about race and heredity.

Regardless of his reasons, Hummer embraced the current system and allowed Canton Asylum to continue as a dumping ground for unwanted Indians. Though he discharged Joseph Louis Bruce, who had recovered from a bout of acute melancholia in December, he had earlier accepted sixteen-year-old Agnes Sloan, an insane girl "afflicted since her birth with extreme idiocy."[10] The difference in the two cases may have been that Bruce's father pressured the Indian Office to send his son home, and nobody wanted Sloan.

Just as Hummer did not break with the past in his indiscriminate acceptance of patients, neither did the new superintendent break with his predecessor's practices in the matter of favoritism. He quickly hired his wife, Norena, as matron of the institution—a position for which she had absolutely no experience or training. Then he did his predecessor, Gifford, one better.

Hummer wrote to the commissioner of Indian affairs about the local

Board of Examiners, which kept a list of eligible people for appointment to the various positions at the asylum. The board was composed of Oscar Gifford, Charles Seely, and Dr. Turner. Hummer asked that the board continue its function and that Gifford and Seely be replaced, stating that he had heard that they were going to resign anyway. He nominated himself as the new chairman and then tendered a new name to replace Seely—Norena Hummer.[11] Empire building began at home, and he grasped authority with both hands.

Power may have been the only comfort the couple had those first miserable months in their new home. Temperatures were frigid and the South Dakota wind blew mercilessly most of the time, part of a radical new environment thrust on an eastern family accustomed to more temperate breezes and temperatures that generally behaved themselves.[12] Toward the latter part of January, a howling sixty-mile-an-hour gale blew down the smokestack of the electric plant that powered the asylum. Hummer and his staff fell back on oil lamps and lanterns, which hindered their ability to care for patients. Hummer couldn't call anyone to complain, because the storm also blew down the telephone wires.

The U.S. Weather Bureau had a substation in Canton, but Hummer didn't need to see a weather flag flapping on a pole to know that he was cold and wretched. He had never seen this much snow in the Mid-Atlantic region around Washington DC, where winters were relatively mild and short. Temperatures in Canton reached twenty-two degrees below zero in January, and the mercury fell below zero on many other bitterly cold days that winter.

The north side of the asylum, where tubercular patients were housed, was especially cold and received no sunshine whatsoever. The epileptic patient Yells-at-Night died November 21, 1908, Hummer's third death at the institution within a month and a half of his arrival.[13] All three deaths were from tuberculosis (TB), a disease ravaging the Native American population.

The tubercle bacillus had been isolated by Robert Koch in 1882, a major discovery that established it as an infectious disease. Though Koch's discovery advanced their knowledge somewhat, doctors still had no cure for the disease and generally could only isolate patients in sanitariums. Treatments consisted of injecting air into the lungs or performing thoracoplasty (surgery to decrease lung size). No effective cures existed until the antibiotic streptomycin became available in 1952.

By 1887, deaths from tuberculosis among reservation Indians had been tabulated in thirteen states, with a low of 45 per 1,000 deaths in Nevada to a high of 625 per 1,000 deaths in New York. On some reservations in the West, tuberculosis accounted for more than 30 percent of total deaths. The prevalence of this and other diseases in the Indian population was reflected in the 1900 U.S. census, the first to differentiate Indians from the rest of the population. Life expectancy for Native Americans was 38.4 years, as opposed to 43 for blacks and 50 to 51 for whites.[14]

The Canton Asylum for Insane Indians had its share of tubercular patients, for whom it could do exactly what other facilities did—nothing. Unlike other facilities, however, the asylum couldn't even try to make them comfortable. The building had four dormitory wings designed to hold ten beds each. Two single rooms and one double were in the cold, sunless north wing, so tubercular patients were put there by necessity to isolate them from patients in the dormitories. Evidently out of desperation, Dr. Turner asked Hummer to procure equipment for a tubercular camp, one idea making the medical rounds because it was a simple and cheap way to separate TB patients from the rest of an institutional population.

Hummer passed along Turner's suggestion to the Indian Office, though he voiced what Turner obviously knew: pitching canvas tents in the bitter South Dakota winter was unlikely to help patients recover. Hummer suggested a hospital instead (at a cost of $60,000 rather than John Charles's conservative $30,000), in which he could actually house the sick, perform an operation should one be necessary, and provide hydrotherapy treatments.

Unfortunately for Hummer, the sickness that Charles had noted in his construction report wouldn't go away just because a new superintendent was in charge; overcrowding, poor hygiene, and patients' weakened immune systems guaranteed health issues at Canton Asylum. Besides acute diseases like colds, influenza, and other typical infections that make the rounds in any enclosed population, some patients showed up with chronic diseases like trachoma, which had also hit reservation populations very hard.

This devastating condition began as a simple eye infection during childhood, but with unsanitary conditions and constant reinfection, trachoma developed into a chronic infection of the conjunctiva (the thin membrane that covers the outer surface of the eye) and the inner lining of the eyelid.[15] As the disease progressed, continued infections caused scarring on the inside of the eyelid. Eventually the eyelids became scarred so badly that they turned inward. The victims' eyelashes rubbed their eyeballs, causing corneal ulcerations that could easily become infected. By their forties or fifties, many victims became blind. Rampant blindness (the disease eventually affected up to 40 percent of some tribal groups) affected the Native American population's ability to be self-sufficient. This was a huge concern for the federal government.

In the early 1900s, several trachoma surveys revealed the presence of a "trachoma belt" across the middle United States, particularly affecting Indian reservations, where rates of the disease in schoolchildren reached as high as 50 to 90 percent. Crowding, poverty, lack of clean water, and poor hygiene were identified as risk factors for trachoma. In 1913 the U.S. Public Health Service earmarked a large portion of its budget to fight trachoma, but doctors and money to fight it were scaled back during World War I. The inflation that followed the war caused a further loss of real funds.[16]

Into the 1920s, the Office of Indian Affairs' preferred method of treating trachoma was through tarsectomy, an unproven operation with a 50 percent success rate. Tarsectomy involved turning the eyelid inside out, scraping away scar nodules with a scalpel or toothbrush, and then cauterizing or disinfecting the scraped area. Follow-up care from the Indian Health Service was abysmal. The operation often left the patient worse off than before, sometimes causing the eyelid to stick to the eyeball.[17]

Hummer didn't have the expertise to perform tarsectomies even if he had wanted to, and he realized early on that the Indian Office didn't want to enlarge the institution. Still, he had to have been appalled at the lack of medical facilities. To a doctor coming from a large, modern institution, the lack of a single hospital bed would have been dismaying. He wasn't just interested in the physical problems he saw, either. Hummer's suggestion for a hydrotherapy room showed that he was conversant with the latest thinking on the treatment of mental diseases, for hydrotherapy baths of all kinds—solid douche, fan douche, perineal douche, spray and sitz baths, showers, and wet packs—were the latest rage.[18] His letter to the commissioner held enthusiasm concerning the subject, an enthusiasm rarely expressed in any of his later official correspondence.

Hydrotherapy in various forms had been a recommended treatment for insanity for many years, and Hummer would have been perfectly familiar with the cutting-edge advice recommended by his ex-boss, Dr. White, in his newly published *Outlines of Psychiatry*. White recommended various hydrotherapy treatments, especially for excited patients, noting that without them, either physical or chemical restraint would be necessary. White also recommended continuous baths for excited patients, praising the sedating effects of warm water.

When patients refused food, which happened often in asylums for a number of reasons, White suggested that they be allowed to refuse it until they became hungry. If they were in poor health, however, they would need to be force-fed through a tube inserted either up the nose or down the esophagus. He cautioned physicians to be careful about prescribing opiates, which could be addictive, and suggested paraldehyde (which had a very disagreeable odor and taste) and sulfanol for the insomnia that frequently afflicted the insane. Similar drugs like chloralamid or chloral could be given as "pleasant elixers." For acutely excited cases, White acknowledged that about the only effective sedative was the alkaloid "hyoscyamus," a potent, dangerous narcotic that could lead to respiratory paralysis; it had similar properties to belladonna. Doctors had to take care in dosing, White warned, as the preparations available "are somewhat uncertain."[19]

In 1907 these recommendations were all that White suggested as particularly required for treating the insane. A hospital was not necessary for any of them, though a dedicated hydrotherapy room would have been ideal. The asylum did not possess hydrotherapy equipment, but Hummer should have been able to manage—at least at times—some form of continuous bath for patients who would have benefited from the treatment. His predecessor had dosed patients with the types of medicines White suggested, so the Indian Office could expect someone with Hummer's qualifications to do as much or more in the way of caring for the insane. Requesting a hospital was an appropriate step, but not an essential one, for maintaining or improving patient care.

The Indian Office's refusal to build a new hospital probably didn't surprise Hummer, who would have been familiar with government budgets and spending cycles. What may have surprised him was the unrelenting detail work that fell to his lot as superintendent. Unlike Gifford, he had a very firm hands-on approach to his duties, and he was reluctant to let (or trust) anyone else to do what he knew he could do better. He threw himself into the minutia of administrative work that accompanied a government, institutional job and apparently didn't delegate one iota of it.

Hummer gradually gave more and more attention to what had probably lured him to the position in the first place—an increased opportunity for power and respect. Hummer wanted more patients, more buildings, and more recognition for himself and his unique facility. He and his staff were already at odds as he endured the long winter, and he concentrated on pursuing expansion while pinching pennies to show the Indian Office that he was careful with its money. His patients interested him as subjects, but he was, at best, indifferent to them as individuals.

A forty-two-year-old Sioux man named John Brown was admitted to the asylum on March 9, 1909, suffering from paranoia and dementia praecox, an early term for what is now called schizophrenia.[20] Hummer examined him and noted several scars, eight missing teeth, and a small external hemorrhoid. Three years later he got around to giving Brown a psychiatric evaluation. He noted that the patient's judgment and reasoning were fair, that his ideation (the process of forming and relating ideas) was slightly diminished, that his self-awareness was good, and that he was self-complacent, indifferent, and well-behaved.

This was the only psychiatric exam Hummer gave this patient during the more than twenty years he remained at Canton Asylum under Hummer's care. The exam showed nothing that even hinted at paranoia or schizophrenia, labels that Brown may have been given before he arrived. Somehow, Hummer was satisfied with the exam and for the next twenty years never gave a thought to the misery he was inflicting on a man that his own examination had proven to be of sound mind.

That indifference spoke volumes about his subsequent years in power.

7. The Reign of Harry Reid Hummer Begins

In the stifling August heat, Martha Smith (Kay-ge-gay-aush-oak), an epileptic Chippewa woman, lay on a mattress soiled by sweat, urine, and feces, restlessly kicking off her bedclothes and her night-dress. She slapped helplessly at the blowflies buzzing over her body. They were laying eggs.

Down the hallways and inside the common areas, cockroaches skittered across the floors and up the walls, feeding and exploring and reproducing. A man, half-slumbering, shifted suddenly at the sharp prickle of a bedbug on his flesh. His fingers plucked the creature free and smashed it against the wall. It squirted blood—*his* blood—as the tiny carcass joined hundreds of other dried splotches on the wall.

In a few days, the blowfly eggs hatched on Martha's bed. Wiggling maggots crawled across the excreta smeared on her flesh, digging deep into the sheets under her body as they followed their instinct to burrow and pupate into adults. The stench of decay clung to her bed, soaked into her flesh, and sweated back out as she continued to lie, unwashed, in her feces. Dr. Hummer pointed her out to his new assistant physician as a "filthy" patient.

The government could do a lot to disillusion an employee, and Hummer may have been disillusioned very quickly. He had dragged his wife and two young children out to a godforsaken bit of country where the wind never stopped blowing and spring didn't know enough to come around at the proper time. Smallpox had broken out in Canton, leaving Hummer scrambling to replace the deteriorated vaccine stock held at the asylum before unprotected patients and staff caught the disease.

Hummer was accustomed to working with trained nurses rather than attendants who received whatever expertise they possessed through on-the-job training. He didn't have a clerk when he arrived, but as the government's special disbursing agent, Hummer was required to requisition all supplies, issue vouchers, render accounts, disburse funds, and maintain files and reports. Rather than allocate any of these tasks to Dr. Turner or someone else on staff, Hummer personally took on all the office work (even down to answering telephone calls) and promptly became buried in details.[1] Actually treating patients and overseeing employees and their work got squeezed out of his schedule. Though he was available to assist Hummer with medical care, by now Turner's honeymoon from escort service was over, and he was back to traveling far afield to bring new patients to the asylum.

Nearly half a dozen patients had died within Hummer's first months of service at the asylum, and many of his charges were very sick with tuberculosis and other diseases prevalent in the Indian community. Other patients had escaped, while the families of patients who were getting along perfectly well pleaded that they be allowed to return home. And always, Hummer juggled lack of beds and space with accommodating the requests for admittance that poured in from the commissioner's office, Indian agents, reservation superintendents, and other sources.

Though Hummer kept a civil face to the community, maintaining friendly ties to newspaper editor Nash and forming professional friendships with a couple of local doctors, he treated his staff—uneducated, inexperienced, and confoundedly independent—with disrespect. He considered it an insult to his judgment for an employee to make a suggestion, and anyone who dared to disagree with him or argue a point got on the wrong side of him in a hurry

Hummer was used to servants and "colored" workers who knew their place. At St. Elizabeths, run somewhat on a military style and definitely on hierarchal terms, Hummer, as a doctor, had ranked just below God. Here in the West, he expected the same kind of master-servant relationship with his staff and couldn't understand why these South Dakotans insisted on acting like his equals. He didn't appreciate their attitude, didn't like any of them, and didn't try to hide his feelings or rein in his explosive irritability.

After Hummer's five-year-old son, Francis, threw rocks and struck two patients and an attendant, Hummer and the attendant engaged in a blistering altercation inside the male ward that left Hummer threatening to "sweep the god dammed ward with you." Even his theoretical equal, Dr. Turner, couldn't escape Hummer's temper. Having been told by his superior to keep him informed of anything Turner thought he should know, the assistant physician approached Hummer shortly after his arrival with the news that the night watchman had told him he was going to resign. In a frenzy of rage, Hummer told Turner that "every damn one of you can resign!"

The asylum would have collapsed had his wish been granted. Never mind that Hummer admitted to Turner that he knew nothing about Indians, their language, habits, or superstitions; presumably, he would learn. Though some written works were sensationalized or colored by cultural prejudice, competent books describing Native American history and customs were available to any interested reader. Additionally, the Smithsonian Institution's Bureau of American Ethnology had just published (in 1908) a lengthy document about Native American culture and continued its study in this area for several decades. Hummer had only to make a slight effort to familiarize himself with his patients' way of life.

What no one at the Indian Office had foreseen was how vast and encompassing Hummer's ignorance was when it came to carrying out the duties involved in running a nearly self-sufficient establishment. Dr. Turner was floored when Hummer asked him what hay and straw were and how to grow onions from onion sets.[2]

Hummer's ignorance wouldn't have mattered so much if he had let someone knowledgeable take over his weak areas and do what needed to be done. Instead, Hummer crippled the asylum's ability to support itself when he told employees to take care of the garden and then wouldn't give them time off from other duties to do it. Consequently, the gardens produced almost nothing; his management style produced similar results with the asylum's dairy farm.[3]

Hummer didn't know how to use the government's ration tables to allocate the correct amounts of food to patients and staff (who received board as part of their wages). Instead, he took the quantity of food he was issued for the year, divided the total by the number of weeks in the year, and distributed that set amount each week.

This method did not take into account the actual number of patients or staff eating each particular week or the number of extra patients the facility was accepting; it undoubtedly did not take into account that food previously supplied in the form of garden produce and dairy products from the farm was no longer available due to his inept management. To further distort the distribution process, when food spoiled or had to be destroyed, he charged the condemned items against his employees' food allowances and made them sign for it as issued to them.

Hummer's system particularly shorted the meat ration for employees and patients, and both groups frequently left their tables still hungry. Employees were a little more fortunate, since they had the means of buying their own food if they chose to do so. The government also provided some types of food as "extras" for the asylum, like canned fruit and sugar. Employees routinely ate these items, and they were not often distributed to patients. Hummer either didn't see it or didn't care; he never intervened.

That did not mean that the Hummers skimped on themselves. As patients went hungry, Mrs. Hummer took plentiful supplies of milk, canned goods, and other foodstuffs for her family from government supplies—so much that employees remarked upon the quantities. Like her husband, Mrs. Hummer did little to endear herself to the asylum's staff. She brushed past both patients and workers as though they were beneath her, stayed mainly in her rooms, sewing, and demanded that asylum staff empty chamber slops and clean her children's playroom as they tidied up the family's quarters. If employees had developed a healthy dislike of Dr. Hummer, they learned to dislike Mrs. Hummer even more heartily.

Norena Hummer, city bred and class-conscious, did not appreciate the western character any more than her husband did. At home in St. Elizabeths, she had depended upon servants to do her bidding. A nurse took care of her children and the couple ate their meals at the officer's club, leaving her with little actual work to do. She was absolutely unqualified for her duties as matron of an insane asylum and performed them with little competence or willingness.[4]

At Canton Asylum, Mrs. Hummer had to do a good portion of her own housework and sewing, as well as take care of her children. Busy with these tasks, she seldom took time to visit the wards, although her position required her to make daily visits. When she did manage to make a visit, she simply breezed through, issuing orders in a patronizing manner that grated on the employees' nerves.

As matron, she controlled much of the institution's daily nonmedical supplies, and she seemed to be deliberately stingy. She refused to issue bedspreads, rubber sheets, bath brushes, dresses, pants, or shirts for the asylum's patients, and the ward attendants patched, repaired, and repatched clothing until it was threadbare and ragged. Many female patients had no underskirts, and few had more than two dresses.

Mrs. Hummer's antipathy for her work was palpable: she scarcely spoke to staff and refused to speak to patients or to even touch their clothing. Attendants complained so vigorously of shortages to Dr. Hummer that he finally asked his wife to go to the laundry and make arrangements to get clothing for the wards and sewing rooms. She replied that she wouldn't touch any of it. Hummer told her she could have an attendant pick up each piece of clothing for her, but Mrs. Hummer still refused to perform the task.

Under her management, patients went barefoot in winter or wore cotton socks and straw hats instead of warmer woolen items, or exposed themselves through patch-holes in their tattered clothing. Meanwhile, the storage rooms held two years' worth of ready-made clothing that could have been issued at any time.

Between the Hummers, the staff and patients were constantly short of every item imaginable: the asylum owned a single, unusable razor (though at least one attendant brought his own to shave some of the male patients), and there were no hair clippers. Towels and soap were at a premium: Hummer allowed two half-pound bars weekly to bathe thirty-two patients in the east ward, and eight towels to dry them with.[5] To save coal, he allowed hot water only two days a week, which guaranteed that nothing would come clean in the asylum's hard water.

On another front, cockroaches and bedbugs—always a problem in institutions—were especially persistent at Canton Asylum. Pinching pennies, Hummer issued two quarts of gasoline or kerosene a week as a bedbug disinfectant for the beds. Hygienic standards couldn't be maintained under the best of circumstances because of the septic problems and range toilets, and many of the patients soiled themselves both inadvertently and willfully.[6] Cold, hungry, ragged, and dirty, the patients were faring worse under a doctor's administration than they had under a layman's.

By February 1909, Dr. Turner had had enough of it. He had endured Gifford's indifference, interminable trips to fetch patients, investigations, and recalcitrant staff who didn't obey his orders. His terminally ill father had died at the asylum after Turner brought him from Pennsylvania to Canton so he could take care of him. Turner had borne the strain of a falling-out with Gifford and Seely, been attacked by a patient and struck in the head with a rock, and now . . . Hummer's rages and incompetence were beyond bearing.

After seventeen years in government service, Turner put in his papers and left the Indian Service at the end of March to begin a private practice in town. Turner set up his office in rooms over the O.K. Restaurant on the east end of what was called the Syndicate block and moved his family from the asylum to a cottage in town. The Hummers were greatly relieved, though the woman who cooked for both the Turners and the Hummers quit when she discovered that Dr. Turner was leaving. Mrs. Hummer either had to add cooking to her chores or accept what the institution could provide but doubtlessly appreciated the extra space; her family had been uncomfortably squeezed by the necessity of sharing space with another family in an area of the facility built to accommodate only one. The downside, of course, was that Hummer now had to take on Turner's duties.

Finally daunted, Hummer asked the Indian Office to provide him with a *single* man to replace Turner. In its infinite wisdom, the office sent him a married doctor with both a pregnant wife and a child. Unfortunately for Dr. L. M. Hardin, by the time he arrived in August, Hummer was already in possession of the asylum's family quarters and had no intention of giving them up or sharing. Hardin also wasn't able to replicate Gifford's and Turner's amicable compromise—unlike Gifford, Hummer and his family had moved to Canton from a great distance and had no home in town, as Gifford had when Turner arrived.

Four corner rooms in the asylum were especially desirable for their light, convenience, and beautiful views. One was taken up as an office, one as a sitting room for the Hummers, another as their dining room, and the last as their bedroom. Two of the three next most desirable rooms were taken by the Hummers as well. The superintendent gave

Hardin's family a back room with two windows and the use of a basement kitchen discarded by Hummer as inconvenient.

Hummer undoubtedly both needed and wanted another physician at Canton Asylum, but he hadn't counted on getting one as stubborn as himself. Hardin was already angry with the Indian Service for a demotion and forced transfer from Leech Lake Reservation, and he wasn't about to accept the quarters Hummer offered.[7] Hardin arrived on August 18, butted heads with Hummer over his rooms, and fired off a letter to the commissioner of Indian affairs on the twenty-second, purportedly with Hummer's knowledge.

After Hardin received a reply that stated Hummer had been told to give him the same or equivalent quarters as his predecessor, the fireworks began. Hummer worked himself into a fury over the issue. "You are insubordinate," he railed. "You are the most insignificant and contemptible pup I have ever had to deal with!"

Hardin left the room, content that the clerk, Fowles, had heard the remarks. The next day, Hummer offered an apology without any apparent show of repentance, and Hardin shrugged it off in silence. Later, Hummer resumed his insults, telling Hardin that he would immediately recommend his dismissal from the Indian Service. Hardin replied that he was at liberty to do so, and from that moment, the two men barely spoke to one another. Hummer ratcheted up the pettiness by appropriating a serving room he had previously shared with Turner and cutting off the dumbwaiter that served it, forcing Hardin's family to use the basement kitchen or pantry to eat in or climb a flight of stairs and pass through two halls and three doors to eat in the dining room.[8]

About that time, Hummer committed the misstep of taking his family on a visit back East.[9] Hardin fired off another letter of complaint to the commissioner on September 4, but now he also listed some of Hummer's more serious shortcomings—patient neglect, overcrowding, and poor sanitation throughout the building. He asked the commissioner to investigate the asylum and Hummer's conduct, as well as to intervene in the matter of his quarters.[10]

Hardin had his back up on his own account, but he was also angry for others at the asylum. He was particularly enraged by Martha Smith's condition. Hummer had pointed her out as a "filthy" patient when

Hardin made his first rounds on August 18; she had been lying in her feces then. Hardin worked for the next ten days helping to oversee the construction of the asylum's new laundry building. When he began making rounds on the twenty-seventh, he found the Chippewa woman still lying in excrement, but now with maggots crawling through it.

Hardin called a female attendant, and together, they cleaned and bathed the young woman as he spoke to her in her own language. Though he felt the attendants shared the blame for Smith's condition, Hardin put the responsibility for the situation squarely on Hummer's shoulders, particularly since the attendants had noted Smith's condition in their daily reports and the matron should have spotted it during her rounds—which Hardin knew Hummer didn't require her to make.[11]

Hardin didn't stop at cleaning up a suffering patient. Now that the Hummers were gone, Hardin issued more rations, had the patients' metal bed frames pulled onto the lawn and fired with gasoline to burn all the bedbugs, and brought patients who had been cooped up in their rooms outdoors into the sunshine. He also took it upon himself to order the potato fields mowed of weeds and grass and then raked and burned, in order to discover the rows and harvest the potatoes. Busy with ward rounds and the other minutiae of running the asylum in Hummer's absence, Hardin still managed to get twelve employees together to petition the Indian Office to investigate conditions at the asylum. He did not sign the petition, but he both urged and engineered it.

His victories during Hummer's absence were not echoed in Washington—no one responded to the petition. On October 12, Hummer came back and Mrs. Hummer put a stop to the increased rations ("over-issue," in her words) at once. She tried to find out what had happened in her absence, but the cook, acting matron, and others did not enlighten her; since she was not on speaking terms with Hardin, he declined to volunteer an explanation.

On October 16, Hardin received a letter from the Indian Office proposing to transfer him to the Haywood Indian School in Wisconsin at a further reduction in salary. On October 29, Hardin and twelve employees swore out nineteen charges against Hummer and his wife and sent them to the Indian Office. With bulldog tenacity, Hardin informed the commissioner of Indian affairs that he had also forwarded a copy of the charges to South Dakota congressman Charles H. Burke. He also gave a copy to Dr. Turner, to show interested parties in Canton.

Within a day or two, Hardin read a brief dispatch emanating from Washington—laying most of the blame for the asylum's problems on him—in the *Minneapolis Journal*. On November 5, the text of the nineteen charges he had leveled at Hummer was published in full by a sympathetic Sioux Falls newspaper, the *Daily Argus-Leader*. Though he would not admit to it, Hardin likely submitted the charges himself or allowed them to be submitted to the paper on his behalf. Someone in Washington hadn't played fair, but the publication of Hardin's charges made an investigation inevitable—he had at least won that battle.

When the supervisor of Indian schools, Charles L. Davis, arrived at the asylum, he found the attendants in such a bitter mood that they would have walked out en masse at the first harsh word; if they had, Davis felt that local feeling was so strong against the superintendent that he couldn't have hired replacements. Davis brokered an agreement between the employees not to quit until he had investigated Hummer and the asylum, and tensions eased.

The nineteen charges he had been called to investigate, in brief, were these:

1. Hummer was ill-tempered, discourteous, disrespectful, and given to abusive language.

2. Hummer issued insufficient rations to the patients and to the employees from government supplies.

3. Hummer required employees to receipt for spoiled canned goods, charging the same against their allowances.

4. Hummer required employees to do personal services for him and his family, even if asylum work had to be neglected because of it.

5. Mrs. Hummer did not perform her duties.

6. Hummer overcrowded the dormitories and misrepresented this condition to the Indian Office.

7. Hummer was guilty of gross neglect in the care of patient Martha Smith.

8. Beds, mattresses, halls, and so on occupied by the inmates were neglected such that they became infested with bedbugs to an extreme degree.

9. Hummer locked up patients without need, to their physical and mental detriment.

10. Soap, warm water, towels, and so on were not provided in sufficient quantities.

11. Hummer failed to provide accessories for the care and convenience of filthy patients and disinfectants for keeping the wards and toilets in proper condition.

12. Patients were not provided with suitable clothing.

13. Hummer failed to provide adequate protection in case of fire.

14. Hummer failed to make needed repairs to the facility.

15. Hummer knew nothing about gardening and farming.

16. Hummer was unwilling to accept the advice or suggestions of his subordinates.

17. Hummer was discourteous when answering the phone.

18. Hummer was inefficient and incompetent.

19. Hummer disparaged the asylum by referring to it as "the joke of the Indian Service."[12]

Davis had his work cut out trying to wade through the morass of allegations and counter-allegations spewing acrimoniously from both employees and superintendent. Hummer denied nearly everything except his ignorance of farming, and he particularly blamed Martha Smith's condition on Dr. Hardin. He said Hardin made the daily rounds and should have seen what was going on. Hardin claimed that when he arrived on August 18, he had gone through the facility with Hummer but had been relieved of ward duties so he could supervise the ongoing laundry construction, having had some experience in that area. He had not seen Smith again until he assumed ward duties on August 27.

This dispute was difficult for Davis to resolve, but the preponderance of evidence suggests that Hardin was in the right. Almost all his other charges were substantiated, and discovering Smith's condition seems to have been a precipitating factor in his calling for an investigation. It would have been like Hummer to give Hardin a time-consuming extra duty while still expecting him to perform another full-time job. Since the two weren't on speaking terms, there may have been some legitimate misunderstanding in that regard, with Hardin thinking his job was to supervise the laundry construction and Hummer thinking it was to supervise the laundry construction *and* make his usual rounds.

It quickly became apparent to Davis, however, that many of the charges Hardin and the employees had made—though sometimes highly colored or exaggerated—were founded in solid fact.

Hummer was indeed ill-tempered and abusive to his employees, whom he threatened with discharge at the slightest provocation. In Washington DC Hummer had been able to speak to servants, hospital staff, and "Negro" workers as a master and expect no questions. Davis believed he had transferred this behavior to Canton, where it was unacceptable.

"He interprets their different way of living, doing, and speaking from what he has always been accustomed, as evidence of their inferiority, and his manner showed every evidence of his feelings toward them," Davis reported.

Hummer's dictatorial methods may have developed during his university days and tenure at St. Elizabeths, but there was nothing in his background to warrant his attitude. The son of a butcher, he had been born on the District of Columbia's K Street SE in a solidly working-class milieu. At the time of his birth in 1879, the street housed two bakers, a boilermaker, a cabinetmaker, two laborers who worked in the Navy Yard, a painter, a machinist, and a bricklayer.

Neither was Hummer an only child or only son, which might have led to misplaced overindulgence: his immediate family at birth consisted of parents, an older brother and sister, and his maternal grandmother. Eleven and fourteen years later the family added a son and daughter, respectively, to the fold. Hummer had risen dramatically in education and career from these roots, and perhaps some shame over his humble beginnings led to overcompensation in his demands for respect. No matter where it sprang from, his attitude was one of long standing and now a part of his character that couldn't easily be modified.[13]

Hummer could not bear to be challenged in any way and told Davis that he "considered it the rankest impertinence for the attendants to make any suggestions as to whether or not the patients needed more out-of-door air and exercise."

At an institution, Davis pointed out in his report, subordinates were expected to exercise considerable discretion in carrying out orders, as well as to show initiative in determining how tasks should be accomplished. Davis concluded that Hummer's attitude toward his employees and his inability to accept suggestions or engage in constructive conversation had precipitated most of the asylum's other problems.

Davis had to show Hummer how to compute food allowances using ration tables, which gave the amounts of food each person should be issued per day or week. He also told Hummer that the government didn't want him to save money by refusing to increase the supplies he had received and that he could contact the Indian Office for additional food. Likewise, his economies on coal were unnecessary. Davis instructed him to supply hot water every day and to get authority to purchase more fuel if he ran out.

Davis attributed many of the substantiated complaints, like Hummer's failure to provide fire protection, to his inefficient management. Fire extinguishers had been purchased nearly a year earlier but weren't charged, and Hummer had simply failed to buy what was necessary to charge them. He couldn't figure out how anybody could safely get up on the roof to repair some shingles, so he left the roof exposed to the elements. And, due to inefficiency, he had shorted the staff of towels and soap rather than put in a request for more.

While he was there, Davis looked into the problems with Hardin's quarters and wrote in his report that "the selfishness of Dr. Hummer was manifest in that he claimed and held every desirable room and offered Dr. Hardin what was left." Davis found other allegations, though true, fairly inconsequential, such as Hummer's practice of making employees receipt for spoiled food rather than going through the process of condemning it. The phone problem lay in the fact that Hummer always tried to answer the phone himself and refused to relay calls for Hardin or his wife.

Asylum staff had to clean Hummer's quarters, but the practice of cleaning the superintendent's quarters had been in effect for several years and was common in asylums.[14] The problem was that Hummer's wife was dictatorial in the extreme and drew no lines as to what needed to be done. The staff resented cleaning up her children's messes and emptying the family's chamber pots. Davis suggested the practice be stopped and that the Hummers hire a servant. Overcrowding existed as alleged, but Hummer had not tried to hide the problem in his reports; the Indian Office was fully aware of the number of patients at the asylum.

Other problems were laid squarely on Hummer's shoulders. Davis found him absolutely guilty of allowing his wife to perform unsatisfactorily, neglecting Martha Smith, stinting the patients of clothing, and needlessly locking up some nonviolent patients.

Inspections are always difficult to sort out, since the accused and accusers are necessarily calling each other's testimony false. However, it is telling that as much as Hummer tried to deflect and attack Hardin's charges, and as sympathetic as Davis was to Hummer's situation, Hummer was found guilty, at least technically, on all counts but one. Hummer maintained numerous times, for instance, that he did not use vulgar language and specifically that he had never used the word "goddam" in his life, but employee after employee quoted explosive diatribes that included the expletive. These statements evidently were too believable for Davis to put the charge down to individual bad blood or exaggeration.

Altogether, Hummer came off very badly in the investigation, even though Davis accepted some of his defenses and cut him slack for not improving conditions that had already existed, such as the cockroach and bedbug problem, the overcrowding, and the filthiness of the toilet areas. (Hardin later retorted that a year should have been sufficient to identify and correct these problems.) Davis substantiated the eighteenth charge, of inefficiency and incompetence, though he stated strongly that it was out of order for the employees to have made it.

Though he differentiated relatively trivial charges, like the phone squabbles and spoiled food disposal, from the shorting of food and clothing for the patients and an abusive temper, Davis did find that as statements of fact, the allegations the asylum employees had made were true.[15] Hummer had also made himself so unpopular that Davis didn't believe he could continue as superintendent. He reported that the verdict should simply be that he is unfit to be at the head of the Asylum, principally by reason of his early life in the City, his lack of training in all practical matters pertaining to the administrative management of the institution, his intolerance manifested toward those working under him, his irascible temper . . . , his utter failure to comprehend the people with whom he must work and the people of the locality where the Asylum is located, and his erroneous notion of institutional management which will not permit him to so much as hear suggestions from one below him in rank. . . . To sum up— his is a case of misfit, and really quite extreme.

Commissioner of Indian Affairs Robert G. Valentine was not entirely satisfied that Davis's suggestion was his only option, partly because Joseph. H. Dortch, who headed the Indian Office's Education Division, thought that Hummer had largely been a victim of the turmoil caused by Gifford's departure. In January 1910 Valentine sent Joseph A. Murphy, the Indian Service's medical supervisor, to Canton Asylum to get a second opinion.

It was either luck or misfortune for Hummer that such an inspector could bring a medical viewpoint to the situation, for the Indian Office had created Murphy's position only that year. The organization had tried to provide health care to its wards for several decades, but its efforts were always poorly funded and more sporadic than effective. After 1877, medical care for Indians had been left to agencies and school doctors, and even now the Indian Office's new medical supervisor fell under its Education Division.[16]

During the asylum's short life, nonmedical inspectors had generally deferred to the opinions of its physician on patient care issues. This approach offered a measure of safety for the asylum and its staff, since a layperson was unlikely to disagree with a doctor's assessments and procedures. A medical inspector was not so easily deflected, since he would be apt to discover whatever shortcomings existed; at the same time, a medical supervisor's stamp of approval for the asylum would be something valuable. Hummer set out to impress the new inspector and rescue his reputation.

Murphy found the same state of tension Davis had and went a little further to take the pulse of the community. Dr. Turner, who had given an affidavit about the conditions at the asylum to Davis, told Murphy that Hummer "is ignorant, bigoted, self-idolized, and of an uncontrollable temper." He further charged Hummer with being responsible for the death of two patients whom Hummer had kept in solitary confinement during the summer and said that "filth and disorder reign supreme" at the asylum.

Several other prominent Cantonites gave varying reports on Hummer's character, and with the exception of the newspaper editor, Nash, seemed to feel that the superintendent would never stop clashing with employees because of his attitudes and failure to understand the western character.

Murphy found that Hummer had made a number of mistakes and misjudgments but said that none individually warranted discharge. As a doctor, Murphy felt that Hummer (with the exception of two or three cases) had handled his patients well. He seemed to accept Hummer's defense that it was Hardin who had allowed the Chippewa patient to lie in her feces but, rather tellingly, did not chastise Hardin for it. Murphy believed Hummer had acted in good faith and tried to do his duty to the Indian Service. He recommended that the Indian Office point out his mistakes to him and give him another chance.

Murphy did have concerns that local prejudice and the unrest among employees could render Hummer useless as superintendent of the Canton Asylum. If the commissioner felt that Hummer should resign, Murphy believed that the resignation should be based "on the present local state of affairs and Hummer's temperamental handicap in coping with it, and not upon professional inability." Murphy could handle the matter of Mrs. Hummer more easily. She was expecting a baby, was asked to resign, and did. The baby, a son, died on February 9, 1910, shortly after he was born, and the Hummers buried him in the Congressional Cemetery in Washington DC.[17]

Commissioner Valentine digested Murphy's report, perhaps looking realistically at the odds of getting someone better than Hummer to accept the Canton post, and in March finally sent the superintendent a stiff letter that particularly chastised him for his abusive temper and his attitude toward Canton Asylum's employees. Valentine said that he believed Hummer had been under a nervous strain because he hadn't arranged his duties so that he wasn't "harassed by the multitude of unimportant matters which you have endeavored to control personally."

Valentine told Hummer to start accepting "pointers" from the employees and to reorganize the hospital staff to create departments with supervisors who would report to him, thereby relieving him "of a great deal of the minor and unimportant details and thus obtain more time to treat the larger matters affecting the institution."[18]

That was that. Hummer's job was safe, even though the asylum was in such a mess that Davis hadn't seen how he could straighten it out. Dr. Hardin refused his transfer and reduction in salary and, after sixteen and a half years in the Indian Service, quit and went to Chicago to pursue postgraduate work. He later returned to Flandreau, South Dakota, and went into private practice, but not before laying the entire case out to the Indian Rights Association in Philadelphia with the exhortation to pursue the matter with South Dakota congressman Charles H. Burke.

Hardin also managed to throw one last public punch. The *Sioux Falls Daily Press* headlined an article "Dr. Hummer Is Vindicated," which Hardin would not let pass. In an open letter to the friendlier *Argus-Leader*, which had printed the charges against Hummer, Hardin made a case for his own vindication.

He stated that Davis had heard the evidence of only a few of the employees who had signed the sworn charges and that he had stated to Hardin that "if he went as fully into the case as it deserved that it would mean that he would have to take charge of the institution, something he did not want to do under any circumstances."

Hummer could be charming when he needed or wanted to be, and he surely wanted to be when Murphy showed up. Hardin claimed that Murphy had spent "nearly a week enjoying the hospitality of the Superintendent, paying [*sic*] whist with him into the late hours of the night, having a good time generally, hearing only his side of the case," and had returned to Washington with a report that whitewashed the real situation.[19]

Two particular items point to the presumption that, again, Hardin was telling the truth. First, Davis himself wrote in his report that he did not interview every employee, because the testimony had begun to be repetitive. Second, the *Sioux Falls Daily Press* wrote in its article that "Official information from Washington . . . gives Dr. Hummer a clean record against every charge made, and brands the charges as malicious and false." This statement was patently untrue. It is far likelier that Hardin's additional claim was true: Dr. Hummer had boasted that his friend at the Indian Office, Walter B. Frye, chief of appointments in the Education Division, would protect his interests at any cost. Combining this with Murphy's good impression and perhaps a bit of professional courtesy, Hummer had survived.

8. Reforms and Canton Asylum

"No incidents of my life have ever impressed themselves more indelibly on my memory than those of my first night in a strait-jacket. Within one hour of the time I was placed in it I was suffering pain as intense as any I ever endured, and before the night had passed it had become almost unbearable," Clifford Beers wrote. "Though I cried and moaned, in fact, screamed so loudly that the attendants must have heard me, little attention was paid to me. . . . After 15 interminable hours the strait-jacket was removed."[1]

In 1908 Clifford Beers spearheaded mental health reform in America after writing his remarkable book, *A Mind that Found Itself*, about his affliction and recovery from mental illness during 1900–1903.[2] A Yale graduate, Beers shocked the nation with his vivid portrayal of the beatings, cruel living conditions, and mental and physical brutality that he and so many others endured at first-rate, nonprofit insane asylums. He wore the straitjacket he mentioned for twenty-one nights straight and parts of each day (in a padded cell) before his doctor decided he could sleep without one.[3]

In the first decades of the new century, asylums were still a popular choice for families confronted with members they weren't able to manage. These institutions offered a range of care and, like Canton Asylum, sometimes stumbled in their choice of staff and services. Scandals popped into public view at inopportune times for their superintendents, who were as unlikely as Hummer to want to air their failures and problems in the open. Food at the New Jersey State Lunatic Asylum in Morris Plains made the headlines in 1908 when a former patient told the director of the county board, "The food at the asylum is something horrible. . . . For instance, sour hash, sour left-over potatoes, dirty hot water for tea and coffee. . . . The lining of the coffee and tea pot cookers is worn off, and therefore the coffee and tea are cooked in poisonous copper cookers."

A widow accused attendants of beating her husband (contributing to his death) at the Manhattan State Hospital for the Insane at Central Islip, New York, in 1911. After three months in the asylum, John Brown's "nose was broken, several teeth were missing, and he had scratches on his face." When she wrote the superintendent, he told her that her husband was being treated kindly, and the assistant superintendent told reporters that "he could not have been ill-treated without the physicians being aware of it."[4]

Mental health care issues did not stir the public the way that trust-busting and the discovery of adulterated foods did, but reform was in the air during the early part of the twentieth century.[5] A sense that life could be better—for the poor, the abused, the forgotten people of the world—spurred the country's conscience. Muckrakers like Ida Tarbell exposed the ruthlessness and greed of Standard Oil Company, the writer Upton Sinclair churned the nation's stomachs with his vivid portrayal of the country's meatpacking industry, and environmental reformers began to check mining and timber exploitation in Appalachia.[6]

The muckrakers and reformers went after child labor, adding power to their rhetoric in 1908 when the National Child Labor Committee enlisted Lewis Hine to take heartbreaking photographs of children working in mills, factories, and mines. Energetic workers Edward J. Barrows and John Collier at the People's Institute in New York conducted field studies on the quality of children's life in the city and the gangs in Hell's Kitchen. The pair also endeavored to bring immigrants' issues to the forefront of municipal concern at a time when newcomers were entering the country in a flood, their numbers increasing from 448,572 in 1900 to 1,041,570 in 1910.[7]

The federal government began to regulate the railroads and the drug industry, broke up monopolies, and intervened in the country's banking system. At the state level, progressives established minimum wages for women and the regulation of factories. Even Native Americans found a victory in a landmark court case that affirmed that Indians had retained their water rights when they moved to reservations.[8]

Just as important, Native Americans' deteriorating health had finally come to the forefront of public attention. In that pivotal year of 1908, the Smithsonian Institution and the Indian Office conducted a survey on tuberculosis within the Indian population. The results were horrifying. Other surveys showed high rates of Native Americans' second scourge, trachoma, and also revealed that huge reservations and the Indian populations on them were covered by perhaps one or two physicians. In 1911 the Indian Office presented this disturbing information to President William Taft, who immediately petitioned Congress for more funds. He didn't get all that he requested, but he did get the attention of Congress: funding for Indian medical services rose from $40,000 in 1911 to $350,000 by 1918.[9] Clearly investigation was in the air and, at the moment, was combined with a desire to do something about the problems investigators uncovered.

Of course, Hummer might have avoided his own investigation altogether if he had reined in his temper and arrogance, but scrutiny and pointed questions had entered America's psyche about the time his failings manifested. Commissioner of Indian Affairs Robert G. Valentine, who had been so lenient with Hummer, soon faced an investigation of his own. In office from June 1909 to September 1912, he resigned just as President Taft revoked a controversial "religious garb" order that Valentine had instituted without consulting the secretary of the interior. (He abolished religious garb and insignia among teachers at Indian schools, a gesture aimed at Roman Catholic priests and nuns.)

Taft called for an investigation into Valentine's stated necessity for the order, but Valentine was already being investigated by the Department of Justice for allegedly bringing liquor onto an Indian reservation in Oklahoma during an official visit. A congressional committee listened to twelve sessions of testimony concerning a number of charges against Valentine, feeling that they were serious enough to warrant investigation even though Valentine had already resigned. The committee found that Valentine "deliberately disregarded, evaded, and violated, in a flagrant manner, both the letter and the spirit of the civil-service law" and that the condition of the Indian Service under his supervision was "one of inefficiency and disorganization."[10]

His own deficiencies aside, Valentine had given Hummer another chance. Even better, Valentine, his private secretary, and inspector

James McLaughlin visited Canton at the end of September 1910, during a tour of the Sioux country. According to the *Sioux Valley News*, the three gave "a thorough inspection of the Government Indian Asylum in this city and found everything in a very satisfactory condition."

On a practical level for Hummer, several troublesome employees had resigned, been removed, or transferred, though Hummer could not escape the animosity that Dr. Turner and others in town held toward him. Hummer began to hire new workers and soon felt fairly confident in his choices, considering the area and the talent pool he dipped from.

Hummer was still somewhat startled by the independent character and transience of his employees, complaining that they often worked only until they had saved enough money to move on. Complaints aside, he had at least learned a lesson about the limits on his ability to replace those who became dissatisfied. He made an energetic case for continuing the practice of offering subsistence to employees when the Indian Office suggested doing away with the practice and simply raising employee salaries slightly. Hummer showed the commissioner that subsistence cost so little (five dollars a month per employee) and that it was so convenient for them to have their food prepared by the asylum's cook that he managed to keep this really desirable perk intact for his staff.

He further unthawed enough to allow employees to hold a masquerade at the asylum around the end of October. They decorated the dining room in black and white, judged costumes, and enjoyed a midnight meal before the festivities wound down. No hard feelings seemed to exist among ousted employees—the paper doesn't mention Gifford, but Charles Seely was one of the costume judges.

Holiday celebrations also extended to patients; the Hummers allowed a decorated Christmas tree and made sure the cook served a traditional Christmas dinner to patients at the asylum. Some type of morale fund must have been available (or Hummer used money he scrimped to save the rest of the year) because patients also received presents and stockings filled with edible treats.[11]

Whether these efforts were merely smart PR or genuine attempts to increase goodwill at the asylum, Hummer still did little to ingratiate himself with the Canton community. Though Dr. Turner had never been as popular as Superintendent Gifford, he was firmly embedded in the town's social structure. Turner was a member of three fraternal lodges and the Canton Commercial Club, enjoyed respect as a physician in private practice, and could be counted on to endorse efforts to move Canton forward.

In contrast, Hummer and his family seemed to consider the East their real home (as it may have been, with most of their relatives still residing there) and visited there as frequently as they could. The local newspaper is conspicuously silent concerning any community involvement or entertaining by the Hummers, and it is clear from other accounts that much of Hummer's social energies were engaged in the larger community of Sioux Falls, approximately thirty miles away.

After his initial period of toeing the line after the investigation, Hummer slipped back into his independent ways. He never followed Valentine's recommendation to divide his workforce into departments but instead continued to make all decisions himself. Hummer required employees to ask permission for almost anything not specifically described as allowable. He had personnel issues to resolve, reports to send to patients' home reservations, inventories to supervise, correspondence of all kinds, vouchers and disbursements to scrutinize, and an endless list of detail work that called for his attention. Inevitably, Hummer once again immersed himself in the administrative side of the asylum's business rather than the medical side.

For someone eager to make a name for himself as a psychiatrist, Hummer's behavior is difficult to understand. Investigations were always a job hazard for asylum superintendents, but Hummer should have been able to run his small institution without drawing undue attention from the Indian Office. Perhaps he could not compete with the sophisticated gym equipment or elegant meals and physical surroundings of an asylum like Massachusetts's McLean Asylum, but the Indian Office didn't expect that from him. Hummer *could* provide a perfectly acceptable poor man's version of asylum care, and if he had only done so he would have had an unremarkable but satisfactory career.

Hummer didn't want an unremarkable career, though—he had come to the asylum hoping to make a name for himself in the psychiatric world and advance rapidly. Hummer *wanted* to be superintendent of an insane asylum. He had thought it would be easier to get promoted to superintendent of a large institution by coming off a position as superintendent of a smaller one, rather than as an assistant physician at St. Elizabeths. He also knew—indeed, made efforts to set himself up as an expert because of it—that his position at a unique facility devoted to Indians was a great strength. And, even though his facility was small and had no funds for hydrotherapy or electrical stimulation treatments, Hummer's regimen for patient care was still not so far from what the rest of the country relied upon to treat insanity. He had a chance to realize his dream and advance his career, but he let it slip through his fingers.

Hummer began well when he advanced his associate membership in the American Medico-Psychological Association to active membership in 1911. Hummer was able to use his position at Canton to advantage at the association's 1912 meeting, when he gave a talk entitled "Insanity among the Indians" in which he presented himself as a uniquely placed expert on the subject. He continued to pursue the latest thinking in psychiatry, purchasing books by Sigmund Freud and his former superintendent, William A. White, and taking a subscription to the *Journal of Nervous and Mental Disease*. One of his pet projects was a planned textbook for the use of physicians in the Indian Service (which was never accomplished).

Hummer was diverted from his main goal and loftier dreams mainly because of the demands he allowed to burden his time. Some of that was justified: he had just been raked over the coals for inefficiency and mismanagement. Hummer also needed to push for improvements in his current buildings and for new construction if he were going to do anything about Canton Asylum's overcrowding, other than refuse to accept new patients. Both issues demanded effort, but once Hummer had satisfied himself with progress on these fronts, he should have pressed his advantage and begun real studies on his patients to follow up on his merely descriptive paper of 1912. Tellingly, "Insanity among the Indians" had only discussed the incidence of Native American insanity and described symptoms of the various dementias at Canton Asylum. Treatment, Hummer told his audience, consisted of "custodial care and attention, together with what encouragement and suggestion we can give in our daily contact."

The time was ripe for Hummer to make a name for himself. He could have conducted some groundbreaking work at Canton Asylum, proved or disproved various theories, or even pointed out failures in current treatment for his unique population or for certain types of insanity. At the very least Hummer could have ramped up his medical rounds and note taking and perhaps discovered something of interest to share with his peers. Instead, he fell into a pattern of taking just a few tentative steps forward, only to fall back almost immediately to the safety and power of his administrative position.

His refusal to step out with original research is both unfortunate and puzzling. Hummer had a great advantage over his peers in that he did not have the stress of a particular "cure rate" hanging over his head as a performance issue. Since the beginning of asylum care, the public had looked to results for their taxpayer outlays—most easily measured or understood by seeing a percentage rate of cures for the patients who sought treatment. The Holy Grail of alienists, high cure rates validated an asylum's existence and justified its superintendent's medical approach.

When asylums were first built, superintendents sought to admit insanity cases that had manifested only recently (acute cases). Early intervention in a patient's mental difficulties during a time when patient populations were low and alienists had time to personally oversee treatment often brought extremely favorable results. Superintendents were justifiably proud that they could so often cure their patients entirely or at least stabilize them to the point that they could return home.

The demands of a burdened public soon changed asylum dynamics. From intimate, well-staffed settings focused on the newly stricken patient, asylums morphed into facilities crowded with patients who had been ill for years. Early superintendents defensively engaged in some inventive accounting methods to make sure their cure rates remained high, but they were eventually thwarted by the public itself.[12]

Most families needed (or wanted) to give up the family members who had exhausted them physically or financially, rather than newly stricken ones whom they believed they could help at home. Superintendents did not want chronic patients, but they began to receive far too many to keep up any pretense that they could cure 40 percent of them (a fairly realistic figure in earlier years). Superintendents weren't necessarily fired for low cure rates, but their prestige suffered as asylums became overcrowded, cure rates went down, and vocal criticism thundered in newspapers.

Hummer did not have to contend with these problems. The *Sioux Valley News* wasn't about to publish anything negative about the asylum, and cure rates were not part of the scorecard inspectors used when they visited. The question never arose when Hummer's management was discussed, and the idea of cures, treatment innovations, and patient contentment does not seem to have been part of his performance objectives. Hummer had the scope to break new ground in his studies and refused to step up to the challenge.

Part of that may have stemmed from his personality. He had just been through an embarrassing investigation that resulted in a poor showing with Davis and Valentine. His ego had taken a blow and he may have been particularly unwilling at that point to do anything that might draw negative attention.

Hummer was frustrated on several other fronts as well. The government would not pay for Hummer's membership in the American Hospital Association or for his attendance at its convention.[13] He also wanted to practice medicine privately in South Dakota, though when he thought he would find the time to do so, only he knew. However, he balked at taking the required exam, declaring that "it's an insult to my position."

The state board of medical examiners refused to let Hummer practice outside the asylum without meeting its requirements, however. Hummer fumed that he would write to the president of the district board—and have that person write the president of the South Dakota board—to have the law set aside for him. Hummer was either offended by the board's position or had no time to study for the exam, because he later decided "to turn down the whole damn state of South Dakota and do no outside practice."[14]

Hummer did relent enough to assist the county insanity commission a few years later by examining cases of suspected insanity and testifying before sanity boards. As he perhaps acclimated to and softened toward his new environment, Hummer began to channel his social energy into the Commercial Club, his church, the Masons, and other groups; he enjoyed singing with the Chanters for close to twenty years. Though a longtime, loyal, and presumably valued member of these groups, Hummer continued to spend as much of his leisure time in Sioux Falls as in Canton.

Other aspects of his new life may have also disappointed Hummer at this time. The weather in South Dakota certainly was a cross to bear: 1912 started at twenty below and stayed cold, finally hitting forty-five below zero on the twelfth. Brutal though they were, at least the freezing temperatures kept the asylum's appalling smell at bay until its deteriorating sewage system—a headache for anyone within range of its stench for the past ten years—could be fixed.[15]

When problems with the sewage first appeared, engineering supervisor R. M. Pringle suggested creating an outlet to channel the asylum's waste into the Sioux River. However, the difficulty of negotiating easements across the properties affected made that solution impossible to implement. More recently, Supervisor Charles had created a plan to carry the sewer line down along the railroad, then through a pasture, and finally into the Sioux River just above Canton. Pringle and Charles thought that this might be the end to their problems, but here Drs. Turner and Hardin managed to throw a wrench into the plan. Pringle noted that some Canton citizens, "led by two disgruntled doctors, former employees of the Asylum," threatened an injunction that the two supervisors thought would be upheld in court.[16]

Finally, Pringle was able to meet with Canton leaders to develop a plan to hook the asylum's sewage to the city sewer. Pringle came to the asylum to look over some details at the end of January 1912, but he was stopped by temperatures of forty below zero and drifting snow. He tried again in March, to be met by ten inches of snow and ground frozen to the depth of two feet. Sometime within the next few months, fortunately, the weather eased up enough to let workers hook the line into Canton's sewer system. Hummer's pleasant rooms in the asylum were now almost ideal.

One of the asylum's major physical drawbacks had been corrected, but a routine inspection by Dr. Jacob Breid in 1912 suggested that Hummer's temper and attitude were still ongoing problems. Breid's report gave a brief overview of the facility, its patients, and their diagnoses and then proceeded to point out several deficiencies. He discussed solutions to the dinginess of the floors, unsafe conditions in the laundry and baking room, and the perpetual overcrowding, while making a case for a separate home for the superintendent.

On the first page of his report, however, he remarked that Hummer "has not been tactful and diplomatic in his dealings with citizens in the community and has at times encountered some difficulties and opposition." Breid must have spoken to Hummer about it, because Hummer assured the inspector that he understood "that his actions in many cases have not been such as to promote harmony."[17] He managed to convince Breid that he was overcoming this particular failing.

Hummer's continued inability to mesh with westerners—aided as he was by a shared heritage and language—boded no good for his ability to understand his patients, with whom he shared little. In the rest of the country, the immigrant population of America had a higher rate of institutionalization than native-born whites. One reason for the inequity was that immigrants often couldn't make themselves understood. Besides language expectations, standards of behavior for anyone in the United States were based on norms prevalent in "white" American society.

An alienist would not have felt he needed to know what was culturally acceptable to a foreign-born patient in order to decide that he or she was behaving oddly. Tragically—or perhaps typically—there was no requirement for the superintendent of the Canton Asylum for Insane Indians to know anything about Indian culture. Gifford had had some familiarity with native peoples, but Hummer's interpretation of patient behavior against his own ideas of "normal" did not make many allowances for culture.

His patients at St. Elizabeths had been mostly of a chronic, quiet class who required custodial care rather than any active treatment. They were also all white men, typically with an armed services background. Hummer had absolutely nothing in common with Indians and made no pretense of understanding the people or their culture. He had admitted this deficiency early on to Dr. Turner and does not seem to have initiated any course of study to correct it.

Native Americans received little forbearance from whites in general, but Hummer's ignorance played out especially badly for the people under his care. Native Americans exhibited as wide a variety of behaviors as other peoples, but certain common values probably worked against them when alienists like Hummer judged their behavior through an Anglocentric lens. Many native cultures encouraged patience, silence, and emotional control, which may have been fallback options for patients who were confused or frightened by their entry into Canton Asylum. Especially if they weren't able to speak or understand English well, patients may have appeared "unresponsive," "catatonic," or "indifferent" to an uninformed observer.[18]

Native American norms regarding eye contact, personal space, body movement, and conversational pace were often quite different from typical American standards. Indians incorporated lengthy pauses and long silences in their speech, minimized body movement, and didn't gaze directly at others. All these behaviors probably marked them as having a lower IQ or mental ability than they really possessed. Even English speakers remained at a disadvantage, since Indian languages do not always have equivalent words or concepts in English.

In spite of his recognition that both westerners and Indians were very different from the types of people he was used to, Hummer apparently believed that sane Indians ought to behave the same way that sane whites did. Whether by intent or indifference, Hummer ignored the waving red flags of cultural differences and language barriers as he began assessing his patients. No stumbling block appeared to give Hummer pause or shake his confidence in his abilities—even the fact that he could not communicate effectively with many of his patients.

In "Insanity among the Indians," his talk before the American Medico-Psychological Association, Hummer said guilelessly, "It is harder to diagnose the condition of the insane Indian because of . . . his reticence, suspiciousness, superstitions, etc., and from the fact that oftentimes our only medium of conversation is the sign language, which with us is very crude."

Despite this admitted handicap, Hummer felt comfortable diagnosing patients who couldn't speak English as imbeciles and morons or suggesting continued treatment for patients whose behavior he didn't understand. In September 1907 Superintendent Gifford had admitted Nakai Yezza, a thirty-year-old Navajo man who came in with a diagnosis of amentia, or extreme mental retardation. He was also a reputed sorcerer—difficult to reconcile with that diagnosis.

Within a month, this man with amentia was able to display a trustworthiness that allowed him considerable liberty and then to contrive an escape from Canton Asylum to Helena, Montana, where he remained at large for nine months. Yezza's admittance paperwork, probably prepared by Dr. Turner, described him as curable. Under Hummer, Yezza was reclassified as a low-grade imbecile.

Alienists, teachers, and other professionals had begun to study both normal and retarded mental abilities after French researcher Alfred Binet, inspired by watching his two daughters grow up, became interested in what would now be called developmental and educational psychology. Binet began to advance new concepts involving intelligence, attention span, and suggestibility for use in measuring intellectual development. Around 1904, Binet and his collaborator Theodore Simon developed the first rudimentary IQ tests, called the Binet-Simon Scale, to determine a child's mental age.

By 1910 this scale was well-known and often used by professionals to test for idiocy (mentality of one to two years), imbecility (mentality of three to seven years), and moronity (mentality of eight to twelve years). Except for a few basic tests to determine the mentality of a one-year-old (move a lighted match in front of the subject to see if he would follow it with his eyes, for example), examiners assumed a common language and culture between subjects and testers.

To determine a subject's mentality above age two, an examiner might ask, "Where are your eyes?" or say, "I'm going to read a sentence (or tell a little story). When I get through I want you to say it word for word, just as I did, without a single mistake. Now listen carefully," and so on. Tests to determine a mental age of eight included asking how much a sampling of stamps would cost at a post office or telling the subject to count backward from twenty to one as fast as possible. Higher mental age tests asked subjects to describe *kindness* or tell the tester which woman was prettier in a pair of drawings.[19]

These kinds of tests would have been well beyond the capabilities of many Indians, even if they spoke English. In 1925 one Canton patient's frustrated cousin wrote to an attorney asking, "Will you please advise I and Emma Frank how we can get Peter Kentuck out of the Insane asilum [sic]." The cousin, John Carpenter, explained the family's situation and then went on, "He was rushed out of here by Supt. Mortsolf and a doctor that ask the Boy if he knew who was the Co. Sheriff also who was the President of the U.S. This boy did not know so he was pronounced insane. Now if this would be the rule there would be many thousands of Indians that could not answer these questions because they did not know and not because they were insane."[20]

Kentuck, who was not quite twenty when he was committed, had already been in Canton Asylum five years before this letter was written. By the time Carpenter wrote, however, Hummer had decided that Peter Kentuck, who spoke very little English, was a moron who needed to be institutionalized for life and refused to discharge him to his relatives.[21]

Even tests for sanity relied on cultural and educational compatibilities between the tester and subject. Dr. White devoted an entire chapter of his *Outlines of Psychiatry* to the best ways of examining the insane. Part of the exam consisted of taking the patient's family and personal history, then moving on to a history of the insanity being manifested. Questions for such an intake included:

Were parents of patient related or did they differ greatly in age?

Was either addicted to the use of alcohol?

Did either commit or attempt suicide?

What is the business, profession, or occupation of the patient?

At the time of birth of the patient did the mother have difficult labor?

Has the patient had any head injuries or convulsions?

Has the patient taken drugs, such as cocaine, morphine, opium or any others for long periods of time?

Did the patient have a physical or mental shock?

Did the attack come on gradually or suddenly?[22]

The physician would next ask the patient how he or she felt: all right, excited, or depressed. He would probe into fears or compulsions, peculiar thoughts, and hallucinations. The next part of the exam, however, would be especially problematic for Indian patients.

The physician would determine if the patient could obey simple commands, like "cross your legs" or "squeeze my hand." Did the patient use the wrong word or have difficulty in understanding the name or word for a thing? Tests for attention involved reading a series of numbers and asking the patient to tap whenever he or she heard a particular number. Other attempts to understand the patient's abilities involved word association, math, and logic tests.[23] These kinds of tests were patently unfair to non-English speakers or to patients from different cultures and levels of education. Hummer probably did not administer these tests, but none of his patients would have done well on them if he had.

Though White's exam was a useful model for his own and other institutions, it created a disservice to special populations. And when it came to deciding the fates of institutionalized "defectives," the ugly specter of eugenics also entered the picture.[24] Sir Francis Galton had coined the term *eugenics* as early as 1883; his intent, originally, was to encourage healthy, intelligent couples to have more children so that society could be improved by their good stock.[25] As time went on, the idea became more negative and was used to support the idea that "inferior" races or people shouldn't reproduce.

In the United States, the biologist Charles Davenport established the Eugenics Record Office at Cold Spring Harbor, New York, and with the office's director, Harry H. Laughlin, began a study of hereditary traits by compiling the "pedigrees" of thousands of families. Davenport by no means represented a fringe movement: the Carnegie Foundation funded his Station for Experimental Evolution at Cold Spring Harbor in 1904. The Rockefellers funded the Kaiser Wilhelm Institute in Germany, whose research laid the groundwork for the ideology of the Nazi eugenics program. John Harvey Kellogg (of corn flakes fame) was on the Advisory Council of the American Eugenics Society, founded the Race Betterment Foundation, and sponsored three eugenics conferences. Other wealthy members of the American Eugenics Society included the banker J. P. Morgan, the tobacco heiress Mary Duke Biddle, and Miss E. B. Scripps of United Press wealth.

Eugenics researchers considered feeblemindedness, shiftlessness, manic depression, sexual immorality, indolence, and even propensities toward dressmaking or a love of the sea to be inheritable traits. The goal of their breeding research was to weed out "defectives" from society and increase the number of "high-grade" people in it.

Eventually, mandatory sterilization of "defectives" became an important goal for the eugenics movement. In 1914 Laughlin introduced a Model Eugenical Sterilization Law that proposed to sterilize a wide range of "defectives," supported by public dollars: criminals; the insane and feebleminded; the blind, deaf, and diseased; and epileptics, among others. A number of states already had sterilization laws on the books by then. Most of these laws were struck down by the mid-1970s, by which time more than sixty thousand "defectives" had been involuntarily sterilized.

Though Hummer did not sterilize patients, his failure to do so was substantially due to the fact that he didn't have the facilities to perform the procedure. He very much fell in with the idea that "defectives" ought not to reproduce. The thinking of the time was that a match between two defectives almost always resulted in another defective and that defective stock degraded good stock. Hummer did not want female patients of childbearing age out in society where they might get pregnant and produce undesirable offspring.

Hummer told the commissioner of Indian affairs that Agnes Caldwell, a Menominee patient who had petitioned the commissioner to release her, "has a splendid home here . . . but is discontented and wants to go home and care for her family. This she is mentally unable to do and the great danger of increasing the number of defective offspring should outweigh her wishes."[26]

Later, in discussing another female patient's possible discharge, Hummer admitted that with the patient in question, Susan Wishecoby, "her attitude is about as near normal as it will ever be. . . . Her actions here are all that could be desired." However, he had an objection to releasing her: "She is but twenty-nine years of age, with good health and the probabilities of bringing children into the world."[27]

Hummer's desire to prevent pregnancies in "defectives" *outside* the asylum did not necessarily guarantee that pregnancies would not occur *inside* it. A twenty-two-year-old Chippewa patient, Isabella Porter, whom he characterized as a low-grade imbecile, suffered a miscarriage on March 20, 1910. She had been given parole privileges until Hummer received a report in December that she had been seen in company with a male patient.[28] Since that time, she hadn't been allowed out unless accompanied by an attendant. Hummer was too late, though, and had to report the incident to the commissioner.

Understandably, Isabella's mother, Josephine Grasshopper, was concerned for Isabella's health and wrote for particulars. She also said plainly that she wanted Isabella to come home. Hummer assured Grasshopper that Isabella "has a splendid appetite and digestion" but that she had not changed mentally and had periods of noisiness and destructiveness. "In view of these facts and the additional fact that she has to be carefully watched on account of her habits, the proposed discharge is not to be considered," he added.

Hummer's words were sufficiently discouraging that he appeared to be comfortable throwing a crumb to the distressed mother, telling Grasshopper that she could "place the matter before the Honorable Commissioner of Indian Affairs."

Grasshopper was persistent, writing again to tell Hummer that her family was in a position to care for Isabella on their farm. "She is lonesome by this time I know and think that she will be better to see her folks once more," she told him.

On June 24, 1910, Hummer forwarded Grasshopper's letters and his reply and asked the commissioner to release Isabella, very much against his own inclination. Hummer wanted Isabella's mother to sign a statement that "she will assume all responsibility for anything that might happen as a result of this discharge."[29]

Isabella Porter's pregnancy was not an isolated case. Earlier, in 1909, Hummer received a Navajo patient named E-nas-pah, who was pregnant before she came. E-nas-pah gave birth about four months after her admittance and died of tuberculosis six weeks after that. Her daughter, Ruth, died two weeks later.[30]

Susan Burch, from the Southern Ute Indian School, was evidently in her first trimester when she arrived at the asylum in 1912. She bore a child on March 9, 1913, about six months after her arrival. Hummer informed the commissioner of the birth, noting that the baby was premature and did not look like it would live long. The baby was taken in as a new admission, but since it did not require a separate bed, was not counted toward the asylum's capacity. The mother died soon after the baby was born, but the baby's fate is uncertain.

Hummer's problems with women still weren't over, but his difficulties soon took an unexpected detour from patients to staff. Hummer had a growing sense that he could do no wrong, and his experience in the Indian Service was proving that this feeling was often justified.

Hummer, too, was a product of his time. Men almost always ran the show, and he was undoubtedly surprised to discover that a woman could cause *him* problems. And as always, an inspector came hard on the heels of an uncomfortable situation that Hummer had created himself.

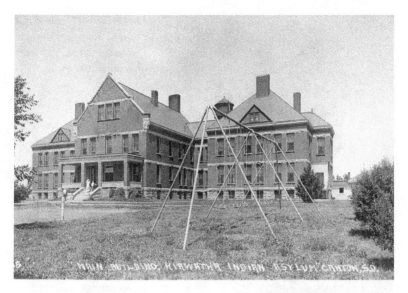

FIG. 1. Front view of Canton Asylum, ca. 1912–18. Courtesy of the South Dakota State Historical Society Archives.

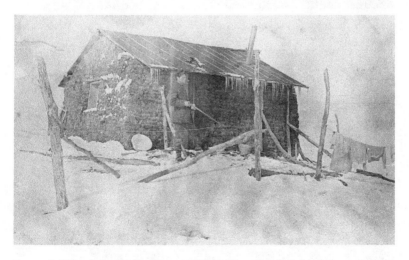

FIG. 2. Cold wash day, sod house near White River, South Dakota, ca. 1910–19. Fred Hulstrand History in Pictures Collection, NDIRS-NDSU.

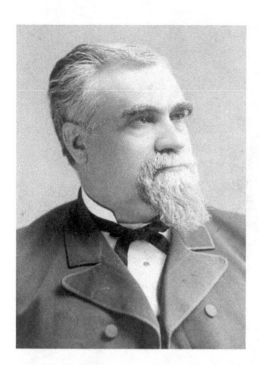

FIG. 3. Cabinet photo of
Oscar S. Gifford, 1885–90.
Collection of the U.S. House
of Representatives.

FIG. 4. Atkins Hall, St.
Elizabeths, 1900. The
Canton Asylum for
Insane Indians did not
have pictures on its walls.
National Archives photo
418-G-26.

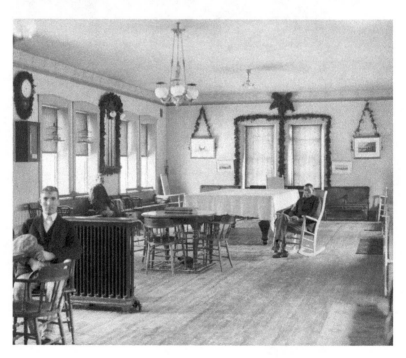

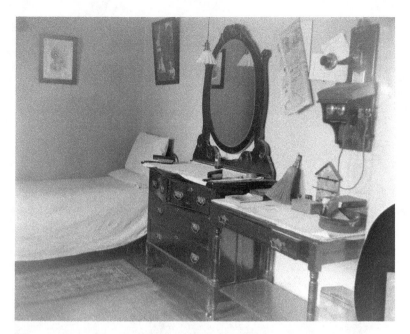

FIG. 5. Attendant's room in Home Building, St. Elizabeths.
National Archives photo 418-G-145.

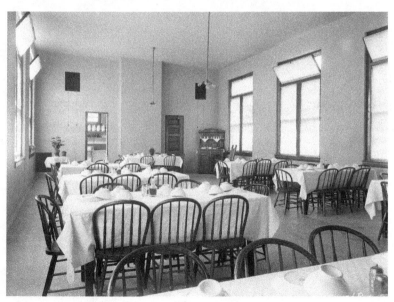

FIG. 6. Q Building dining room, 1905, St. Elizabeths.
National Archives photo 418-G-258.

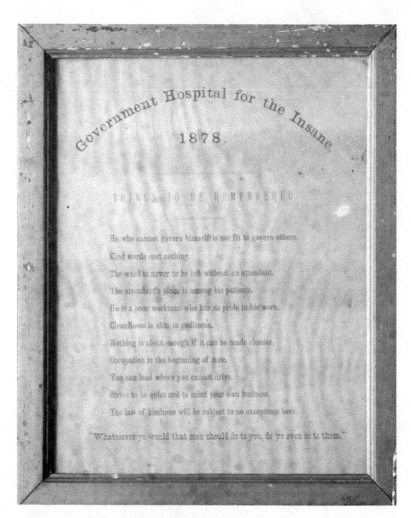

Fig. 7. "Things to Be Remembered," 1878, served as a reminder to all St. Elizabeths staff on how to treat patients. National Archives photo 418-L-2-2.

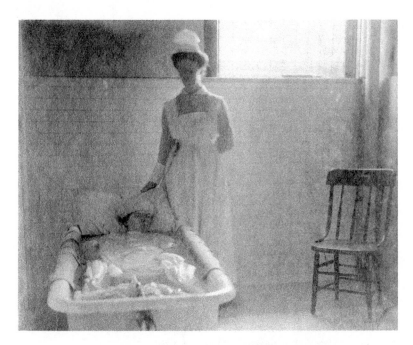

FIG. 8. Hydrotherapy, St. Elizabeths. National Archives photo 418-P-127.

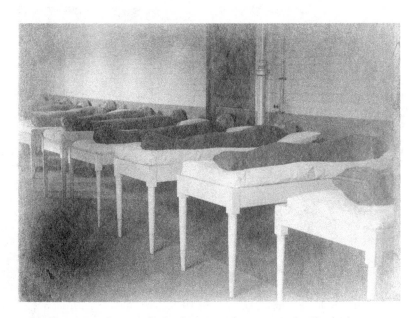

FIG. 9. Patients undergoing hydrotherapy pack treatment, St. Elizabeths. National Archives photo 418-P-129.

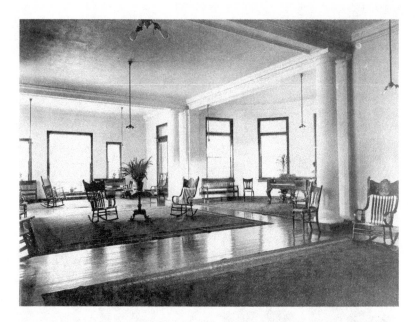

FIG. 10. The common room at St. Elizabeths was probably not duplicated at Canton Asylum. National Archives Photo 418-P-179.

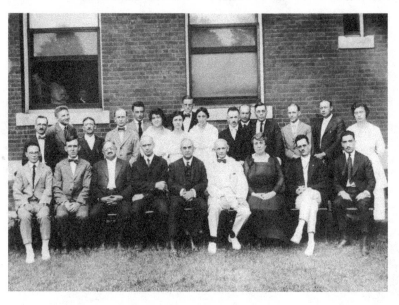

FIG. 11. St. Elizabeths staff, ca. 1919 or 1920. Dr. Samuel Silk is in the front row, far left. Dr. William A. White is in the front row, fifth from left.
National Archives Photo 418-P-394.

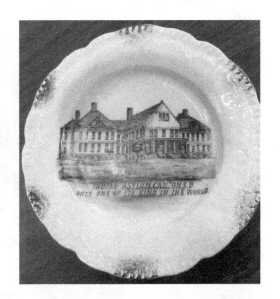

FIG. 12. Tourist plate.
Courtesy of Dr. Anne
Dilenschneider,
photographer.

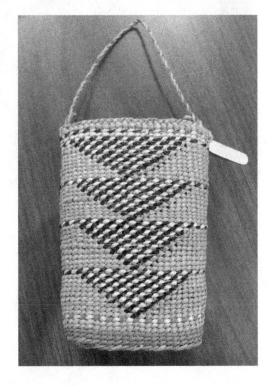

FIG. 13. Patient craft.
Courtesy of Dr. Anne
Dilenschneider,
photographer.

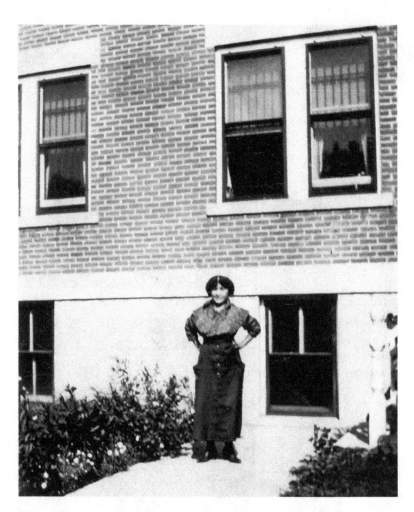

FIG. 14. Canton patient Susan Wishecoby
sent this picture to the commissioner of
Indian affairs in 1922. National Archives
photo HD1-211375496-2015-001.

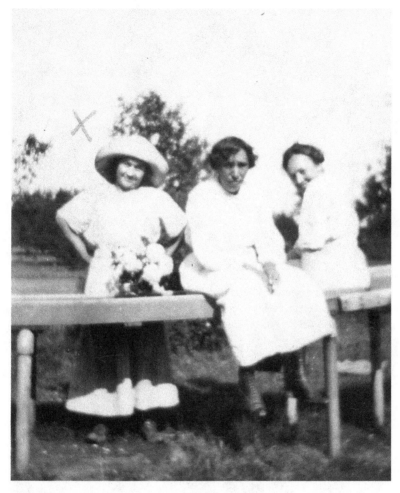

FIG. 15. Susan Wishecoby with two friends, 1922; photo sent to the commissioner of Indian affairs. National Archives Photo HD1-11375552-2015-001.

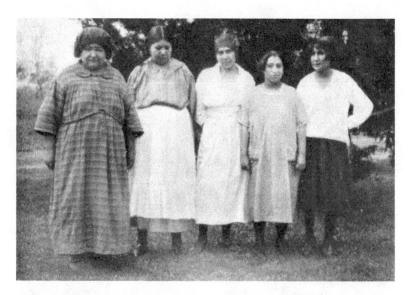

FIG. 16. Female patients photographed during Professor Kraepelin's visit to Canton Asylum in April 1925. Photo courtesy Springer Publishing Company from *Paralysestudien Bei Negern Und Indianern*, by Dr. Felix Plaut and Professor Emil Kraepelin (Berlin: Verlag von Julius, 1926).

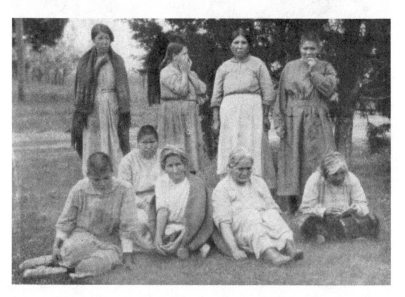

FIG. 17. Another group of female patients. Photo courtesy Springer Publishing Company from *Paralysestudien Bei Negern Und Indianern*, by Dr. Felix Plaut and Professor Emil Kraepelin (Berlin: Verlag von Julius, 1926).

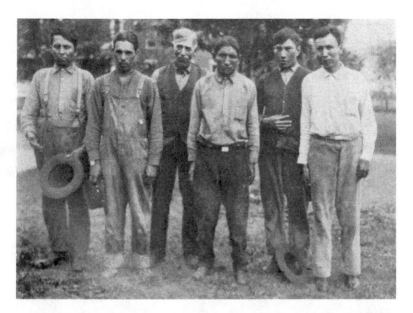

FIG. 18. A group of male patients. Note that all patients are wearing "citizen" clothing. Photo courtesy Springer Publishing Company from *Paralysestudien Bei Negern Und Indianern*, by Dr. Felix Plaut and Professor Emil Kraepelin (Berlin: Verlag von Julius, 1926).

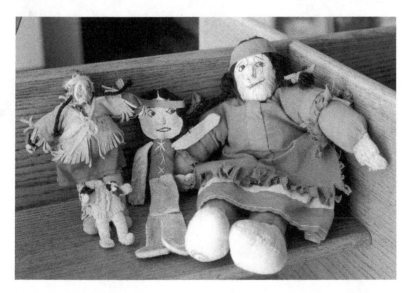

FIG. 19. Dolls made by patients at Canton Asylum. Reprinted with permission from the *Sioux Falls Argus Leader*. Photo by Elisha Page, lead photographer.

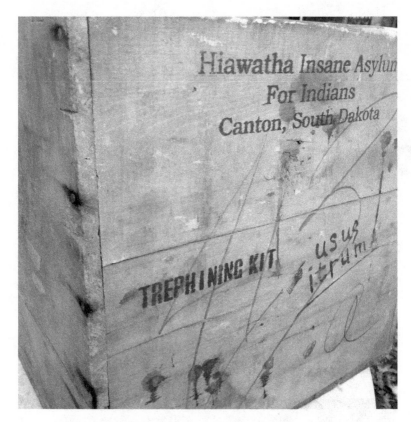

FIG. 20. Trephining kit. Courtesy of Dr.
Anne Dilenschneider, photographer.

9. Let the Investigations Begin

A mos Deere had taken ill that evening and then steadily grew worse—something in his abdomen was giving him tremendous pain. Two of the ward attendants carried him onto another patient's bed and fetched the doctor, but Hummer didn't think he had an emergency on his hands. He gave instructions for attendant Martin Van Winkle to medicate Deere himself. The medication Hummer had specified needed to be administered via syringe, but the attendant didn't want to go get one.

Van Winkle muttered that he had already asked Miss Hendricks (the matron and acting nurse) for a syringe once and had been told it was for use on the west ward. "I'll be damned if I'll go in and ask her for it again," he added.

His fit of pique didn't help his patient, though, and Deere's pain grew worse. "Please get the doctor," he finally begged. "Please get the doctor."

Van Winkle refused. "Here's some ice—put that over your pain."

The ice didn't help, and Deere endured the agony as long as he could. "I can't stand the pain! I can't stand the pain any longer," he finally cried. "*Please* go get the doctor!"

"Lie still there, you'll be all right—what the hell's the matter with you?" Van Winkle snapped.

It was a long night for Deere and he both screamed and cried. Finally he called for the help of another attendant, pleading, "Please go get Mr. Smoots. Please go get him! I need him to send a telegram to my brother—I'm dying."

"There's no danger of you dying," Van Winkle replied scornfully. "Hold that ice over you."

The other patients listened to Deere moan and cry the rest of the night, though Van Winkle either was unmoved by it or simply left Deere by himself so he could go elsewhere in the building. Relief came in the morning when more sympathetic workers immediately took Deere upstairs to see Hummer. The superintendent was furious to discover that Van Winkle had not obeyed him and began snapping out orders—including one to fetch the neglected medicine and syringe. The attendants worked hard, but it was too late. Deere, thirty-seven years old, died at noon.[1]

Spot Omudis, a Chippewa who was characterized as an imbecile and mischievous, was also an epileptic. One night Omudis had a frightening seizure so violent that he fell from his bed. He thrashed and jerked on the floor, which probably woke another patient, James Two Crows.[2]

When Two Crows found him, Omudis lay face down in a pool of blood. Two Crows ran to get Van Winkle, but Van Winkle merely said, "Oh, he will get up." He was right. Omudis lay quietly for a few more minutes, regained consciousness, and crawled into bed, dripping blood.

The callousness of Van Winkle is unnerving. Nighttime in the asylum could be frightening under the best of circumstances, but Van Winkle often turned off all the lights so that the wards lay in complete darkness. One repercussion—which he didn't seem to mind—was that patients who needed to use the toilet often wandered frantically, knocking over chairs or stumbling into beds as they tried to find their way to the facilities. Others simply urinated on the floor or in bed. Van Winkle then called them "damn Indian sons of bitches!" and, if other incidents are anything to go by, left the mess for the morning crew.

Van Winkle opened all the ward windows—no matter how cold it was—rather than flush and clean the range toilets often enough to keep the odor from accumulated waste at bay. The smell drove some of the patients to do his job for him, though the day attendants often came in and flushed the toilets in the morning.

Van Winkle beat some of the patients regularly, particularly a man called Papa. When the unfortunate patient went into the toilet room, Van Winkle would instigate Spot Omudis to help him tease and pound the man with a broom or mop stick until Papa became so overwrought he would grab and break the toilet fixtures.

Van Winkle wasn't the only employee with a hard heart. During a card game, a patient nicknamed "Colonel" had some sort of seizure or "fit" in the presence of Van Winkle and the other card players and urinated in his bed.[3] None of the players assisted him, but instead they laughed and made disparaging remarks. Van Winkle said that "it was good for him" to lie there and left Colonel in his soiled condition all night. For a spot of amusement during another card game, the players threw an old man named Walker out of bed and then ran upstairs, laughing. Apparently it was so much fun that they came back down and did it again.

As superintendent of an insane asylum, and even as a mere physician at the very large St. Elizabeths asylum, Hummer had to know that patient abuse occurred, whether it was sanctioned or not. Rather than encouraging an open dialogue with his employees, however, Hummer had them so cowed that the decent ones were afraid to let him know what the bad ones were doing. Even worse, his bad temper sometimes affected patients. One employee stated during the Hardin investigation that Hummer ordered Omudis handcuffed and shackled when he wouldn't give up keys the staff thought he had. The patient remained thus for seven hours, with one hand eventually released so he could eat. Many of Canton Asylum's staff and patients must have been glad when Hummer's job went on the line again just four short years after his first major investigation.

Life was actually going pretty well for Hummer at this point. He and his family enjoyed lengthy stays in the East to visit family, and though they likely traveled there by train, Hummer had purchased a spiffy new Ford motorcar in 1912. He had also cemented the goodwill of at least one citizen of Canton by taking a subscription to the *Sioux Valley News* (as noted in its December 6 edition). Finally, *finally*, his affairs were being reported like those of any other Canton citizen, rather than as terse notes that seemed little more than fillers for the Local Mention column. His wife had joined the ladies' Reading Circle and entertained the club at the asylum; the friendly paper reported Hummer's jovial, but inept, attempts to make whipped cream for the festive luncheon that followed. Further, it told how the men who had come to pick up their wives enjoyed "the congenial" doctor's cigars and conversation in his study.

Life was going pretty well for Oscar Gifford, too. Bailey, Gifford's married son, and his wife were able to break away from their own routines to visit fairly often. Gifford was a prized speaker who offered his talents freely to clubs and churches, lodges, and fraternal halls, and his name appeared frequently in the *Sioux Valley News* in connection with community events. Even Jenny Gifford had her successes, and she surely enjoyed her appointment as librarian of the town's new Carnegie library.

In the summer of 1912, Gifford received the tremendous honor of being elected commander of the Grand Army of the Republic, Department of South Dakota. A crowd of his fellow citizens, members of the Grand Army, and the city's band serenaded him enthusiastically for one more accomplishment that he—and through him, they—had received because of his popularity and talent.

A quiet few months allowed Hummer to catch his breath in time for another Christmas at the asylum. He and his wife did their best to make it festive with their usual decorated tree; whether they allowed patients to help put up ornaments is unknown. Special Christmas candies were on sale at the grocer's for eight to fifteen cents a pound, or the asylum cook might have made them herself from sugar she could buy at less than five dollars for a hundred pounds. Even though Christmas was not a holiday celebrated by non-Christian Indians, any kind of festivity accompanied by candy and treats would have been welcomed. Even the Hummers, separated by many miles from their own close relatives, surely enjoyed the chance to immerse themselves in the holiday season.

The grippe (influenza) made its rounds as usual that winter, and it fairly prostrated Gifford and many others by January 1913. Gifford was robust and active, though, and the paper wished him well in his recovery. It later reported that he just couldn't seem to shake off the infection, which had settled in his kidneys. The paper noted in the second week of January that Bailey and his wife had come from Massachusetts to visit Gifford, which cheered him considerably. On January 16, the seventy-year-old Gifford was dead.

The community sincerely mourned his passing, remembering Gifford as the statesman and visionary, loyal South Dakotan, and Canton booster that he had been since joining his fate with Dakota Territory's in 1871. He had been an influential politician, a popular businessman, and a trusted official; his service at Canton Asylum was remembered in his obituary, without any note of his failure there. Gifford's Episcopalian service was generously attended by friends and colleagues from all over the state, and included a Masonic liturgy. His lodge was draped in mourning for thirty days following his funeral.

It is improbable that Hummer had liked, admired, or socialized with Gifford, and he had his hands full with concerns other than the passing of the man to whom he could credit much of the town's antipathy toward himself. He had his own tragedy to mourn: the Hummers' infant daughter, named Norena after her mother, died January 16, 1913, after a short week of life. Hummer's aunt came west during the harsh winter days of February, presumably to help the family cope while Mrs. Hummer recovered. A month later, Hummer came down with a bout of measles—a serious disease for an adult—though he recovered with no apparent ill effects.

Whether he made a special effort or simply enjoyed some good luck, Hummer created few ripples over the next few months. The Indian Office installed playground equipment at its boarding schools during 1912 and 1913; Hummer managed to get a giant slide, six swings, and a seesaw for his asylum, which patients thoroughly enjoyed.[4] Data from the commissioner of Indian affair's annual report showed that a total of 156 insane Indians (of which only 55 were currently being treated at Canton Asylum) had been tabulated by reservation superintendents, ensuring that Hummer could justify even further expansion once the hospital filled. Things were definitely looking up.

Hummer's continued push for a hospital had finally met with success, and in October 1914 most of the work on it had been completed. Almost as gratifying, Hummer had actually received public credit for all his efforts, with the newspaper saying in black and white for the whole town to read, "The entire enterprise owes its inception, development, and consummation to Dr. Hummer who is ever alert to serve the interests and advance the well being of the unfortunate beings confided to his care."[5]

With the new hospital going up, he had hopes that visitors of importance might stop by to give their approval of his work. He had opened the asylum's doors to the public, pushing for sightseers and publicity in a way Gifford never dreamed of doing. Almost nine hundred visitors toured the facility in 1911, and in 1913 over eleven hundred people came to see the unique facility.[6] Small papers in other parts of the country often mentioned that citizens who had gone to Canton to visit relatives had also visited the insane asylum there. An Iowa paper reported in 1912 that when Edith Baker visited her aunt, she also visited the Indian insane asylum; more than a decade later, another Iowa paper noted that a family who had been visiting relatives in the region also "visited the Grotto of the Redemption at West Bend, the New State Park at Oak Groves at Hawarden, Ia., and the Indian insane asylum at Canton, S. Dak."[7]

Few notable visitors toured the asylum, and the academic world had yet to take notice of this unique facility. The doors remained open to just about anyone else who cared to come, though some visitors were undoubtedly more welcome than others. When the editor of the *Hudsonite* and his niece dropped in during a tour of the countryside, they found Dr. and Mrs. Hummer on the lawn "watching over their charges, who were playing like happy children everywhere on the grounds." The good doctor, said the piece's writer, "has made a splendid record during the five years that he has had charge of the institution."[8] Those would be the last kind words Hummer would hear for a while.

Whatever cease-fire with his staff the superintendent had managed after Breid's 1912 inspection had now gone by the wayside. The *Sioux Valley News* reported that a couple of employees had "severed their connections" with the asylum, an unusual citing in that the paper did not routinely mention the hiring or departures of employees.[9] In a later revolt of some sort, Hummer had to explain to the commissioner of Indian affairs why thirteen employees refused to get vaccinated.[10]

Hummer himself remained as overworked as always, which did not improve his notoriously short temper. In his defense, the administrative tasks Hummer faced each day could be mind-numbing in detail and scope. He had to account for every penny he spent—including thirty cents for friction tape, the dollar he needed to repair an icebox, and the twenty-two cents that were unexpended from a hundred dollars in 1914's general purpose funds.

In one letter to the commissioner of Indian affairs, Hummer recommended the sale of some calves and asked permission to shoot a sick horse that was discharging pus and was too weak to stand. After

Washington decided that the horse would probably get well and refused permission, Hummer had to send another letter, informing the commissioner that the horse had died.

One spring Hummer got a sharp letter from the assistant commissioner, E. B. Meritt, which went head-to-head with any example of micromanagement Hummer himself could offer: "This Office is in receipt of a letter from the Bureau of Mines stating that [the] sample of coal recently received from you in unnumbered container is not prepared in accordance with Appendix A, Method of Sampling Coal Deliveries, as pieces of coal over ½" in size were found therein."

Hummer was directed to immediately see that those charged with preparing coal samples (possibly himself) "familiarize themselves with the above mentioned Appendix A and especially Secs. 5, 6, and 7 thereof. You will note that all impurities and pieces of coal must be crushed and shall not contain any pieces larger than 3/16 of one inch in size, screening out of the larger pieces will not be allowed."[11]

This kind of relentless detail work would have driven more saintly men to distraction, but Hummer had now accepted the additional, incessant demands of construction. As much as Hummer wanted the hospital and embraced control, he felt himself wearing down under the sheer volume of work. Home was just more of the same, since he couldn't get away from the asylum's environment.

He undoubtedly craved both sympathy and support from his staff and family, but he was drawing a blank with the former. He didn't like many members of his staff and felt that only one or two of them were actually "loyal"—a favored term for employees who either didn't cause him problems or actually aided him in his agenda by reporting on the others. His family may have worn him out more than their presence refreshed him. His sons marred the surface of the hallways—so difficult to scrub—by roller-skating down them, and the two boys generally teased and annoyed the patients. Whether he noticed, cared, or made them stop is unknown, but they were obviously rambunctious and somewhat insensitive.

Norena Hummer's attention was taken up with the care of her household (she *did* know the boys roller-skated, and didn't stop them), and she was unsupported by any close family member who might have offloaded some of the demands on her time. Norena had a sharp temper and quick tongue and, if fatigued and stressed from her own burdens, may have used it without restraint on her husband.

Perhaps that's when Hummer's eye began to roam. There does not seem to have been any hint of impropriety until this particular period, and Hummer may have only wanted a little companionship and mild courting or the admiration of someone still in awe of his authority. Eventually, he settled on the only acceptable outlet he could find to meet his unfulfilled needs—the help.

It began with the matron, Randy Hendricks. Hummer was not as circumspect as he should have been, because his affair—whether the details of it were correct or not—soon became common knowledge. In a letter to a former employee, Raymond Smoots (the attendant Amos Deere trusted) said that "everyone in town knows about the love affair out here."[12]

Someone must have made a specific allegation to the Indian Office, because in February 1914 the commissioner sent a special agent named Dorrington to investigate the charges. Two former employees swore an affidavit to support the allegations. One was specific: Mrs. Charles Sheppard said that in October 1913 she had been walking around the building and happened to look in the office window. There she saw Hendricks talking to Hummer, who had his arm around her. She leaned over and kissed him; he rose from the chair, put his left arm around her, and turned out the light.

"They both stayed in the dark room for about fifteen minutes," Mrs. Sheppard concluded. If her statement is true, she obviously found salacious pleasure in the possibilities the situation presented and stuck around to see if something else would happen. Inspector Dorrington, however, could not substantiate any of the charges made by Sheppard, and Hummer was not reprimanded.

The episode may have given him a jolt, for he evidently dropped the matron as a potential dalliance. He resumed his old habit of taking out his frustrations on his staff, who in turn made his life miserable. When Hummer raged to the chief engineer about the hot water not working, the employee told Hummer to go to hell. Hummer fired him, and the man's wife quit as well.

Smoots, in regaling his friend with these details, characterized the situation by saying, "Things are going to the devil in general." He added, "The girls knocked off a $35.00 parlor lamp for Doc and broke it." In that same period, Katherine Knox, whether by intent or mistake, gave the female patients lye instead of coffee.[13]

Part of Hummer's difficulties can probably be attributed to a plain old case of cabin fever on the part of his employees. Most of them lived on-site and could not get away from one another during the unrelenting winter weather. Their work was stressful and distasteful in the extreme. Employees had little leisure, even fewer diversions, and nowhere to go; gossip would have been the prevailing source of entertainment.

Hummer's activities would be a natural subject of conversation among employees under the best of circumstances, but in the closed world of the asylum, he could not get away from their scrutiny. Likewise, in that environment, any slight or unkindness would have been picked apart, resented, chewed over, and nurtured. Hummer's temper and genuine disregard for his employees' feelings only gave them better scope to bear him ill will.

At least in the summer, employees could get out in the fresh air. They could walk or hitch a ride to town, visit with friends, and in general, catch their spiritual breaths away from the asylum. On a hot day in mid-July, the laborer Ione Landis accepted a ride into Canton from Hummer, whose wife was out of town. On the way, Hummer became somewhat overfamiliar, complaining at the same time that he didn't know what he was going to do if his wife didn't come back.

They stopped near the Rudolph Hotel in town, Hummer saying that he had company to take out. The Rudolph was Canton's most luxurious hotel, with a spacious lobby, marble tiles, a grand staircase, and a telephone in each of its forty-four guest rooms. Landis decided to walk back to the asylum, but Hummer told her to go ahead and ride back with him. Landis either thought she had put her employer in his place or decided she couldn't manage the trip back on foot, because when his visitors failed to show, she got back in the car. Instead of returning to the asylum, however, Hummer took another road.

"This isn't the way to the asylum," Landis protested.

"There are more ways than one," Hummer replied. "Let's go to Sioux Falls."

"No, I don't care for shows," Landis replied, finally catching his drift and endeavoring to deliberately misunderstand him.

Hummer drove north for another mile or two, then turned east onto a road with no houses. Here he began to more forcefully caress and draw the girl to him.

"You're a married man!" Landis exclaimed, but nothing stopped his roving hands. "Please—I'm only a poor girl with nothing but my self-respect," she pleaded. Eventually she grabbed his hands so that he would stop using them to touch her, and she screamed as the car almost rolled.

"My God, girl, you are going to kill us both!" Hummer shouted. Landis had gotten his attention, but now that they were stopped, he pulled out a contraceptive.[14] "I've bought this and had several chances to use it, but haven't," he told Landis. "You are in safe hands."

"I'm going to walk!" Landis retorted.

Hummer had enough sense to know he could never get away with outright assault. Defeated, he told Landis, "Why, I was just joking with you."

Landis told her friend, Mary Wiggin, about the incident, but Hummer preempted any complaint she could have made to Mrs. Hummer by telling his wife at least some version of the escapade. Mrs. Hummer, always haughty, became especially cold to Landis.

Soon after her return, Mrs. Hummer—knowing the staff was short two women—told Landis that she would have to begin working in the Hummers' rooms, cleaning. She forced Landis to scrub the toilet on her hands and knees instead of with the usual broom, and in one instance, hid a half-burned matchstick on the baseboard to see if Landis would find it. When she didn't, Hummer called Landis into his office and told the matron to watch her because "she was a decided shirk."

Landis had wanted to keep working at the asylum to earn enough money to educate herself for a higher position, but she had had enough. She had tried to please the Hummers and especially tried to avoid running into the superintendent if she could help it. Hummer sought her out for reprimands, sometimes in front of others, and Mrs. Hummer made snide remarks to Landis in private about not taking "too many rides in an auto." Hummer apparently provoked Landis once too often, and she called him a liar. He promptly dismissed her, and four months later (May 8) she sent a complaint to the commissioner of Indian affairs.

Investigations into Canton Asylum's affairs were becoming prompter, and in June the Indian Office sent Dr. L. F. Michael to investigate this latest incident. When faced with Landis's charge, Hummer exploded, saying that "the entire statement is a scurrilous fabrication, given by an ex-employee, having been discharged."

He didn't stop there, and Michael stated, "My only regret is that I had no stenographer to make a complete report on what he said." The gist of it boiled down to Hummer feeling that he was overworked, unappreciated, and tired of answering charges from dismissed employees.

While Michael was there, patient James Herman and chief engineer Norman Ewing approached him with their own charges of patient mistreatment.[15] Additionally, Ewing complained to Michael about Hummer's management. Hummer couldn't immediately do anything about Herman because he was a patient, but he could do something about Ewing. Michael filed his report June 12, and on June 16 Hummer sent a letter to the Indian Office, charging Ewing with spying, perjury, neglect of duty, tasting whiskey on the premises, and stirring up discontent among patients and employees. According to Hummer, Ewing was "out of harmony with the Office," and he recommended Ewing's immediate dismissal.

A few days later, Hummer sent another letter to the commissioner, stating that he had given Ewing a copy of his charges and that when Ewing came to the office to hand in his reply, Hummer read part of Ewing's letter and "called his attention to his misstatements which did not improve his humor." Ewing and Hummer had words at that point, which did not improve Hummer's own humor. Hummer analyzed Ewing in his letter to the commissioner, coming as near as possible to calling Ewing insane without actually saying it. He further accused Ewing of falling in love with a white woman and of becoming angry when his charges to Michael were not supported.[16]

In a remarkable jump in reasoning, Hummer went on to say, "The next step in these cases is 'what can I do to get even.' This thought is responsible for the numerous murders, suicide, etc., which fill the daily press and results in trials, and, usually the incarceration of the individual in an asylum." Following his groundwork to undermine Ewing's character, Hummer said, "I consider that, with this man at large and in his present frame of mind, and furnished with a master key for the institution, there is no certainty as to what he will do. Remembering the assassination of Supt. Stanley *I shall arm myself and use my weapon in self-defense*, if necessary. . . . I sincerely and earnestly recommend his immediate removal before some crime is committed. This is not said through any fear, though I expect an attack in the dark, rather than the open." After it received such a letter, Michael's report must have given the Indian Office plenty of food for thought.[17]

Michael had heard rumors of patient mistreatment in the women's ward but could find no one who would talk. He had interviewed another former employee, the clerk who had replaced Seely, who didn't say anything of material value except that "he had had his differences with Dr. Hummer and that he was through at the Asylum." Jacob Fowles said that he had seen more than one employee called into Hummer's office and given a severe "going-over" in his (Fowles's) presence and that of anyone else standing by. "The worst thing I can say, is that the Doctor has an ungovernable temper; its [*sic*] dynamite and liable to go off at any time," Fowles concluded.

Michael made a telling comment at this point: "This matter of temper, has much to do in keeping employees shy of the Asylum office and in reporting things for fear of being subjected to a 'going-over.'"

Among recommendations to convert ward laborer positions to attendant positions and to fill the vacant physician's position, Michael formally stated that Van Winkle should be separated at once from the service and that two of the attendants who could have reported his and others' misconduct should be reprimanded themselves for not doing so. Since Hummer did not make a sworn statement in rebuttal to Ione Landis's charges, Michael submitted that case without recommendation.

Someone at the Indian Office made his own rather severe recommendations after reviewing Michael's report. In a twelve-page document titled "Statement Regarding Harry Hummer, Superintendent of the Canton Insane Asylum," the unsigned author (perhaps Assistant Commissioner E. B. Meritt) reviewed Michael's and Dorrington's reports concerning Hummer's suspected dalliances, as well as reports from Davis's 1909 investigation and other notes about the asylum, and came away with a much harsher picture of Hummer's conduct.

The writer brushed aside Hummer's defense that Landis's allegations had been made nearly a year after the incident and zeroed in on the fact that Landis had sworn an affidavit and Hummer had not. Furthermore, he saw that Michael had interviewed nearly all the staff and found that even those who didn't get along with Landis had nothing specific to say against her; most of the staff, as well as a few townspeople Michael spoke to, gave her a spotless character reference. The writer's conclusion was that the charge *was* substantiated. He wrote:

> The case of Miss Landis is pathetic. Here was a girl who bore a good reputation, as testified to by all who knew her. Dr. Hummer tried to take advantage of her, and failing in his purpose he has apparently attempted in every way to get her in a position where she could be dismissed. He required her, a Government employee, to scrub his private rooms in addition to her work at the institution, and when she failed to so much as to locate a burnt match on the washboard in the bathroom he called the matron to his office and told her to watch Miss Landis as she shirked her work. There have been other cases of a similar nature, in which it is plainly apparent that when he did not want an employee longer he resorted to similar means to get grounds upon which to dismiss them. His acts in this respect are little short of persecution.

The writer recommended that Michael be instructed to take temporary charge of Canton Asylum, that Hummer be suspended and given an opportunity to submit his resignation, and that the vacant physician position be immediately filled by a competent alienist of Michael's choosing. The writer's anger is evident throughout the statement. He says flatly that Michael had not done his duty when he refused to make a recommendation based on his report and scrawled a note at the bottom of the last page for the reader he was addressing to see Dorrington's report.[18]

After reviewing all the reports and this forceful statement from either Meritt or someone else high enough in the Indian Office to prepare such a document, the commissioner of Indian affairs, Cato Sells, wrote to Hummer,

> It is suggested that you keep a more careful watch on your conduct and especially control your temper so that this Office may not be subjected to the necessity of investigating charges of that character.

You must be aware of the fact that, while charges of immorality may not be proven, the fact that such charges are made should indicate to you the necessity for an extremely careful watch on your conduct in relation to the female employes of the institution.

I dismiss these charges and trust that in the regulation of the internal affairs of the institution there may not be cause for any further investigation along these lines.[19]

In December 1915 Hummer was elected vice president of the Seventh District Medical Society of South Dakota. On January 20, 1916, Dr. R. E. L. Newberne, the Indian Office's chief medical director, completed a general investigation of Canton Asylum. He was suitably impressed with Hummer's various arrangements and even managed to find humor in the sanitary arrangements. Flies were kept under control through suitable methods, like keeping stable waste from collecting, using screens, and applying a concoction of formaldehyde and molasses as a deterrent. However, Newberne was amused by the extra assistance from the patients. "In the summer time one of the principal amusements of the patients is swatting flies," the inspector noted. "And if they had their way the screen-doors would be left open in order that the flies might enter for the swatting contests."

After giving a rundown of his own credentials and training in hospitals for the insane, Newberne pronounced the Canton Insane Asylum for Indians a well-managed institution. He further said, "The thorough training of Superintendent Hummer . . . is reflected in every department and no where to a greater degree than in the sympathetic treatment of its unfortunate patients committed to his care."[20]

10. Life among the Indians

Agnes Caldwell was a Menominee Indian from Keshena Agency, Wisconsin, who was admitted to Canton Asylum at age twenty-six. Her admittance may have been brought on by the stress of sleep deprivation while she cared for a sick relative, but Hummer promptly labeled her with feeblemindedness and a weakness for sex. Her husband frequently added to her stress by sending her letters full of bad news and asking her when she was coming home to take care of their children.

In turn, Caldwell wrote many plaintive letters to the commissioner of Indian affairs: "I got a letter from home I show it to him [Hummer] the letter I heard about my little Boy he was very sick we all like to see are children I am feeling just Blue from that day. . . . O Dear my poor children I wish I could see them I think of them ever day and night my little Boy asking me if I am ever coming home."[1]

She wrote the commissioner because Hummer had told her—as he told other patients—that he couldn't release her without the commissioner's permission. Caldwell's letters revolved around concern for her aging parents and her children and her belief that she was well and should be released. Hummer likely took her poor sentence structure and spelling as an indication of her feeblemindedness, without considering her considerable accomplishment in learning to speak and write English. By the time Caldwell arrived in 1917, Hummer was especially loath to release anyone he could justify retaining.

Hummer didn't feel Caldwell could care for her children properly, but he had additional qualms. "Owing to her weakness for the male sex and her feeble-mindedness, I fear there would result feeble-minded, epileptic or idiotic children, if she were permitted to be at large," he wrote in response to one of her letters to the commissioner of Indian affairs. Going through the motions, however, he asked the commissioner's advice concerning her possible release, knowing from experience that his superior would not contradict his own feelings on the matter. Caldwell may or may not have been mentally deficient, but Hummer eventually allowed her to do general housework in his own home.[2]

Coupled with his desire to keep patients at the asylum, either from genuine concern about their welfare or to expand his institution—or a little of both—Hummer faced pressure from other powerful forces. His institution was considered both a haven and a holding tank, and various interests wanted to take advantage of its mission.

When Canton Asylum first opened, reservation agents were appointed by the president and required confirmation by the Senate. In turn, these agents appointed reservation clerks, millers, mechanics, blacksmiths, and other subordinate employees, including the superintendent of reservation schools. By 1908, appointed agents had been phased out and replaced by civil service superintendents, but the latter were equally powerful.[3] Though they controlled what sometimes amounted to fiefdoms, these men were nearly overwhelmed with administrative details and responsibilities. Anything they could do to make life easier—like getting rid of a troublesome Indian—would be attractive.

Canton Asylum had been built to accommodate forty-eight patients, who had at first just trickled in.[4] Soon, though, reservation superintendents took advantage of it as a place to funnel unwanted charges and clamored to get their most exasperating or time-consuming inhabitants out of their hair. That is not to say that the need for some type of institutional care was not often genuine, but merely that its necessity was based on factors other than insanity that had been confirmed by qualified—and objective—medical men.

Hummer had fifty-eight patients by February 1912, with another forty-nine applications from agents on file that he could not accept; his capacity usually fluctuated between full and overflowing. Hummer— with the full knowledge of his superiors—kept a perpetually overcrowded asylum. Caught in a vicious cycle of needing more patients to justify more buildings and staff and needing more buildings and staff to ease the stress and discomfort of the added patients, Hummer perpetually walked a delicate line, trying to expand his territory without overloading himself to the point that he failed completely. He took whoever the Indian Office wanted to send him, so long as he could possibly squeeze another body into the crowded facility.

Ironically, the only official letter that seems to have been offered in protest to the "dumping" of Indians at the asylum had come from the energetic Dr. L. M. Hardin. During Hummer's absence in September 1909, Hardin, as physician-in-charge, had to decline accepting two insane Arapahos because of overcrowding. In his refusal letter to the commissioner, he added, "As long as the institution accepts imbeciles, cripples, harmless old people, etc., and the place made a refuge for all kinds of defectives it is not possible to care for all who seek admission."[5]

Hummer had never protested as Hardin did, and the start of 1916 found his accommodating ways beginning to pay off. His long-desired hospital had been constructed and fitted out (though not yet with the showers and hydrotherapy equipment he had so desired) so that he could accept occupancy on the first day of that year. Along with the increased capacity came increased staff and a wider scope of authority.

He also had a home of his own—a spacious and well-appointed cottage—at last. His $6,000 estimate for it had been reduced to a couple of dollars short of $4,000 but it still bought him beamed ceilings, red oak throughout the interior, a built-in icebox, a range, a fireplace, and a large basement. It was a dream come true to get away from the constant presence of his patients and staff.

His new dairy barn had been approved and was under construction, and Hummer had already offered enthusiastic plans for further construction: a long-desired epileptic cottage. After that, he wanted to remodel the old laundry building and build a chapel/amusement hall so that patients didn't have to hold church in the dining room. The hall would hold moving-picture equipment for the enjoyment of patients and staff while also acting as a convenient place for employee dances—employees "whose life here is not one continuous bed of roses," as he told the commissioner.[6]

He was certainly right concerning the challenges employees faced. Easy as it is to blame attendants for neglecting and abusing their patients, these poorly paid men and women lived under conditions almost guaranteed to make them fail at their duties. Most occupied a single room in the main building and ate food that was institutional and sometimes sub-par at that. They adhered to the same tiresome schedule as the patients, often working into the late evening and then rising early. Attendants had little leisure time unless they took it on the sly during slack periods, and they were on constant call while off-duty without additional recompense.

Even disregarding their limited personal space and leisure time, the workplace itself was unpleasant in the extreme. "Filthy patients" were so called because they frequently soiled themselves; attendants did not have the luxury of latex gloves or face masks to limit contamination when they began to clean up after the accidents.

Inspection reports and statements from Hummer himself indicate that many patients were extremely careless in their toilet habits, threw or smeared feces on the floor and walls, and otherwise created disheartening conditions for attendants to work in. When an inspector wrote that the asylum had no radiator covers to prevent possible burns, Hummer explained that he had originally placed wooden covers with wire-cloth screening over the radiators for safety. However, patients used the wooden frames for weapons and "would expectorate on them and urinate through them" to such an extent that they became unsanitary. He was probably just being practical in deciding that the radiator covers were best removed, especially since burns had proven to be infrequent.[7]

The stench in such a place would have been almost palpable. Routine maintenance couldn't be performed because the asylum lacked trained personnel who had the time to perform it, and the asylum frequently looked rundown and shabby. Fights between patients were so frequent that even pictures on the walls had to be taken down so they could not be used as weapons. The workload was overwhelming. Added to the other problems, Hummer offered no training whatsoever to new staff. In a small town out West, these new hires were almost certain to know little about institutional protocols or patient management. With no training in how to handle common institutional problems, little time off, and a lack of opportunities to decompress, attendants undoubtedly snapped at times.

Under these dismal conditions, anything Hummer could do to make the workday easier was well worth doing. To his credit, the superintendent did try to lighten his employees' burden with what amusements he could furnish inexpensively.

Hummer invited the Canton Band to play at the asylum, which it did occasionally, undoubtedly entertaining the staff as much as the patients. He tried to install moving picture equipment and a radio—for years an ongoing effort with the Indian Office—and allowed dances and other entertainments. Hummer subscribed to several popular consumer magazines—*Good Housekeeping, Ladies' Home Journal, Literary Digest,* and *National Geographic,* among others—that his employees (and perhaps patients) could enjoy. He even dismissed a cook whose skills were so abysmal that employees complained to him about their meals. But, though he was delighted with his new buildings and was perfectly willing to make life easier for his employees when he could, Hummer still had to be careful with funds.

The fly in his ointment—and one that could bite and fester if ignored—was the niggling problem of per capita costs. Hummer knew his costs were exceptionally high compared to those of other institutions because of Canton Asylum's small size. The facility's remoteness also figured into the prices he had to pay for necessities, particularly fuel and rations. His payroll was proportionally higher than at other institutions because it simply took a set number of people to operate the place—farmer, laborers, cook, seamstress, and so on—whether he had one patient there or a thousand. Dividing his base expenditures by forty-eight or even fifty-eight patients just couldn't give him a price for housing each patient that compared favorably with other institutions. Hummer knew he could ill afford to let anyone leave the asylum, let alone a woman like Agnes Caldwell, who was liable to turn out defective children. She, and others like her, would stay.

Hummer had long ago told his first assistant, Dr. Turner, that he intended to "make a record of economy for himself" at the asylum. Though Inspector Davis had reproved him in 1909 for his excessive penny-pinching, Hummer still contrived to return money to the Indian Office from his allotted funds each year. This year was no different: out of the $45,000 that had been appropriated for Canton Asylum in 1916, Hummer told the commissioner he would use only $33,000, leaving $12,000 available for other uses. Coupled with the $8,000 he expected to save from his support fund, Hummer estimated he would have $20,000 available for the construction of his epileptic cottage and amusement hall.

Hummer had to tread carefully, though. In 1910 the average per capita cost for the institutionalized insane in the United States was $175, with a high of $230 in New Jersey and a low in New York of $160. At Canton Asylum, per capita costs had been $366 in 1907 and $394 in 1908. Hummer had brought these figures down to $323 in 1909 and a triumphant $300 in 1911.[8] However, with new construction and added personnel, costs were bound to rise again. Hummer also knew that Canton Asylum's costs exceeded those of keeping patients at St. Elizabeths, an institution that remained a very real threat to him even though Indians were not its targeted patient group.[9]

Hummer had spent eight years fighting for a home and a hospital, and he wasn't about to surrender these triumphs so his patients could stay at cheaper facilities. Keeping his patient count high was imperative—especially as the assistant commissioner, Edgar B. Meritt, had begun to ask pointed questions about finances. In February 1916 Hummer had sent the commissioner of Indian affairs a letter announcing he could accept forty new patients now that his hospital had opened, but he did not receive the expected flood of bodies. He must have been nonplussed when Meritt wrote back to say that most of the cases of insanity his office had recently investigated had turned out to be unfounded.

Then, in March, Meritt asked a question that must have chilled Hummer: "In this connection it occurs to the Office that in many instances it has been able to place Indians in state institutions at less per capita than would have been the case had the patients been sent to the Canton asylum. It is not uncommon for the Office to get a rate as low as $20. per month. Please inform the Office why in your opinion the per capita cost at Canton should exceed that figure."

Acting both on a recommendation from Dr. Newberne's otherwise glowing report and to relieve the relentless nature of his duties, Hummer had actually requested another physician (who would also be a property clerk) to help him at Canton Asylum, less than two months earlier. Now he hastily reminded the commissioner of Indian affairs that his payroll would have been even higher than it was, except that he had assumed the duties of both superintendent and physician to save money.[10]

Hummer went on to explain that his personnel, currently at a ratio of one employee to every two and a half patients, created a high expense that would go down with the admission of the forty new patients. He stated that if he could increase capacity to three hundred patients, he would be able to get his per capita costs to between $250 and $275.[11]

It had taken fourteen years to acquire the capacity for eighty-eight patients—any expectation that expenditures for an additional two-hundred-plus bodies would suddenly materialize was just pie-in-the-sky dreaming. Hummer likely spent some time fretting over the situation, though he must have also realized that the Indian Office could not really be anxious to abandon over $100,000 worth of land and buildings to the sparsely populated state of South Dakota.[12] That this was so became evident when Congress approved an additional $7,500 in 1917 to "repair and improve the road leading from the said asylum for insane Indians to the city of Canton, South Dakota."[13]

Despite that bit of reassurance, Hummer and the rest of the country had plenty of things to worry about in 1916. The United States had retained its neutrality during Woodrow Wilson's "he kept us out of war" presidential campaign, but the possibility of staying that course looked grim by the end of the year. In April 1917 the United States did join the European conflict. Hummer soon received a communication from the National Committee for Mental Hygiene (Clifford Beers's organization) asking him what facilities he had to accommodate the expected influx of mental cases resulting from the war.

The committee estimated that 20 percent of patients requiring treatment in military hospitals would have mental and nervous disorders. Superintendent White at St. Elizabeths had frankly told them that his facility couldn't absorb many of these patients, and the committee was now trying to discover which hospitals *could* accommodate mental cases, for its report to the Council of National Defense.[14]

Hummer wrote to the commissioner of Indian affairs, saying that he couldn't give a definite answer about his capacity to handle patients until he knew what would be required. Would Canton Asylum set itself up as a general hospital to care for the extra cases expected as a result of the war, or only for the mental cases? He stated emphatically that the asylum was ready and willing to do its share and more. Then Hummer slipped in a sly jab: "I am sorry that your Office decided that we should not build the proposed epileptic cottage, as this would have given us additional beds which might have been used for the purpose now in question."[15]

Whatever he may have anticipated, Hummer never received a great influx of patients due to the war. He received twenty patients in 1917 and another twenty-nine in 1918, bringing his total to eighty-one patients at the end of fiscal year 1918.[16] Uncharacteristically, Hummer discharged two female patients nearly back to back in 1918. The first was Mary Walking Day, who had developed "a small spot on the little toe of the right foot, which developed into gangrene . . . and I suggested amputation of the right leg above the knee," Hummer began in explanation.

Somehow, Walking Day's family got hold of Hummer's diagnosis and proposed course of treatment. Her husband and uncle showed up on Hummer's doorstep, saying they wanted to take her away immediately. There is no record of the confrontation, if any, but Hummer acquiesced immediately. He then had to write the commissioner after the fact, to ask if he had done the right thing. All Hummer would say about it was, "It appears that the Indians are opposed to amputation."

The second woman discharged, Mary Mann Fisher, had improved considerably since her admission in June 1917, though Hummer cautioned the commissioner in July of the following year that Fisher's husband was trying to get her to sign a "certain paper" and he didn't know whether it was in her best interest or not to sign it. In December Fisher was much improved, but Hummer still said, "These cases frequently relapse and I fear a relapse in this particular case unless the home conditions are quite favorable." Despite his concerns, he did release Fisher later that month.[17]

A touch of gangrene aside, Hummer wrote proudly of his patients' excellent health during the war years, even though several had died from meningitis and tuberculosis. He had nipped a case of "liberty measles" in the bud by quarantining the patient, and though measles, chicken pox, and smallpox had prevailed in Canton and the immediate vicinity, no one at the asylum had become infected. The Canton library had closed for two months during the war because of the flu epidemic, so Hummer may have felt justified in his accomplishments. With so many of his patients in poor health to begin with, a wave of influenza within the asylum could have been disastrous—and that had not happened.[18]

Though he may have enjoyed relative freedom from infectious diseases, no insane soldier would have enjoyed the food at Canton Asylum. Supplies at home were rationed so that soldiers overseas could get enough to eat, and the pickings could be slim this side of the Atlantic. Hummer, along with the rest of the country, had instituted "one beefless, one porkless and one wheatless days each week and six extra wheatless meals per week, in addition to which we purchased a quantity of wheat flour substitutes, the net result being a material falling off of the appetites of some of our patients and employees resulting in a perceptible loss of weight for practically everyone here and a considerable degree of grumbling and discontent among the less patriotic of our employees."[19]

Despite employee grumbling, Hummer supported the government's recommended measures to help the war effort. He served as a major in the Army Medical Reserve and his fourteen-year-old son, Francis, received a trophy cup from the National Agricultural Association for Best War Garden raised in Lincoln County, South Dakota, in 1918.[20] Patients also did their part to help the war effort. In May 1918 Hummer reported holding $1,350 in second Liberty Loan bonds for nine of his patients. Patient Susan Wishecoby (and perhaps others) knitted sweaters for "our soldier boys" through the Red Cross.

However, the war drained the Indian Office of medical men as physicians resigned to join (usually) the Medical Department of the Army. This exodus left the Indian Office at 60 percent strength for its physician positions in 1918; the shortage was difficult to remedy in years to come, since many doctors accepted civil positions after the war ended.[21] Hummer was thirty-nine in 1918—still a relatively young man—and could have chosen to make the same career move many of his peers were making. He may have stayed at Canton because he felt he was needed there, felt himself too old to join the army . . . or because he realized the physician shortage made him more valuable than ever to the Indian Office.

Whatever his reasons for staying, Hummer did the best he could during the war, even though projects and equipment like hydrotherapy apparatus had to sit on the back burner. Still, he had been promised an addition to the laundry room, which was welcome news. His dairy herd was increasing nicely, even if his cattle for meat and his sows were not multiplying as they should.

However, Hummer's most pressing problem concerned his workforce. Because of the war, he had vacancies he couldn't fill, and Hummer complained that he had to retain staff that he would have otherwise discharged. Hummer suggested increasing the salaries of the ward attendants to forty dollars a month for men and thirty-five dollars for women or resorting to using Indian labor. He qualified the last suggestion by saying, "I must confess that neither of the three Indians formerly employed here gave any satisfaction."

In July 1918 Hummer made a plea "for the admission of such Indian soldiers or sailors as may be unfortunate enough to become insane in the service of our Country in this terrible war," even though he was down to one male attendant and one female attendant for the eighty-one patients he had.[22] How Hummer and the asylum managed during this time is not on the record, but in December the superintendent was back to requesting more buildings: his prized epileptic cottage and his chapel and amusement hall.[23]

Agnes Caldwell continued to suffer from loneliness and homesickness and wrote another fruitless letter to Cato Sells: "I try my best to be good out heare there is nothing is matter with me. . . . My girl she is died now. . . . My little Boy is pretty sick to. . . . I feeling Blue that I well never see my little gril [sic] again [I] feel bad enough to heare my little boy is sick and please let me go home and see my boy I do like to see him now this [daughter?] she is gone I will never see her no more I feel bad to day."[24]

Assistant Commissioner Meritt told Caldwell not to worry about her children, for they were in good hands. "In the meantime you should attend carefully to your own health and keep yourself in good condition, so that you may be able to return when Dr. Hummer decides you are well enough."

Such crumbs of hope sustained Caldwell for years.

11. Another Sort of Prison

World War I ended on November 11, 1919, but America's war with its Indian population still raged. Since colonial times, some battles had always been overt with bloodshed and bitterness on both sides, but later battles became systemic wars on the Indian psyche.

The United States had originally treated Indian groups as sovereign nations but found it difficult to annex their land under this system or to administer it afterward. Congress solved the problem neatly: buried within the Indian Appropriations Act of 1871 was the statement that "hereafter no Indian nation or tribe within the territory of the United States shall be acknowledged or recognized as an independent nation, tribe, or power with whom the United States may contract by treaty."

That ended treaties and sovereign nations. The Supreme Court had already decided in 1823 that Indians could occupy lands within the United States but could not hold title to those lands—their "right of occupancy" being trumped by the United States' "right of discovery." Given their tenuous legal hold on land, it was easy enough in 1887 for the Dawes Act to divide communal reservation land into 160-acre parcels called "allotments" and dole them out to individuals who had a blood quantum of at least one-half (later changed to one-quarter).[1] Millions of acres of surplus reservation lands were then opened up for settlement, which tended to greatly benefit whites and impoverish Indians. Even before the Dawes Act passed, cavalry officer Richard H. Pratt had created his model off-reservation boarding school in Carlisle, Pennsylvania, so that the work of erasing Native American culture could begin.

Anglo-style education for Indians was not a new idea; in the 1600s

British colonies had organized "praying towns" for Indians to receive so-called civilizing Christian instruction while being separated from their own communities. In 1775 the Continental Congress appropriated $500 to educate Indian youth at Dartmouth College in New Hampshire, and a statement for educational expenses in 1789 shows that $425.51 was incurred "in equipping George M. White Eyes, an Indian youth of the Delaware tribe . . . he having been educated by order and at the expense of the United States."[2]

Mission schools, run by religious organizations and financed partially by the Indian Office, became common during the nineteenth century. The government also established its own Indian schools, operating 76 reservation boarding schools and 147 day schools by 1900 as it phased out mission schools.[3]

However, children going to schools on reservations could still be corrupted by the continued influence of parents and the surrounding culture, said Pratt. If they could be sent *away* to schools where parental or home influences couldn't undermine the process of teaching students how to be white, assimilation would proceed more quickly. Time and distance would break the bonds children had to their heritage, Pratt argued, and shift their path toward "civilization."

Assimilating Indians through education was an attractive proposition. Secretary of the Interior Carl Schurz (1877–81) believed it would cost $1 million to kill an Indian in warfare and only $1,200 to school a child for eight years. Beyond that, said other enthusiasts, by educating children so they could enter the larger white society and earn their own livings, the government would gradually escape the heavy costs associated with annuities, food, clothing, and social welfare programs provided to Indians.[4]

The Indian Office embraced the ideas and methodology Pratt instituted for assimilating schoolchildren but went a step further. Agents condoned and aided the forcible removal of children as young as five or six from their parents or engaged in outright kidnapping to send young Indians hundreds of miles away to attend the government boarding schools.

As soon as they arrived, students were thrust into a different world. Teachers cut the boys' hair, replaced both sexes' Indian names with new Anglo-Saxon ones, forbade them to speak even a single word in their native language, outfitted them with "citizen" clothing, and then set them to work learning a trade. The attitude of the Indian Office was reflected in the words of John B. Riley, the Indian school superintendent: "Only by complete isolation of the Indian child from his savage antecedents can he be satisfactorily educated."[5] It goes without saying that the children were forbidden to practice their spiritual customs.

Homesickness plagued the students, but runaways, or "deserters," were usually arrested and sent back to the schools they hated when they were caught. Ten- and eleven-year-old girls who escaped from Rice Boarding School in Arizona were forced to walk with heavy cordwood packs on their shoulders while being beaten with a club once they were recaptured. Runaways there were chained to their beds and marched to meals with chains fastened to their necks.

Indifference to their students' feelings often ran to downright cruelty on the part of school staff. The superintendent at the Walker River Agency School in New York ordered ten girls to be publicly stripped to the waist and then flogged with a buggy whip for stealing a can of baking powder. Senate inquiries into boarding school discipline in the 1920s showed that Indian Service employees whipped children with leather straps and sometimes struck them until blood ran from their faces to their knees.[6]

Physical abuse and starvation were common, and diseases like tuberculosis and trachoma were rampant; in 1912 a congressional study found that nearly 70 percent of Indian children in Oklahoma boarding schools were infected with trachoma. Children died (and were buried) at schools, while parents received infrequent reports that did nothing to allay their misery at the loss of their children.

Reformers faced huge fights over funding for such basics as food and clothing for these Indian children. In 1929 the powerful chairman of the House Appropriations Committee, Louis C. Cramton, positively refused to increase food allowances from 20 to 37.8 cents a day for children at boarding schools. Publicity stirred up by a vocal John Collier pushed the Senate to restore the original request, but Cramton won when he managed in committee to check the increase to only 28 cents per day for food.[7]

Despite these issues, many in authority considered boarding schools great successes. In 1910 the superintendent of Indian Schools, Estelle

Reel, said that "76 per cent of the pupils who came out of the Indian schools were worthwhile," which "speaks volumes for a system of education which can, in so short a time, develop from an uncivilized race 76 per cent of men and women capable of taking their places in the body politic of this Republic."[8]

Years later, the Indian Office underscored its approval. In 1926 Assistant Commissioner of Indian Affairs Edgar B. Meritt published an explanatory bulletin, *The American Indian and Government Indian Administration*, which attempted to put most of the Indian Service's actions in a positive light. In it, he lauded the service's school system, saying, "The Indian Bureau is conducting one of the most efficient school systems among the Indians to be found anywhere in the United States or the civilized world."

As though that were not enough, he quoted Dr. Samuel A. Eliot, a member of the Board of Indian Commissioners: "I wish I might send my children to an Indian school. There are no finer in the country, public or private."[9]

The Indian Office's refusal to look at its weaknesses, along with the government's official policy of assimilation, guaranteed that Indians would be forced to do whatever white authorities felt was best for them. Even relatively benign paternalism had the strength of the correction rod behind it, and Indians everywhere knew that disobedience to government mandates would mean trouble. At least schoolchildren had an end to their term in (virtual) prison: they could go home when they graduated. Crazy people, however, had no such term limits.[10]

James Herman's father was German and his mother was a halfblood Cheyenne with rights to the Rosebud Reservation in South Dakota. A little gout ran in the family, but no insanity. Herman began to drink when he was twenty-one, by all accounts just about whenever he could conveniently get his hands on an intoxicant. Otherwise, he worked hard as a carpenter and was credited with helping build most of the schoolhouses and farmers' stations on the Rosebud Reservation. Through his mother, he had a land allotment and, because of it, cattle and money.

Herman was born at Fort Randall and attended a post school there. His father had not adopted his wife's culture, and the only time that Herman participated in reservation life was on issue day—if the pickings were good, he drew rations, and he skipped them if they weren't to his liking. He lived as a white child and later as a white man in a white community, where he had a good reputation.

Herman married a pretty, sixteen-year-old white woman when he was thirty-three, but he continued drinking heavily. This led to domestic difficulties, and at forty-four, he promised his dying mother he would stop drinking. He kept his promise for five years; however, continuing problems at home led him back to alcohol. He and his wife had seven children, five boys and two girls, and having a drunk for a husband undoubtedly colored Blanch Herman's attitude toward him. As he grew older and more feeble, as well as afflicted with gout and rheumatism, he became less and less attractive to his young wife. In 1914 he went on a drinking spree that was his undoing.

After seventeen years of marriage, Blanch had had enough. She called the insanity commission in Gregory County and initiated proceedings to have her husband declared insane. They obliged with a diagnosis of alcoholic insanity and were ready to send him to the state hospital in Yankton. Before they could commit him there, they discovered that Herman had Indian blood in him. The commission sent him to Canton Asylum instead, where he arrived on February 28, 1914.

It was the rock-bottom experience Herman needed. He sobered up, toed the line at the asylum, and tried to get out.[11] Initially, as sometimes happens in domestic cases, Blanch Herman relented and appeared willing to work toward a reconciliation. She visited her husband at the asylum and in June wrote the commissioner of Indian affairs saying that she would accept responsibility for her husband if he were released. Hummer told the commissioner that Herman was "far from being a well man" but that he had displayed no harmful tendencies. He was willing to release Herman, since Blanch had offered to take her husband to a hospital in Hot Springs, South Dakota, as well as pay all the expenses of the transfer.

Early in August, after Assistant Commissioner Meritt had authorized Herman's release, something interfered with Blanch's support. She either became involved in an affair with a local man or decided she enjoyed her freedom. She not only refused to sign the all-important release of responsibility form for the asylum but also began to actively campaign against her husband's attempts to gain his freedom. As a white woman with access to Herman's land and money, she presented a formidable obstacle to his efforts.

When Herman's relatives realized that his wife was not going to take him to Hot Springs as planned, his brother offered to accept responsibility for him in March 1915. Frank Herman sent Hummer a notarized statement to that effect, which was acceptable to the superintendent. Before Herman received his liberty, though, his wife fired off a letter to the commissioner of Indian affairs, objecting to the release:

> [I] will say that I do not think Frank Herman is in [a] position to care for James Herman for the reason that Frank Herman is an invalid and is forced to use crutches all the time and he is not financially able to care for him.
>
> Besides Frank Herman has two sons who are both addicted to the use of intoxicating liquor and since this was the cause of James Herman's present condition, I am sure that it would be unwise to place him in touch with persons where he might get liquor.

She tightened the screws further by stating that she had visited her husband at the asylum and thought he would be better cared for there than with relatives. Meritt rescinded his authorization to release Herman in April, and by June the asylum was enmeshed in the investigation that revealed Van Winkle's cruelty and other lapses in Hummer's management.

Hummer had fired his chief engineer for daring to speak against him during that investigation, and now he knew that James Herman's testimony had gone a long way toward putting his management in a bad light. When Herman wrote the commissioner in November, asking for permission to visit his relatives at Christmas, Meritt denied his request—almost certainly after putting the matter before Hummer for guidance. The superintendent had evidently revised his opinion that Herman "displayed no harmful tendencies."

Herman had many friends who continued to agitate for his release, and Hummer undoubtedly got a shock when he received a carbon-copied letter that Supervisor of Indian Schools Davis had sent to the commissioner. It turned out that Herman was actually a citizen of South Dakota and not a ward of the government. Hummer surmised that Herman was in the asylum illegally and wrote, "Under these circumstances, I respectfully beg your Office to take steps to protect me from the law, as now I appear to be in the position of breaking the law by holding this man."

His fear at the injustice done Herman did not keep him from adding, "James Herman is far from being a well man, mentally, and should not be given his liberty, as dangerous or criminal actions may result." Hummer suggested sending his patient to Yankton, Herman's original destination.

The Indian Office seldom moved quickly, and certainly not when the matter before it was only the release of a patient. In February 1916 the insanity commission of Gregory County, which had originally found Herman insane, sent Commissioner Cato Sells a request for Herman's release. Signed by both the commission's representative and a county judge, the document stated that the commission believed Herman had sufficiently recovered from the alcoholic insanity he had been suffering at the time of his commitment. They absolved the Indian Office of liability and asked that Herman be released.

Whether Blanch Herman notified him or he heard it through the grapevine, Dr. M. H. Clagett, who had examined Herman during his original sanity hearing, wrote the commissioner on March 2, 1916, in protest. According to Clagett, two years earlier Herman had suffered from alcoholic hardening of the brain and a permanent cure was out of the question. Clagett sealed Herman's fate by saying that "there is no way to tell when a brain storm could occur, and during these storms he would be very dangerous. " The commissioner took Clagett's opinion, coupled with Hummer's statement that Herman was a dangerous man, and refused to release him.

P. J. Donohue, a friend of Herman's and the attorney who had told the Indian Office that Herman was a citizen, now brought in a friend from Congress, Representative Harry L. Gandy, writing to Gandy:

Harry, this is one of the worst frames up [sic] that ever happened by any body. Jim Herman is half breed Indian and his wife is a white woman and she is tired of him. . . . I can show by white neighbors that this woman has a white lover that has been a steady caller.

I have seen Jim Herman and I know him for twenty five years and he is no more insane than he was twenty years ago, he was crazy with alcohol when they sent him, but he had two years to get it out of his system.

Donohue was willing to go to court to get Herman released but hoped that Gandy could accomplish the task more easily. Donohue sent Gandy a petition to the commissioner of Indian affairs that was signed by fifty-three local men who stated that they knew Herman, or had visited or received letters from him, and were convinced he was no longer insane. They requested an investigation into Herman's situation and that he be released.

Meritt replied promptly to Gandy after the congressman duly forwarded the petition. Meritt again refused to release Herman, because the superintendent of the Canton Asylum "has so far always reported that this man is of unsound mind" and because Herman held great ill will toward his wife, whose safety might be endangered by his release. Meritt further stated that an Indian's wardship was not terminated when he became a citizen, thereby underscoring the Indian Office's right to do as it pleased.

James Herman escaped in March 1919, having had parole privileges for the previous four years—Hummer apparently finding nothing inconsistent in giving a man he characterized as unsound and dangerous unrestricted access to the outdoors. Herman made his way to a brother-in-law's home and then went on to visit his children. The brother-in-law didn't turn Herman in to authorities—his wife did.

Hummer dispatched an attendant to fetch Herman and later forwarded a letter to the commissioner from Herman's brother-in-law, requesting his release. Hummer again brought up the question of law and whether Herman, in fact, should be detained at Canton Asylum; he asked that either Herman be sent to the Yankton asylum or the Indian Office assume responsibility for holding the man at Canton.

Meritt replied that the office would assist Hummer in the event of habeas corpus proceedings and told him to take Herman's transfer up with the superintendent of the Yankton asylum. In any event, Herman had to pay for his own return to Canton Asylum.[12]

Back at the asylum, Herman wrote to the commissioner in September to ask again for his release, promising to work to provide for his family and not to "behave as before in the way of drinks or harming any one in the least." In October Meritt wrote to Hummer, asking about his progress in the matter of transferring Herman to the Yankton facility.

By that time, Herman had escaped once more. He had again gone to his brother-in-law, and Meritt told Hummer to find out if the man would accept responsibility for Herman. If so, Hummer could parole him to his in-law.

Another attorney, Josiah Coombs, had now gotten involved and wrote Hummer to ask if he still thought Herman was insane. In his letter, Coombs had x-ed out "had been" confined at Canton Asylum and inserted "is," which led Hummer to write a note to the commissioner stating that "Mr. Coombs could probably furnish information as to Herman's whereabouts."

Hummer merely replied to Coombs's letter that Herman had been admitted in 1914 for mental disease, which existed at the time and "continuously hereafter." Hummer stated that "as superintendent, I know that he was insane at the time of his departure and therefore cannot recommend his release and discharge as sane."

By the end of October, Blanch Herman telegraphed Hummer that her husband was in custody of the sheriff at Butte, Nebraska. Hummer, in turn, telegraphed the commissioner to ask what he should do, as Blanch wanted someone to go get her husband and return him to Canton Asylum.

Meritt must have realized at this point that Herman was no ordinary patient; he wired Herman's brother-in-law, Christ Anderson, to ask if he would assume responsibility for Herman if he were paroled. Anderson replied in the affirmative but requested an inquiry into Herman's sanity. Meritt wired back, telling Anderson to ask his own local board to look into the question.

Meritt also took the time to inform Josiah Coombs that Herman was now "in the jurisdiction of the State of Nebraska, therefore, whatever legal action you may decide to take does not concern the Bureau of Indian Affairs nor the Canton Asylum for Insane Indians."

In Nebraska, the Boyd County Board of Commissioners of Insanity met to examine James Herman and on December 31, 1919, declared that he was not insane. Commissioner Sells wrote to Representative Gandy of the board's decision but told Gandy that "after a thorough review of the whole case" he wasn't satisfied that Herman was a sane man. Sells also referenced Hummer, "our recognized authority upon this subject," who had stated that he couldn't recommend Herman's release and discharge as sane, either. Sells must have received some push-back from Gandy, for Meritt directed medical supervisor Dr. R. E. L. Newberne to immediately divert to Bristow, Nebraska, to examine Herman.

Blanch Herman obviously saw the writing on the wall and had sometime during this period arranged a property settlement through her attorney. Dr. Newberne's visit settled the question of Herman's sanity, for the doctor found in his favor and declared him competent to handle his business affairs. He dismissed Blanch's stated fears that her husband might murder her and supported the property settlement under negotiation.[13]

It had taken six years, two attorneys, a congressman, two insanity boards, a petition by fifty-three men, and a special investigator to free James Herman from confinement for a drinking spree. The commissioner was finally convinced that the case was at an end and told Hummer to strike Herman's name from the list of patients.

Herman's property was released to him by the Department of the Interior, even though allotted land was supposed to be held in trust for Indians for twenty-five years under the Dawes Act. (It was presumed that after twenty-five years, Indian allotment holders would have assimilated into American culture and be able to earn their livings from the land.) The deed, or "patent," would be conveyed to the Indian as a "patent in fee." An amendment to the Dawes Act (1906) allowed the fee-patenting process to be shortened if individual allotment owners were found competent to manage their affairs. Unscrupulous people sometimes persuaded Indians to try to get their land early, through "competency commissions" that would affirm they could handle their affairs. Allottees who spoke little English or were confused by smooth-talking land speculators soon lost their land. Before the twenty-five-year trust period had ended, two-thirds of these lands had passed out of Indian hands.

Herman got his land early but promptly hired an attorney to protect his interests. During his confinement, Herman's original attorney, Josiah Coombs, had told him that before he could be released, he would have to deed his wife half of his allotment. Herman would then pay Coombs his attorney's fees by deeding him half of the remaining half. Under this deal, Herman would retain one-quarter of his original allotment as a result of his confinement. Herman's wife had already taken out a mortgage on his 240 acres of land and had sold all his cattle for several thousand dollars. While he was confined, she received all of Herman's annuities from the Indian Office and all the income from his allotted land.

Herman now faced old age, crippled with rheumatic arthritis and gout, as a nearly penniless man. His only hope was for his new attorney's success in preventing his pending divorce settlement from absolutely impoverishing him.

The divorce settlement did not go as smoothly as Blanch Herman and Coombs had anticipated. In 1921 Coombs finally applied to the Indian Office for help in getting paid for his work to free Herman. Meritt's position, stated plainly to both James Herman's current attorney and later to Coombs, was that Coombs had done nothing on Herman's behalf that warranted payment.

Meritt said that *other* people, like Herman's brother, his brother-in-law, and attorney P. J. Donahue, had brought Herman's affairs to the attention of the Indian Office. Meritt went further in discussing his position with Herman's new attorney. "Mr. Coombs has been advised that the contracts made with the Indian previous to his receiving a patent in fee are void so far as they affect his land," said Meritt. He added self-righteously, "The Government would resist any attempt to illegally attach the property or to compel the Indian to convey according to the alleged contract."[14]

Coombs got his own congressman, M. P. Kinkaid, involved. Kinkaid told Cato Sells that he remembered taking Coombs to Congressman Gandy's office to introduce them and that consequently, Gandy had introduced Coombs to Sells. Kinkaid said he was convinced that Coombs had come to Washington solely on behalf of Herman and hoped that Sells would consider Coombs's case.

Sells finally squelched the affair once and for all. He told Coombs that he hadn't performed any service for Herman that warranted a fee because Coombs had not submitted anything—ever—as proof of Herman's sanity. Sells followed that barb with the somewhat galling assertion that it was the *government* that had resolved the issue by designating officers to investigate Herman's mental condition. Sells flatly told Coombs that the government had a duty to deliver patents (the land held in trust) to Indians, who didn't need attorneys to help them make applications.

Sells also pointed out that any contract made before the patent was issued was void and that the land couldn't be attached for any debt or contract entered into or made while the land was held by the government. He underscored the point by informing Coombs that "the act of June 25, 1910 (36 Stat. 855), provides a penalty for inducing an Indian to sign a deed or a contract affecting the title to his land, and also for offering the same for record."

After another couple of paragraphs that continued to put Coombs in his place, Sells finally concluded, "It seems that you do not fully take into consideration the relations between Indians and the Government, and the duty of the Government toward its wards."

Coombs was undoubtedly dissatisfied with this reply, but there was no mistaking Sells's veiled threat. Herman, who had been imprisoned six years in an insane asylum for drunkenness, was finally receiving protection from the Indian Office.

The records in the Indian Office end here so far as James Herman's fate is concerned. His property settlement presumably ended up more fairly distributed than originally designed by his wife and Coombs, and his many friends likely helped him settle back into working life. Herman was undoubtedly a changed man from his stint at Canton Asylum and, after six years of sobriety, a successful recovering alcoholic. During Newberne's visit to ascertain his sanity, Herman had told the doctor that he would never drink again.

Newberne told the commissioner of Indian affairs: "I believe him. His spirit is broken."[15]

12. The World Outside

R owley Johnson was troublesome, indeed—immediately after his epileptic seizures, he became confused and fought with anyone around him. For the good of the other patients and for his own protection, he spent much of his time in his room at Canton Asylum. Although most Indian families did not like to send loved ones to an asylum, they often found that it was the only viable course if the person became unmanageable or violent. Rowley's parents recognized that his condition made his care both time-consuming and physically draining, but they still wanted him home. They insisted that they were his guardians and ought to be able to have him released and, in the summer of 1920, pleaded with Klamath Agency superintendent Walter West to intercede on their behalf.

Johnson's mother was a determined woman. Besides offering to hire a full-time attendant for her son, she visited the agency's superintendent often enough that he finally wrote to the commissioner of Indian affairs about the case. As her letters and West's finally made their way through the bureaucracy, Hummer grew tired of Johnson's drain on his manpower. By the time he had a chance to weigh in on the issue, Hummer was ready to discharge Johnson.[1]

His staffing problems encouraged the decision—discharging a time-consuming patient would make way for an easier one from the backlog of applicants. Patient Susan Wishecoby, an epileptic who was otherwise well oriented and observant, seemed to feel this distinction very keenly. She wrote to Commissioner Sells in 1920 that "I don't think if I keep on trying to be good. the gooder we be the longer we stay. The ones who miss carry on they seem to be the ones who go home first."[2]

Hummer must have been shocked when the acting assistant commissioner, C. F. Hauke, rejected his recommendation to discharge Johnson. In a letter to West, Hauke mentioned Hummer's recommendation to let Johnson return to his family if they agreed to accept responsibility for his conduct, but he added that it was "a recommendation that the Office is not disposed to accept."[3] It seemed to Hauke that Johnson's was exactly the kind of case that required institutional care—not a return to the reservation.

Dismayed at the refusal or not, Hummer still got his way. Three months later, Hummer wrote the commissioner that Johnson was ill with pulmonary tuberculosis and feared likely to die. Hummer had written to Johnson's mother, inviting her to visit her son, and recommended that she be allowed to take him home.[4]

Allen Owl, a Cherokee admitted to Canton Asylum at the age of twenty-seven, felt the weight of Hummer's preference for less troublesome patients. Like Johnson's, his family also made frequent requests to have him returned home. Owl himself asked the commissioner for his release, stating that his health was fine.[5]

"He is about as well as he ever will be," Hummer told the commissioner in reply to an inquiry. "He has a good home here, is well taken care of, is well-behaved and trusted with parole privileges of the grounds and an occasional pass to town to the picture shows, in addition to which he was permitted to work with neighboring farmers this season, earning about one hundred and fifty or sixty dollars."

Hummer recommended against Owl's request to go home and hoped that the Indian Office would write Owl a "nice letter" to that effect. Hummer's concern was that Owl perhaps wouldn't do as well once he left the asylum. "I believe that it would be but a comparatively short time before there would be a return of more active symptoms which would necessitate his re-incarceration in an institution for the insane." Hummer got his way with this easier patient and kept Owl.[6]

He received few other challenges to his judgment or his authority. In fact, Hummer had received an additional measure of that authority in 1919, when the Indian Office told reservation superintendents to submit their requests for admission directly to Hummer rather than to the Indian Office. Hummer could unilaterally accept anyone whose legal eligibility and mental status gave him an opening to do so.[7]

Perhaps simply because he could, Hummer told a requesting agency in 1920 that he would accept eleven-year-old David Lovejoy, an epileptic who, the reservation doctor assured him, was otherwise in good health. Someone may have intervened, however, because Hummer indicated later that Lovejoy's application had not been acted upon. In 1922 he did accept six-year-old Amelia Moss, a Caddo child. These children may have represented "easy" patients to him, or he may have simply felt that their superintendents' recommendations were sufficient.

The notion that children this young could be insane was not merely a matter of convenience or cover for Hummer; it was an accepted fact among alienists. In a 1915 article in the *American Journal of Insanity*, "Insanity in Children," the author, John W. W. Rhein, noted that the literature included such studies as "a case of insane fury in an infant of 9 months of age" and that the author himself was currently treating seven cases of child insanity. Some cases of insanity in children originated from unexplained causes, but other cases were a result of infectious diseases like diphtheria, pertussis (whooping cough), and typhoid fever.

Hummer surely recognized that he wasn't going to swell his rolls with insane children. Instead, he had to cling to the patients he had and bring in as many others as possible. To do that, though, he had to have more buildings, and to get more buildings, he had to have more patients—it was the same old two-step that he had been dancing for years.

Hummer became increasingly reluctant to release patients, even though he had a myriad of employee problems that made managing the asylum supremely frustrating. At the end of March 1920, two male employees, William Juel and Louis Hewling, abruptly left the asylum after being turned in for sneaking into the female ward to talk to patients. Just a couple of months later, one of his female attendants, Hazel Lane, resigned and, upon leaving, loaded her trunk with supplies from the asylum.[8]

Hummer weathered the turmoil, but the situation could, and did, get worse. The ward attendants, who were always stretched thin, simply could not keep an eye on everyone all the time. Hummer had already revoked parole privileges for all females for a number of years to prevent any sexual contact between male and female patients. Nevertheless, Agnes Caldwell became pregnant and delivered a girl on March 26, 1921.[9]

Caldwell had been one of the females that the male ward attendants had visited the previous year.[10] According to both men, Caldwell, and her roommate, they had only talked through the keyhole of the women's locked door, though the women said upon further questioning that the men had once come into the room to talk.

Hummer had locked Caldwell in the female ward for several weeks after the incident but later allowed her to work in the hospital dining room. Employees (probably without Hummer's knowledge) also allowed her to help them with laundry work in the basement, undoubtedly so hard-pressed with their duties that they risked disobeying Hummer to allow Caldwell to work on her own. She and Allen Owl met in the basement about twice a week until he was discharged on October 26, 1920. Hummer told the commissioner that the ward attendants, Juel and Hewling, had left the facility too early for either of them to be the father of Caldwell's child; thus he deduced that it had to be Allen Owl.[11]

The pregnancy was not only an embarrassment for Hummer personally, as the asylum's superintendent, but it was also a failure on a higher level: a failure to prevent the procreation of defectives. Hummer's draconian solution to female pregnancy—denying all women parole privileges—spoke loudly about his feelings on the subject, which echoed those of other administrators in charge of Indian morals.[12]

Hummer was not outside the realm of mainstream thought in his desire to prevent patients from bearing children. Though many psychiatrists did not embrace his attitude—St. Elizabeths' superintendent, Dr. William White, emphatically denounced the sterilization of institutionalized patients—many lawmakers and ordinary Americans believed the country should vigorously protect its genetic stock. Thirty-three states eventually adopted eugenics-based laws, many of them calling for the sterilization of the insane. Oregon performed the last compulsory sterilization in 1981.

Hummer didn't perform sterilizations, but he still managed to fail his patients at a fundamental level. Hummer seldom displayed empathy with anyone, but he particularly lacked insight into his female patients' feelings. Their desire for relationships led him to label them as "nymphomaniacs" or as having a "weakness for men." Such labels made it easy for him to justify harsh measures that were a matter of convenience rather than treatment: denying parole privileges for all females condemned the guiltless on the grounds of infractions that had not yet been committed.

He never addressed the real issues driving what he considered "illicit" relationships between patients: loneliness, homesickness, and isolation. The human need for companionship was as great for Indians at Canton Asylum as it had been for them on the reservation. Try as he might, Hummer could not stop men and women from wanting to meet and become friends or lovers or from desiring more than the sometimes harsh words of an attendant.

Hummer never seemed to consider that many of his violent or quarrelsome patients likely acted out of frustration and anger rather than insanity, as they snapped under the pressures of asylum life. Unless his patients already spoke English, they were guaranteed isolation and misunderstanding after they arrived, from both attendants and other patients who could not speak their language. With so many tribes represented among a relatively small number of patients, finding someone to talk to and become friends with was a challenge for non-English speakers.

Of course, not all tribes were friendly toward each other, and traditional hostilities may have been a factor in some of the patients' fighting and aggressive behavior. Normal personality clashes, present in any group of people, were never sorted out among the Indian patients. Some patients may have considered themselves akin to prisoners of war and on principle refused to cooperate with attendants or other patients; trying to escape would have been a mandate for them, as well.

Because he did not understand Indian culture and wasn't sensitive to even white people's psychological needs, Hummer found it simple to assume that all his patients' negative behaviors resulted from insanity. That allowed him to take what measures he thought necessary to rein them in, without much concern for his patients' feelings.

Hummer casually condemned many of his patients to almost dungeon-like conditions because he would not get involved with his attendants and the care they gave. When Dr. Hardin created so many issues for Hummer back in 1909, one of his many complaints was that Hummer locked up nonviolent patients simply for convenience.

Hardin was appalled to find that patients were kept inside for months or years at a time. Hardin recognized one patient, Frank Starr, as a former pupil at the Indian school where he had worked. Because he had been locked up for so long, the boy had begun to lose his physical health. Hardin allowed him to go outside, and during Hummer's five-week absence, Starr gained sixteen pounds and worked daily.

Another patient, Baptiste Gingras, had spoken English, played ball, and engaged in other sports, but Hardin revealed in a deposition that he "has lost all his energies and will not in my opinion live but a few months on account of having been kept too closely housed."[13]

Fortunately for Hummer, ill-advised patient confinement did not typically draw the Indian Office's attention. Despite Caldwell's pregnancy and his pervasive employee problems, Hummer had just put in a couple of good years. Nothing had brought the superintendent to the special attention of the Indian Office, and any inspections he had were apparently routine. Hummer could not prevent thirteen of his staff from joining the National Federation of Federal Employees in January 1921, but he did have the opportunity to ensure some degree of loyalty by hiring his sons as laborers.[14] Hummer also brought his parents to live with him for a period, and Levi Hummer, born in 1848 and in his seventies, was on the payroll as a laborer in 1923.[15]

In 1919 Canton Asylum had finally received its precious hydrotherapy equipment. There are few patient notes available from the institution, so it is unclear what kind of hydrotherapy (if any) Hummer tried to use. Even if he had employed this new equipment extensively, it would have been about the only nod to modernity he could have managed. Regardless of his new buildings and other institutional improvements, except for the hydrotherapy, Hummer could offer little more than he had over the past ten years.

This was not entirely Hummer's fault. Alienists had continued to study and care for mentally ill patients but had generated few resounding breakthroughs. Phototherapy had its day around the turn of the twentieth century, and facilities like the Peoria State Hospital in Illinois flooded sun parlors with different-colored lights (blue, violet, amber, or opal) intended to match and somehow treat various psychoses. Leucodescent lamps with globes of various colors allowed attendants to administer these light sessions even at night. Not a resounding success, phototherapy had the advantage of being relatively inexpensive and harmless.[16]

In 1921 the American Medico-Psychological Association changed its name to the American Psychiatric Association and renamed its mouthpiece, the *American Journal of Insanity*, as the *American Journal of Psychiatry*. To avoid negative connotations, psychiatrists also moved away from terms like *asylum* and began to call their institutions hospitals. Still, recreational activities and occupational therapy of various kinds along with traditional sedatives, tonics, and antiseizure medications dominated as core treatments for mental patients. The first significant new psychotropic drug, chlorpromazine (Thorazine) wasn't FDA approved until 1954.[17]

Other professionals interested in mental illness were now competing with psychiatrists. Neurologists, who had been treating traumatic brain injuries since the Civil War and considered the brain's relationship to mental illness well within their scope of expertise, particularly disagreed with psychologically based theories on the origins of most mental illness.[18] They sought to connect insanity to physical roots and seemed vindicated by early treatments like the Bergonic chair. This device delivered electroshocks to soldiers who had been traumatized (shell-shocked) during World War I; however, electroconvulsive therapy for major depression did not develop in its present form until 1938.

Advances in the germ theory of disease and bacteriology led other medical men to ascribe the cause of mental illness to curable physical conditions. They would be proven correct for conditions like pellagra, a niacin deficiency created by the 3-M diet (fatback *m*eat, corn*m*eal, and *m*olasses) then prevalent in the South and poor rural areas. Pellagra's symptoms included confusion, memory loss, depression, mania, and hallucinations, which had led alienists to believe pellagra caused insanity. Public Health Service physician Joseph Goldberger investigated pellagra in 1914 as part of the service's research team and eventually found a preventative factor in dried yeast; in 1937 a chemist at the University of Wisconsin found the actual cure for pellagra to be nicotinic acid.[19]

Despite their deteriorating status as supreme experts, psychiatrists did make progress. They had previously focused on patients who exhibited the extremes of behavior that indicated acute or chronic insanity.

Doctors now considered *spectrums* of behavior, which ranged from what might be considered normal to various degrees of extremity.[20] (Mere eccentricity could now be accommodated by a spectrum system and life behavioral analysis.) Experts were also beginning to look at patients' life histories and behaviors so they could analyze current behaviors and perhaps intervene *before* a crisis occurred. This preventative interest led to outpatient treatment in offices and clinics rather than asylums and intrigued professionals who found treating chronic mental illness in institutions discouraging and unrewarding.

Sigmund Freud had initiated psychoanalysis in the late 1800s, but his "talking cure" didn't become popular in the United States until after World War I. Typically, only wealthy and well-educated people had the time and money to delve deeply into their subconscious this way. Such long-term, intensive treatment would have been hopeless at institutions, with only a few staff physicians spread among hundreds or thousands of patients. And even if Hummer had been inclined to try psychoanalysis, the method would have been impossible at an institution with nearly insurmountable language and cultural barriers.

Hummer bought the latest edition of White's *Outlines of Psychiatry* as well as books like *Epitome of Hydrotherapy, Principles of Mental Hygiene,* and *Nursing Mental Diseases,* but he did not have access to the amenities of larger hospitals. Canton Asylum was decades behind St. Elizabeths in every area—research, professional staffing, and medical capabilities—and would never have the money and attention that an institution for the care of the military in Washington DC could command.

St. Elizabeths had been on the forefront of forensic psychiatry when Superintendent William Godding hired neuropathologist Dr. Isaac. W. Blackburn in 1884. Godding created the first pathology laboratory in a U.S. mental hospital, while Dr. William White later created the first psychotherapy department in a mental hospital in 1907. In 1919 St. Elizabeths was the first psychiatric hospital in the United States to use pets as part of therapy. The facility included a training school for nurses, gave instruction courses for students of the army and navy medical schools (as well as George Washington, Georgetown, and Howard Universities), and provided lecturers for welfare groups and other organizations. And it had used hydrotherapy since the 1880s.[21]

The luxurious McLean Asylum in Massachusetts had established a training school for nurses in 1882 and established pathological and biochemistry laboratories before the turn of the century.

Some medical hospitals had begun attaching reception centers for the insane to their main buildings to house patients during the commitment process. These reception centers later developed into psychopathic hospitals that treated only acute cases of insanity or specialized in only certain disorders. Doctors tried innovative treatments and published their results. Institutions that couldn't keep up with new strategies for patient care and asylum management often became custodial in nature, warehousing patients rather than treating and curing them. Canton Asylum had already fallen into this category.

Hummer's real problem lay in that he wasn't doing what he *was* able to do. Literature of the period emphasized accurate and detailed record keeping on patients, and as always, asylums across the country presented extremes of compliance. Several demonstrated best practices, though many others offered more mainstream and realistic efforts. The private Channing Sanitarium in Brookline, Massachusetts, accommodated twenty-five patients with a staff of two physicians and thirty nurses, as well as a clerk to type records. The much larger state hospital in Clarinda, Iowa had a patient population of around one thousand but still had a purposeful records program. Patients remained in bed the first few days after admission so that staff could get to know them, and they contacted friends, colleagues, or other persons for additional information about patients if their records were incomplete at admission. The Peoria State Hospital, burdened with more than two thousand patients, held a staff meeting every morning at which a case history was presented, discussed, and the patient reexamined, giving at least one patient each day the in-depth care that the institution's size made impossible for all.[22]

Paradoxically, as documentation became an increasingly important tool for case management, Hummer's efforts in this area went steadily downhill. He had once modeled his record keeping on St. Elizabeths' standards, but in later years a lackadaisical approach toward exams and patient records earned him constant criticism. No one at the Indian Office ever offered a consequence for his neglect.

In 1911 Hummer processed Lucy Gladstone (also known as Lillian

Gladstone), a thirty-seven-year-old manic-depressive from the Flathead Reservation in Montana, as a patient. Hummer gave her a physical exam and wrote short, but comprehensive, notes about her condition. He diagnosed her mental condition on a second, detailed exam sheet.

Though it probably wasn't a typical part of his psychiatric exam, Hummer asked Gladstone to write a family history. The five-page result was a clear rendering of a life marred by ill health, marriage at eighteen to a morphine-addicted husband who habitually threatened her life, poverty, and hopelessness. After years of stressful marriage, her husband aimed a gun at her and their baby. The gun jammed, and he stormed away. Gladstone went to an aunt and returned to her husband as he lay on his deathbed. He died refusing to speak to her.

Gladstone worked while she raised her three children, but she had to send her two oldest ones to school while she kept the baby. In her words, "times were hard, and wages were low." She lived with a man for all of three months before he was arrested for murder, but her bad luck continued and she found herself pregnant. The baby died after two years, and Gladstone left home again. It was after that, she said, "that all the trouble started."

She married a jealous man who made her afraid to speak to anyone, and Gladstone ended up so nervous and frightened that when she became pregnant, she drank oil of hemlock to abort the child. She worked in a logging camp while her husband drank up his own wages, and eventually rumors began to make their way around town, to her detriment. She began to "take spells" that left her fainting and exhausted and unable to work anywhere.

Gladstone went to a former employer and asked for some carbolic acid. She tucked the bottle under her pillow and spent the night thinking over her past life and troubles. In the morning, she swallowed the acid. Five minutes later she felt like she was strangling and then knew nothing until she woke up in her brother's home. After sixteen days of bed rest, she was committed to Canton Asylum.

Hummer's original diagnosis for Gladstone was manic depression with hysterical symptoms, and he attributed her attacks to some emotional event she had previously experienced.[23] He maintained short, but reasonably comprehensive, monthly reports on her state of mind and physical health. He wrote in April 1911 that Gladstone conversed intelligently and assisted in the sewing room and with laundry work. In May she was depressed for a short period after receiving some letters from home but had stopped having seizures.

Throughout the next few months, Hummer's case notes indicated that Gladstone was occasionally depressed but was not delusional or demented. He also noted that Gladstone was neat and tidy and caused no trouble—attributes that he came to cherish in his patients. She was very likely helped by the change in her environment, and Hummer considered her recovery complete by August of that year. He released her without qualms to the care of her brother, confident enough of her recovery to send her there unescorted.[24]

Less than twenty years later, Hummer had formally ceased to even make monthly patient reports to reservation superintendents, though he maintained that he included weekly progress reports in patient files. The notes that are available are terse and sketchy and usually change little in wording. Rather than Hummer, the asylum's attendants made them.

Dynamic psychiatry required the study of a patient's life history, and Hummer didn't have the time or ability—or apparently even the desire—to gather accurate and detailed information about his patients. He couldn't be expected to speak their many languages, but Hummer didn't seem to make an effort to enhance the scanty information he often received, or even to ask the Indian Office for the occasional interpreter for an alert and responsive patient. He did not review the records that he had and either correct or change diagnoses, even when they conflicted with behaviors he discussed with the Indian Office.

Hummer sometimes expressed frustration when he couldn't attend an important medical conference, but otherwise he appeared comfortable with his books and periodicals and occasional interactions with the medical men in the Indian Service. Canton Asylum had lost any edge it ever had, though, and had become little more than a warehouse.

Shrugging off these considerations, Hummer began 1921 with a new commissioner of Indian affairs, Charles H. Burke. Author of the Burke Act, the new commissioner was a strong proponent of both assimilation and a paternal government policy toward Indians. The act he wrote (as an amendment to the Dawes Act) attempted to both protect Indians from unscrupulous whites while simultaneously pushing them into white society. The act prevented Indians who received land allotments from becoming citizens for twenty-five years, which kept them under at least nominal government protection. At the same time, the act gave the secretary of the interior the authority to decide Indian competency and release allotments early.[25]

Hummer never let an opportunity slip by and, soon after Burke took office, wrote to him about a matter "very near my heart." It was expansion, of course; Hummer called his "little plant" entirely inadequate. Hummer needed several new buildings, more dairy cows, more acreage to grow grain for the cows, and more room for the patients he had to regularly turn away. "Will you not, in the spirit of humanity, give some consideration to the proposition of securing additional land for us," Hummer wrote.

After explaining that state institutions wouldn't take insane Indians and that he could provide them with the best possible care, Hummer ended with the exhortation "but I also believe that if you make a plea to Congress for us . . . that your conscience will mark this act as one of the best of your administration."[26]

Commissioner Burke made it clear that he did not want to expand the asylum, though he did ask Hummer to present any information he had to support his assertions that Indian patients were being turned away at state institutions. More ominously, he wanted to know the status of Hummer's patients, including information about their tribal relationships, enrollment, and allotments. Even worse, he asked Hummer which patients could be returned to their homes "with a reasonable degree of safety and of those who may be committed to State Institutions."[27]

Hummer must have sucked in his breath at this point—it was not hard to see where Burke's inquiries were headed. Hummer had only ninety-two patients—far too few to his mind—and he had no desire to go backward.[28] He was finally realizing the results of many years' worth of cajoling: new buildings, a hospital, modern equipment, and a private cottage for his family. Hummer even had his much-requested moving picture equipment, though without an amusement hall, he had to show movies in the dining room. (These were usually slapstick comedies or movies in which Indians appeared.) He had managed to raise enough pigs to be able to cut his beef bill in half and had squirreled away $2,000 in his supply fund to return to the government.[29]

No matter what he did, though, he could not reign in his per capita costs: $405 per patient.

Hummer doggedly set about trying to save his institution. Statistics seemed to be on his side, if he could somehow use them effectively. Between 1910 and 1918, the number of insane men and women in U.S. institutions had risen from 187,791 to 239,820—an increase of nearly 28 percent, though the population as a whole had increased only by about 14 percent.[30]

The Indian population in the United States (exclusive of Alaska) was 336,337 in 1920.[31] Surely there had to be hundreds of insane Indians who could come to Canton Asylum. The commissioner of Indian affairs had reported only 102 insane Indians in the United States in 1910, but Hummer either didn't think those figures were correct or thought that "civilizing" Indians over the past decade had resulted in many new cases. He was determined to drum up all the business he could, and in June Hummer wrote to various reservation and school superintendents in order to gather his own statistics.

He began, "The management of this institution, believing the same is not fulfilling its entire function because it is not caring for *all* of the insane Indians in the United States, has prepared a tentative program of expansion." Hummer then asked the superintendents for a count of their patients needing care at his asylum.[32]

Hummer did not receive the flood of names he undoubtedly expected. The Turtle Mountain School offered him a sixteen-year-old who had been deserted by her husband and was now followed by "worthless boys" (no mention of mental problems); a twenty-year-old woman who already had three illegitimate children and was in a state institution; an eleven-year-old boy with violent spells; a partially paralyzed, troublesome woman; and a seventeen-year-old with an illegitimate three-year-old child. The agency superintendent pronounced this young woman "feeble-minded" and a nuisance.

Other agencies were even less helpful. The superintendent of Southern Pueblos Indian Agency in Albuquerque, New Mexico, told Hummer that the Pueblo Indians "for the most part are adverse to the removal from their villages of Indians suffering from the various phases of incompetency" and that there were no insane Indians on the reservation.[33]

Another agency had three names for him, stating that the Indians were not insane but merely feebleminded and not competent to earn their own living. Another also offered up its imbeciles, along with an epileptic and a "deaf and dumb" man.

The superintendents' responses were undoubtedly frustrating, but nothing could be worse than the next blow from Burke. In August the commissioner told Hummer to transfer all patients who were not actual wards of the government to the appropriate state institutions. These non-wards were Indians who either were not under the allotment system or who were citizens of a state. Hummer was dismayed—he needed his patient count to go up, not down. However, a light touch of agreement and compliance had always worked well in the past, and Hummer graciously accepted Burke's request while he looked for maneuvering room elsewhere.

In reality, Burke had dealt Hummer a setback rather than a death blow—Hummer otherwise remained in a relatively safe spot. Muckrakers were exposing Standard Oil's corruption, the tragedy of coal mining conditions, and the fraud in patent medicines, but they were not looking at the plight of Indians in insane asylums. If Hummer could keep on Burke's good side, he was sure to weather any tentative challenges to his desires for the asylum.

Despite their lack of attention to Canton Asylum specifically, social progressives *were* looking toward groups of people that the general public usually ignored, and that included Indians. As money dried up to support the People's Institute in New York, for instance, social workers and other progressives like John Collier did not simply wither away.

From a solidly upper-middle-class background, Collier had rejected the pursuit of financial and social success after seeing his parents destroyed by it. His father became involved in a financial scandal that led to his suicide; his mother had become addicted to laudanum after the scandal and died from the complications of her addiction. As a young man, Collier found healing in the outdoors and in wilderness areas. In rejecting typical American success, he began to lean toward idealistic socialism, in which communities helped each other and worked through cooperation and reciprocity. When he later became acquainted with Native American societies, Collier found much to admire.[34]

Collier eventually moved from New York to California and began work in adult education for immigrants. Still naïve or exceptionally bold, Collier began to lecture in circuit tours between Los Angeles, Fresno, Berkeley, and San Francisco to discuss significant contemporary issues. The issues under consideration touched on community action and public policy, and during these days of the Red Scare, his well-attended discussions soon brought him to the attention of federal authorities. The Justice Department lobbied through the Better America Federation of California to have the appropriation for Collier's program cancelled.

He received an invitation from an old New York friend, Mabel Dodge, to join her at Taos Pueblo, New Mexico, where she lived with her Indian husband, Antonio Luhan. Collier packed up his wife and children and went to stay there a while in December 1921. He was shocked and appalled at the living conditions he found among Indians as he worked and studied in the area and, when he later returned to California to teach, kept those memories close to his consciousness.

In 1922 President Warren G. Harding's corrupt interior secretary, Albert B. Fall, proposed to take sixty thousand acres of land from the New Mexico Pueblos without adequate compensation, through the Bursum Bill. Introduced by New Mexico senator Holm O. Bursum, the bill proposed to allow the land claims that non-Indians who had settled on Pueblo land were requesting, as well as to divert Indian water rights. Collier was dismayed when Stella Atwood, a powerful member of the General Federation of Women's Clubs and chairman of its Division of Indian Welfare, notified him about the pending legislation. Both were solidly opposed to the measure.

Collier, as well as others, had begun to believe that if Indians were going to be able to retain their ethnic identities and preserve their way of life and traditions, their land would have to be protected. The Bursum Bill would force the Pueblos to prove their land titles—a mishmash of old treaties and Spanish and Mexican land grants that were now obscure or never recorded and of arrangements that gave unreasonable protection to people who had purchased or squatted on Pueblo land.

Pueblo land titles were a vastly complicated affair at this time, since they had owned their land independently after the Treaty of Guadalupe in 1848 and the Supreme Court had ruled in 1876 that they were not wards of the government. Some non-Indians bought land that both parties thought the Pueblos were free to sell, while many squatters simply moved in to claim land by encroachment.

When New Mexico became a state, however, the federal protector-ward relationship came up: if Indians in New Mexico were not considered federal wards, then the state would enter the Union under different conditions than other states. The United States regained its jurisdiction over the Pueblo Indians in the 1912 Sandoval case, concerning the sale of liquor in two pueblos. In 1913 the Pueblos were officially declared wards of the federal government, and all non-Indian Pueblo land titles came into dispute. The actual amount of land under question was about a tenth of what the Pueblos owned, but it was valuable irrigated land that whites badly wanted. Other provisions of the Bursum Bill also affected the Pueblos adversely, but the near-automatic transfer of disputed Indian land into non-Indian hands remained the greatest issue.

Under the Bursum Bill, Anglo and Spanish settlers would receive actual title to Pueblo land if they could prove continuous possession of the land before or after 1848 and had some sort of written documentation—regular, irregular, disputed, nonregistered, and so on—for it. Additionally, anyone who could prove continuous possession of Pueblo land since June 29, 1910—even without documentation—could claim title to it. (This group would include squatters.) Those who couldn't manage to claim land under these provisions could appeal to the courts or to the Department of the Interior for a favorable special ruling—which, under Fall, they were likely to get.[35]

Collier and other progressives decided to take on the Harding administration. It was a fool's fight, of course, but a friend arranged financing for Collier to leave his job and organize a defense for the Indians. A superintendent at the Indian Bureau's Espanola, New Mexico, office gave Collier a copy of the Bursum Bill, which almost no Indians in New Mexico even knew existed.[36] Collier went back to Taos Pueblo and, with Antonio Luhan, informed all the Pueblos from Taos to Zuni about it. The Pueblos organized and took their case to Washington.

Collier and seventeen Pueblo representatives—with little power and money to sustain the fight—started off on a journey to raise consciousness about the bill and whip up opposition to it. Collier apparently donated seven thousand dollars he had received from the sale of his house to the cause and gathered both money and momentum from sympathetic supporters as he and the delegates crossed the country. His friend Stella Atwood rallied the nearly two million women of the General Federation of Women's Clubs to help lobby against the bill. She and Collier persuaded periodicals like *Sunset Magazine* to give them a mouthpiece for the Pueblos; its editors also distributed articles about the Bursum Bill to Congress. By the time the two friends and their fellow activists were through, over one hundred newspapers and periodicals had given them favorable publicity concerning the bill and their protest against it.

Commissioner Burke decried Collier's and Atwood's efforts, saying that it was like "going to a lot of children to stir them up." In his opinion (he supported the Bursum Bill) there was nothing wrong with what the bill proposed. "Propagandists are touring part of the country with a company of dancing and singing Pueblos in full Indian regalia, in order to awaken people to the 'crime' in New Mexico. There is no crime in New Mexico," he said.[37]

In 1923 Collier and the Pueblos representatives finally ended up in Washington DC before the House Committee on Indian Affairs. There Collier took the witness stand, testifying with information taken from two confidential Indian Bureau reports that had been given to him by the bureau's farm agent in Espanola.[38] The reports showed that the per capita income of the Tesuque (Pueblo) people was $14.66, including the farm goods and livestock they raised and consumed. Indians testified—old men who were poor and had never been in front of such an audience—and they deeply affected the congressmen attending the hearings. Collier and his cohort had already garnered a groundswell of popular sympathy.

During testimony, the Fall-appointed government attorney for the Pueblos, Colonel R. E. Twitchell, admitted that the Bursum Bill did not favor Indians. Fall refused to discuss the bill and instead attacked its opponents, saying that propagandists had twisted his words and misled the public about it. Though the bill and alternative versions remained active for several more months, the Bursum Bill was eventually killed in the House. In Collier's account of that fight, he said that Senator Bursum's rage was huge. "We all went to see him, the Indians and I, and he was shaking with humiliation and rage—at us."[39]

Burke had to be similarly outraged by the efforts of a vocal group of muckrakers gaining steam during the early 1920s. Empowered by his recent victory over the Bursum Bill and passionately dedicated to helping Indians retain their cultures, John Collier attracted various Indian interest groups that were willing to work with him despite some of their philosophical differences.

Collier and a number of other progressives, like Harold Ickes and Hamlin Garland, founded the American Indian Defense Association in 1923, with Collier functioning as its executive secretary. The organization was praised by supporters of Indian rights and dismissed as a bunch of romantic do-gooders by others. Despite his critics, Collier's energy got results. He formed a team of lobbyists who regularly pushed Congress to recognize Indian culture and tribal organizations. In 1925 Collier became editor of *American Indian Life*, a newsletter that kept Indian concerns in front of the public.

The rhetoric from this increasingly active band of Indian-rights supporters was shaming and inflammatory, and it spilled beyond the confines of niche publications. Besides articles with titles like "The Red Slaves of Oklahoma" and "The Accursed System," which appeared in *American Indian Life*, Collier and others wrote in national magazines like *Sunset Magazine*, *Current History*, and the *Forum*. The writers didn't mince words, calling the government's treatment of Indians a disgrace, legalized robbery, and shameless. For the first time, dissenters focused on the Indian Office as an entity, rather than pointing out one particular corrupt or incompetent individual. The Indian Office's usual method of pushing out a particular disgraced employee and moving on was losing its effectiveness, though public and even congressional backlash seemed equally ineffective to actually change the department's methods.

These increasingly strident challenges to Indian policy did not affect life at Canton Asylum, which continued to roll along with its usual ups and downs. Hummer discharged several patients under Burke's directive, finding that some of them had recovered quite nicely.[40] However, Hummer had already waited out several commissioners and knew that Burke would probably decrease his scrutiny if nothing untoward occurred at the asylum. He didn't challenge Burke, who philosophically was in his camp, and his correspondence to the Indian Office continued in his usual gentlemanly language.

Burke didn't stop Hummer from taking in a few patients, and Hummer did so without discrimination. He relied on Rosebud superintendent James McGregor's assessment of James Black Bull ("it is plain for anyone to see by just looking at him that he is not sane") for one diagnosis.[41] Another superintendent, C. H. Gensler of Lac du Flambeau, wrote to Hummer about Edith Schroder: "We have a feeble minded woman here aged about 29 years who is having a baby every year. We must get rid of her as she is a nuisance and a menace to society. She was married at one time but is now divorced. The man was forced to marry her. She has babies just the same whether married or not."[42]

Schroder was packed off to Canton. When a man named B. Fitzgerald protested that a woman with a nursing baby should not have been sent to an insane asylum without an examination or court hearing, Meritt pointed out that Schroder was not committed to Canton Asylum because she was insane, but because she was feebleminded.[43] "The Office believes that if you are a true friend of this woman you will be glad that she is now in a place where she will be protected," Meritt finished.

Meritt's name is on much of the correspondence and reports concerning Canton Asylum at this time, and he had obviously changed his stance on the relative expense of housing patients at the federal asylum versus state institutions. His position in 1916 that Canton Asylum was a drain because state asylums charged only $20 a month (for a per capita cost of $240 annually) had reversed to a belief that Canton Asylum was far cheaper than state institutions.

World War I had changed everything. St. Elizabeths had reached a peak per capita cost of fifty dollars per month during the war, double its prewar rate of from twenty to twenty-five dollars per month. With thirty-seven hundred patients, the hospital couldn't farm enough land to keep expenses down. In this respect, Canton Asylum was in a better position, with its significantly lower population and proportionally greater acreage. Other institutions, in New York and Massachusetts, were struggling with greatly increased costs as well, and Canton Asylum now looked almost like a bargain.[44]

In hearings before a subcommittee of the House Committee on Appropriations in 1922, Meritt told Chairman Louis C. Cramton that Canton Asylum was very efficient.[45] The average cost per year for everything—employees, transportation, hospitalization, burials, upkeep of the buildings, and so on—came to a little less than $400 for each patient.[46] The costs at state hospitals, in contrast, ranged from $480 to $600, exclusive of transportation, clothing, and burial expenses. Meritt's new insight undoubtedly influenced Commissioner Burke, who now allowed Hummer the same free rein with patients as had his predecessors.[47]

Things were looking up for Hummer. Friendly Dr. Newberne, who seldom found anything amiss at Canton Asylum, urged the construction of an epileptic cottage in his July 1922 report. His next words were music to Hummer's ears: "If all the imbecilic and epileptic patients that ought to be in custody were hospitalized, room would be needed at this asylum for 500–600 more patients." He continued, "The asylum is a modern psychopathic institution which the Indian Service may 'point with pride.'"[48]

Hummer was once again comfortable in "placing the matter entirely in your hands," when it came to recommending discharges to the commissioner. He no longer received challenges to his judgment, and when patient Frances Espinoza begged for her release, she was met with a united front. In her letter to Burke, Espinoza complained of fighting with another patient because of the other's lack of manners. She wanted some money she was apparently owed, so that she could get out and go home. If she couldn't, she told him, she would "be in the next world."

A friend of Espinoza's, A. R. Manby, wrote to Hummer on her behalf, explaining that Frances had made two enemies on her home reservation. She had evidently seen something there and spoken about it, and "his people used their influence to take her out of his country," according to the writer.

If Manby's statement was true, Frances's fear and aggressiveness, though natural under the increased stress of confinement, would tell against her. Hummer told the commissioner that "paranoia is the most dangerous form of mental affliction" and that great harm might result if Espinoza were discharged.

Espinoza wrote to Burke again, telling him how much she hated the asylum. She hated the nurses and employees, saying that from what she knew, the place "might be a red light house." Espinoza added, "The meals are very poor, half cook. They feed us just like pigs on roots."

Hummer forwarded Espinoza's rant with a short note that said, "This should give you a fair idea of the workings of this girl's mind."[49]

Still on a winning streak, Hummer received another inspection. Though not quite on par with Newberne's report, the visit from the chairman of the Board of Indian Commissioners, George Vaux Jr., to the "shire town of Canton" was still extremely gratifying. Vaux found it "touching to observe the devotion" that some of the patients displayed toward others with different afflictions. Few patients were violent. Now and then some had to be kept locked up in a protected room, but in the main they "were not difficult to control." This is in contrast to Hummer's statement to a reporter for the *Sioux Valley News* that "the patients do fight a good deal" and that the women were worse than the men because "they picked up anything handy and hit without a thought of the consequences."[50]

It is a tribute to Hummer's skill at positive spin that Vaux's inspection went well, because it could have been disastrous. For years, Hummer had been trying to get more land so he could increase his livestock holdings and save expenses, but his requests had fallen on deaf ears. When Vaux visited, Hummer allowed his cows to graze on the asylum's front lawn and along the roadside, citing lack of acreage to grow grain and provide adequate pasture for the cows. Vaux was suitably shocked, and he wrote to the commissioner that Hummer should be authorized immediately to improve his herd quality by purchasing Holsteins. And, just as Hummer wanted, Vaux recommended additional farmland as the institution's top priority.

Vaux pointed out that, in addition to the savings Hummer realized with his livestock program, Hummer saved the asylum a great deal of money by having the inmates do all the house and farm work. He also saw that Hummer was a great believer in getting patients out of doors in good weather and, as a result, most patients, "given the type of patients under consideration," were in good health. Cheerfulness reigned everywhere, Vaux said. Lacking a medical background, the chairman could only parrot Hummer's version of the asylum's condition.

Vaux undoubtedly took Hummer's rose-colored version of asylum life at face value. But the grounds probably did look inviting in the pleasant June weather, and Vaux probably did see patients enjoying themselves on the playground equipment Hummer had procured. They could exercise on the sturdy swings, merry-go-round, slides, and turning bars, stroll the grounds if allowed some sort of parole, or sit and rest in the settees and lawn chairs that typically dotted the lawn. Trusted patients like Susan Wishecoby and John Brown could go into town to enjoy themselves or take automobile rides with the staff.

Men and women alike had allowances for tobacco, which they smoked with relish, though men seemed to employ smoking as a pastime more than the women. Female patients often engaged in stringing together bead necklaces, making handbags with beading, and weaving baskets from strong grasses to sell to visitors as souvenirs. A few men might whittle wooden items as souvenirs, but they didn't seem to engage in crafts as much as the women did. Indoors, pool and billiard tables provided amusement.

Though Vaux had not visited any state or county hospitals, he didn't believe Indians could receive better care in them than they could at Canton Asylum. Hummer had recently purchased $1,500 worth of hydrotherapy equipment and added an operating room and a sleeping porch to the hospital. He had increased his livestock to twenty cows and eighty-three pigs—cost-saving measures that reduced his need for government funds for subsistence. Vaux's visit fortunately occurred before hog cholera wiped out Hummer's pigs in September.

Vaux was clearly in Hummer's corner. He recommended funding for an epileptic cottage, amusement hall, and central heating and lighting plant—all projects Hummer badly wanted. Among Vaux's many other suggestions was one to purchase gravestones for deceased patients. "There is no excuse imaginable," Vaux said, "that would justify the failure to put up a simple inscribed marker at each grave."[51]

Unfortunately, Vaux received as little sympathy for this suggestion as Hummer and Gifford had. The graves remained unmarked.

13. Hummer Can't Keep Up

America was dancing to its own mad tune during the heady Roaring Twenties. Though the Volstead Act had served up a dry glass of Prohibition, the nation's citizens instead developed an unquenchable thirst for speakeasies and illicit booze. Al Capone flourished, F. Scott Fitzgerald wrote *The Great Gatsby*, and even shoeshine boys had money to invest on margin in the stock market. Americans could buy a Model T for $299 in 1924, though radios were still pricy at $50 to $100. Flappers danced the Charleston, listened to jazz, and wore dresses with hemlines that almost showed their knees. Men sat on flagpoles, carried hip flasks, and sang "Yes, We Have No Bananas." Everyone, it seemed, was having a blast.

The operative word was *seemed*. Groups of forgotten people—blacks in the cities, poor whites in the Appalachians, and sharecroppers of both races—couldn't manage to climb on board the party wagon. Canton Asylum residents might watch a movie once a week, but it was a meager tidbit of entertainment in a bleak life. Good times, not social causes, were on the agenda, and the little guy had to fight for himself. Excepting a few determined individuals, concern about the plight of Native Americans seemed to be a particularly distant afterthought—especially for their guardians.

Certainly President Warren Harding's secretary of the interior, Albert Fall, cared nothing for his department's mandates to conserve natural resources and (through the Indian Office) to protect the country's Indian wards. Fall had received his post as a reward for helping Harding win the 1921 presidential election. Under his leadership the Interior Department became an indifferent champion of anything, let alone Indian rights or welfare. Passionate articles and an isolated victory like that of the Pueblos over the Bursum Bill rattled few cages there or in the Indian Office.

Though Hummer's desire for power was on a petty enough scale compared to the corruption of his superiors, he was a good fit with the Interior Department and its supervisors, who looked either to their own interests or to outdated social policy to guide them. Hummer thrived on the lack of oversight afforded by his distance from Washington, and he usually managed to swat away unfavorable inspection comments like pesky flies.

Hummer continued to present an erudite face to the world, managing to hold his own as an expert on the workings of the Indian mind. During a 1923 controversy about peyote use during religious ceremonies, Commissioner Burke turned to Hummer, as the bureau's Indian psychiatrist, for illumination. Hummer was unable to enlighten the commissioner on the topic beyond a description of peyote's effects but weighed in with his opinion that "if we are only capable of properly evaluating religion when under the influence of such a drug, then we had better be without religion."[1]

Though he could not attend symposiums and conferences, Hummer kept up-to-date with medical knowledge by buying books and journals. His failure to implement new or better practices resulted from his managerial style and decisions rather than lack of information. By 1931, Hummer reported to the American Medical Association's survey of mental institutions that he didn't have staff meetings, had no systematic psychotherapy, did not conduct research, and gave no training to nurses or attendants or for any kind of therapy (like the hydrotherapy he said he used).

Hummer conducted only urinalysis for patients, didn't engage patients in any kind of diversion or occupational therapy, held no dances or theatrical shows, and had no patient library. He was ready to read about psychiatry but apparently grew less and less willing to actively practice it. He was also comparatively silent about the asylum's hospital—a building he had championed for years. Presumably he treated his most gravely ill patients there, but nowhere did he specifically say he performed surgery or treated patients in a way he couldn't have treated them without the benefit of a hospital building.

Hummer's lack of active involvement in either psychiatry or medicine makes his possession of a trephining kit all the more odd and disturbing. Trephination is a procedure that uses a cylindrical, saw-like instrument to drill a hole in a patient's head. The seriousness of the surgery makes it extremely unlikely that Hummer's predecessor, Dr. Turner, had ordered it, since Turner had no hospital facilities during his time of service. It is equally unlikely that the arrogant Hummer would have kept a useless piece of equipment favored by a perpetual thorn in his side like Turner for a couple of decades.[2]

In ancient times trephination may have been used to release evil spirits or in an attempt to alleviate symptoms associated with the skull and brain, like convulsions or headaches. It is used today to relieve subdural hematoma, a collection of blood under the skull (but outside the brain) that occurs most frequently with head trauma. Doctors make a trephining hole in order to suction out the blood and relieve pressure on the brain, which can otherwise be life threatening to a patient.

Hummer did not likely foresee too many life-threating brain traumas requiring trephination in his patients, so the question is why he ordered a trephining kit. Hummer would have been exposed to the practice during his time at St. Elizabeths: records show that between 1905 and 1908 at least three trephinations had been performed for reasons like treating a "cortical hermorrhage [sic]," a cerebral cyst, and localized meningitis. However, St. Elizabeths housed skilled surgeons and a large hospital, which the Canton Asylum did not.

Around the time of Hummer's arrival at the asylum, a certain amount of investigation into trephination to relieve epilepsy had begun. A 1904 article in the *Boston Medical and Surgical Journal* discussed eleven cases where the procedure had been tried. The doctor who reported on these cases, John C. Munro, was not terribly enthusiastic about the practice, saying, "I know of no more discouraging field for the surgeon than trephining for epilepsy."

He did go on to offer a bit of hope, saying, "I cannot but feel instinctively that there is a small class of unfortunates suffering this disease which can be helped, probably in a way at present unexplainable." Munro urged a larger study with comparative data on what types of patients benefited from the treatment. He speculated that patients who could potentially find relief would be those who had lesions in the "viscera and other organs" that had contributed to or caused their convulsions.

With no more encouragement than that, Hummer made quite a leap to acquire a trephination kit if he planned to perform the procedure to relieve epilepsy. Since he made no mention of such surgery, he may have had second thoughts and never used his kit. But Hummer considered epileptics his most troublesome patients. Later medical inspections show that he overdiagnosed epilepsy, and other documents underscore that it was clearly a condition Hummer focused on. Could he have performed trephining secretly or experimented on some of his epileptic patients? Could he have used the kit for something else entirely? A trephining kit was removed from the Canton Asylum for Insane Indians when it closed—that is all anyone knows at this point.

In only one respect did Hummer appear to be a step ahead of some of his peers, and that step was actually beyond his control. The *American Journal of Insanity* had applauded St. Elizabeths' ratio of physicians to patients (1:133) in a tribute to Dr. White's twenty-fifth year of tenure there, but Hummer's ratio was lower at roughly 1:90. Of course, he couldn't match St. Elizabeths' eleven-thousand-volume library, nursing department, and training clinics. He also couldn't parlay his patient-to-physician ratio into above-average care.

However, Hummer's paper at the 1912 American Medico-Psychological Association had given him a veneer of expertise, and he still tried hard to exploit it. Early on, Hummer had thrown open Canton Asylum's doors to the public in an effort to drum up publicity and, hopefully, prestige for his work. He continued this practice through the years despite the paucity of professional credit he got from it.

The Canton Chamber of Commerce joined Hummer's publicity efforts, and at some point, tourists could actually purchase Canton Asylum souvenir items well beyond Indian beadwork. Postcards featuring the asylum were available at any town drugstore, and though there seems to be no surviving official documentation about their origin, commemorative plates, spoons, teacups, and similar items with Canton Asylum's picture were available for purchase.[3] Presumably, the city and the asylum made money from these purchases.

The odd tourist or two were always welcome, but newspaper reporters were especially so. Their articles typically mentioned the uniqueness of the asylum and its patients before moving on to discuss the asylum's history, its beautiful grounds, and Hummer's wonderful care. Many times, writers added interest to their pieces by focusing on patients who were particularly colorful or peculiar in their eyes: "Wahbesheshequay is one of the Indian patients, and foremost among the most audacious to greet visitors at the institution. She is short and fat, and as jolly as one of this type would imply. . . . She has the toddle and shimmy and several other of the more Americanized dances in her repertoire, and every male visitor passing through the corridor to the women's ward becomes a noble chieftain to her, capable beyond all protests and excuses of making an ideal dancing partner."[4]

Besides describing male patients in ribbed corduroy suits and women making their own dresses, the writer told about a patient, Luke Stands By Him, who thought he was the owner of a farm with sixteen hundred white elephants on it. Other writers described patients like a Choctaw girl who told visitors about her experiences scrubbing floors for George Washington and Abraham Lincoln. Some patients may have been oblivious to a lone reporter touring the facility, but others were surely uncomfortable when groups of curious outsiders came to gawk at them as though they were exhibits.

Schools found insane Indians interesting on a number of fronts. Sociology, home economics, civics, and democracy classes frequently asked for permission to tour the asylum, and students often wrote to Hummer to gather information for class reports. Even children young enough to require their parents' accompaniment passed through the asylum. Occasionally Hummer received a request from medical school faculty to allow their students to see the patients; Hummer tried to personally guide these tours. For all others, he wrote a standard note of reply that visiting hours were from 1:00 to 5:00 p.m., Wednesdays and Fridays. The superintendent never lost his ardor for publicity and personal prestige, but Canton Asylum remained a small institution with a narrow field of study for its activities despite his best efforts.

Disappointed perhaps at the lack of personal and institutional renown, Hummer at least was the asylum's master. He diligently guarded his power and authority both *at* and *over* the institution with an effective combination of passive-aggressive tactics that usually defeated anything that challenged him. In August 1921, patient Susan Wishecoby wrote a long letter to the commissioner of Indian affairs explaining her homesickness and the way she felt she had been tricked into entering the asylum: "I certainly set down for a few moments before I go to bed and think of the days that has passed when I was at home. Mrs. Marbles was the one who got me to make up my mind to come out here. That wasn't fair of her to do. . . . If I would of known I was coming to an asylum I couldn't of come at all. But Mrs. Marbles said I was coming to a hospital."[5]

Wishecoby's other primary complaint was the amount of unpaid work she had to do at the asylum. Besides caring for their own rooms, able-bodied patients scrubbed the asylum's wooden floors with hard well water (which even male inspectors noted made them difficult to keep clean), did laundry, helped in the kitchen, and assisted with farming chores. None of these tasks was simply busywork to keep patients occupied—it was hard physical labor that also served the institution. In Hummer's efforts to keep operating costs down, he found unpaid patient labor an excellent resource.

The commissioner's office routinely forwarded patient communications to Hummer for his reply, and Hummer did not fail to respond promptly to Wishecoby's complaints. "She . . . is actively homicidal (probably the result of auditory hallucinations) at other times and cannot be trusted for any length of time," Hummer replied.

He admitted that Wishecoby did a fair amount of ward work but recommended against paying her for it. Hummer justified his decision by saying, "The work she does is for the double purpose of helping her physical condition, keeping her out of trouble and distracting her attention from what she believes is persecution at the hands of her (imaginary) enemies."[6]

Evidently, neither Hummer nor the commissioner found it strange that someone with active homicidal tendencies would be allowed to work freely within the wards. Since Hummer actually did try to separate violent patients from others, his contention that Wishecoby was homicidal seems a deliberate falsehood. He also doesn't state why being paid for her work would invalidate the benefits she received from it, but the commissioner did not question that, either. (Patients received profits from the sale of their beadwork.) Hummer simply dismissed

Wishecoby's complaint with an attack on her mental status—a practice he always found effective—and continued to do what he wanted. Unfortunately for patients, what he wanted to do seldom included letting them go home.

Within the psychiatric field, however, entrenched attitudes were loosening, and superintendents had begun to approve long trial furloughs to feel out the suitability of discharges. They sought to reeducate the insane for tasks that they *were* able to do, rather than give them up as hopeless because they didn't have their former abilities or could not pursue their old careers. These changes held out much greater hope that a patient could eventually be released.

Hospitals were also beginning to move away from huge warehousing facilities to smaller cottage plans that allowed patients with similar needs to be grouped together in a homier atmosphere. Doctors still believed that architecture was an important influence for patient treatment and arranged these cottages as either small "villages" with a mix of patients or along occupational lines so that one cottage might contain farmworkers, another workers doing construction jobs, and so on. The cottage plan had the advantage in that small cottages accommodating six to twenty people were cheaper to build and more easily authorized than facilities for hundreds. Besides being more homelike, cottages could be added almost indefinitely so long as the asylum compound did not run out of acreage on which to build them.

In Germany, Dr. Emil Kraepelin was conducting groundbreaking work in identifying symptom clusters in mental patients, with the hope that he could create a better classification system for mental disorders than currently existed.[7] He also introduced a view that certain conditions of insanity (such as melancholia) were caused by outside factors and could be successfully treated, while others (like dementia praecox) were caused by organic problems within the brain and were incurable. Kraepelin eventually identified what are known today as schizophrenia and manic-depression and, with his colleague Alois Alzheimer, co-discovered Alzheimer's disease. By the 1920s Kraepelin had gained worldwide renown in the world of psychiatry and had published an influential textbook that he revised annually until his death in 1926.

These new attitudes and discoveries embraced innovations in psychiatric treatment. A report in the April 1923 issue of the *American Journal of Psychiatry* discussed a new treatment for mental disorders: infecting patients with tertian malaria.[8] In this procedure the blood of a person infected with malaria and not yet treated with quinine would be injected into the mentally afflicted patient. That patient would be allowed to have eight or nine attacks of malaria before receiving quinine, during which time his or her blood was drawn so as to infect another patient. The article concluded, "It may be that every large hospital for mental disorders may have to maintain one or more malarial patients as sources of infectious material."

Dr. Julius Wagner-Jauregg pioneered research into this therapy, which became better known as "fever therapy."[9] He had observed that mental symptoms sometimes ceased in patients who had survived typhoid fever and began to experiment with controlled ways to induce fever. By 1917 he was working with malaria, which could be treated with quinine, as a viable fever inducer. In 1927 he earned a Nobel Prize (in the category of physiology or medicine) for his work in fever therapy.

Wagner-Jauregg focused on patients suffering from general paresis, the psychiatric condition resulting from the brain and nervous system damage that syphilis caused over time. Bizarre as it might sound today, his innovative treatment was highly welcomed. General paresis was nearly always fatal, and fever therapy enjoyed reliable success rates of around 60 percent if one counted remission as well as cure. Fever therapy remained popular until the 1950s, when penicillin brought relief from syphilis's devastating consequences.

On another positive note, that same 1923 issue of the *American Journal of Psychiatry* also carried an article about epilepsy, which discounted some of the stereotypes associated with the disease: the "epileptic disposition," marked by brutality, evil, and destruction; hyperreligiosity; and the psychosis associated with epilepsy. The authors pointed out that many of the psychotic or violent episodes attributed to their patients were committed right after their convulsions, when they were confused. Though they did not explicitly connect the dots to the notion that perhaps epileptics shouldn't be sent to mental institutions on the basis of something they did during or after a convulsion, their study at least planted the seed.

Both study doctors did explicitly state that they did not see the "epileptic personality" that authors of textbooks reported. Since insanity had been linked historically to epilepsy, this changing view offered hope that epileptics might someday find a more compassionate approach to the treatment of their illness. On another encouraging note, these authors also observed that the drug Luminal controlled epileptic convulsions very well.[10] Hummer embraced this new medicine wholeheartedly, as epileptic patients remained his cross to bear throughout his tenure as superintendent. By 1925 he was ordering eight thousand tablets at a time from the Winthrop Chemical Company.

Along with psychiatry's progress in treatment and perception, and a new focus on record keeping and patient evaluations, patient reforms had also begun to creep into the field. In 1909 Clifford Beers and others had created the National Committee for Mental Hygiene, the precursor of today's National Mental Health Association. One of the organization's first steps had been to draw up a set of model commitment laws, which were slowly being adopted during the 1920s.

In this, as with other progressive steps, Hummer's institution had not changed with the times. Commitment procedures still followed the same easy pattern: a reservation superintendent somehow determined that an Indian was insane and asked if Hummer had room for another patient. If he did, the process was complete and everyone was happy except the patient.

Superintendents or agents probably didn't spend much time sifting through the nuances of mental health. When they were alerted by staff or doctors that certain people were unable to care for themselves or weren't receiving adequate care from their families, they looked for a remedy. Rather than see a mentally challenged, ill, or physically handicapped person suffer, they turned to the only institution they could easily access for long-term care. Superintendents were unlikely to make critical distinctions between something like "feeblemindedness" and "melancholy." That was Hummer's job—and he failed miserably.

With that caveat, it is also undoubtedly true that Indians who constantly got into trouble or seemed unable to follow behavioral expectations were sent to Canton Asylum as punishment or as an easy way to get rid of them. Families also misused the asylum. John Brown was a patient who displayed so few symptoms that the nurses and attendants at Canton Asylum did not consider him insane. Brown enjoyed nearly unlimited ground and city parole privileges and must have been both reliable and self-sufficient to a great extent. But his wife did not want him released when a visiting inspector suggested discharge, stating that he "might give her some trouble at home."[11]

Commitments were complicated affairs within Indian families, just as they were for white families. Violent or uncontrollable behavior made the decision easier, but many families held on until they were exhausted or too old to care for someone who needed extensive oversight. Records show that some patients were discharged and then returned to Canton Asylum, evidence that the patients' families were willing to care for them but simply couldn't. Some families undoubtedly wanted a break from a family member's incessant care and didn't protest the commitment. Others were not happy at all with a commitment and agitated faithfully for their loved one's return. From the content of some of the letters available, some families may have willingly allowed members to go to the asylum, perhaps after a drunken spree or other disturbing episode or as a substitute for a hospital. Many thought their relative would stay a short time and get well, and letters also show their second thoughts about prolonged commitments.

Amos Red Owl wrote a number of times to the commissioner of Indian affairs on behalf of his daughter, Lizzie. In one letter, he explained that Lizzie had been treated at Hot Springs (ailment unspecified) and that she had been operated on without his knowledge. Red Owl said that the operation caused his daughter to have "spells" and that he had sent her to Canton for help: "And she was same condition when she was home she got the same spell yet, at the asylum. I therefore respectfully and earnestly request of you to grant me a permission to let her come home. . . . I could take care of her at home she just have that same spell, no better in asylum."[12]

Red Owl's attitude was not unique. Families that had willingly relinquished a family member to the asylum expected a cure. When they discovered that their loved one continued to have the same problems, they often wanted the person back. But by that time, discharge was out their hands and in Hummer's. For him, patient and family protests were scarcely worth entertaining, and he usually squelched any desire for a discharge as quickly as he could. Since all psychiatric decisions flowed through Hummer, he had nearly absolute control over the fate of his patients. As the 1920s rolled on, he conducted business as usual at the Canton Asylum for Insane Indians.

It wasn't business as usual with his superiors, however. Secretary of the Interior Albert Fall resigned from the cabinet in 1923 amid the turmoil of the Bursum Bill protest and the Teapot Dome scandal. In the latter affair, Fall had convinced the secretary of the navy to give him control of large western oil deposits, which were for the navy's emergency use in wartime. However, Fall secretly signed leases with oilmen from Harry Sinclair's Mammoth Oil and Edward Doheny's Pan American Petroleum companies, in exchange for $400,000 in loans he wasn't required to repay. Fall did not mention Teapot Dome or the Bursum Bill when he resigned but instead cited the unwarranted public attacks against him and the failure to discuss important issues in the way he wished as the most important factors in his decision. Harding replaced Fall with his postmaster general, Hubert Work.[13]

Work had served as a colonel in the Army Medical Corps during World War I and in 1920 served as the president of the American Medical Association. Having a medical man as head of the Interior Department changed its focus somewhat. Work took his duties far more seriously than Fall had, immediately convening a Committee of One Hundred, composed of Native American leaders as well as prominent white men, to survey government policies and make recommendations on them.

Whether Hummer appreciated or feared having a medical man as the head of the Interior Department is unknown. Hummer considered his position as an expert on Indian psychology to be unshakable, and he perhaps relied on the buffering effects of Burke and Meritt to protect him from any radical changes at the top. About the worst fallout for Hummer in the new appointment was the knowledge that Work could scarcely be expected to adopt the degree of indifference that Fall had maintained. Nonetheless, Hummer had no reason to believe he couldn't outlast whoever entered the arena—as secretary of the interior or commissioner of Indian affairs—just as he had in the past. Besides, Hummer suddenly had his hands full with his own institutional drama.

On July 12, 1923, Hummer accepted Jerome Court into Canton Asylum. Court had a documented history of violence and had been judged insane by his local medical board. He protested bitterly that he was not. No one cared what Court thought, and authorities at the reservation viewed his departure with considerable relief as good riddance to a troublemaker. Hummer was accustomed to patients who didn't think they were insane and had learned to ignore their protests. This time, however, he faced someone as intent on getting his own way as Hummer himself.

Court proved to be a handful. He was articulate, strong-willed, and determined. He escaped shortly after arrival but was captured and returned to Canton. He then turned his attention toward an attendant named Ava Dunn, flirting with her in the laundry room and the basement coal room, and even in the dormitories. He was a quick worker. After plenty of note passing and stolen kisses, Court's seduction was complete and the two eloped just a little over a month after his arrival.

Dunn resigned from the asylum on August 24 and that night returned in a taxi with a key to the main building's side entrance. She and Court traveled in the waiting taxi to Sioux Falls, where they took separate rooms at the Albert Hotel.[14] When they met the next morning, Court told her that he had been approached by a policeman and needed to leave town. Since they had arrived at the hotel after midnight and were meeting at six in the morning, this tale does not ring true—Court had probably used the woman simply as a means to get out of the asylum.

Dunn hired an automobile to take them across the state border to Dell Rapids, Iowa, where she stayed for a couple of days before taking a train back to Sioux Falls. Unfortunately for her, Hummer received a tip that she was there. He and the Lincoln County sheriff drove the thirty miles from Canton to Sioux Falls and cornered Dunn in the Sioux Falls Western Union telegraph office.

Hummer filed charges against Dunn with the assistant district attorney two hours later and, between himself and the lawmen, obtained her confession and a promise of assistance in capturing Court if they would be as lenient with her as the law permitted. That same night, Hummer, the sheriff, the Sioux Falls assistant U.S. marshal, and Dunn piled into the sheriff's car and drove to Dell Rapids, where Court was sitting in jail after being picked up for trying to sell a pair of Dunn's shoes. Hummer and the sheriff left Dunn's prosecution in the hands of the assistant district attorney and returned to Canton with Court.

Her affection apparently undiminished, Ava Dunn wrote to Court afterward, saying, "I can't see why it's so aful [sic] for me to love you? Many white men marry Indian women so why not white woman Indian Men." She seemed to realize that the affair was over but reassured "Jerry" of her continued love and support. "I won't help you to run away again but I'll write and will send you little things each week that I can."

For his part, Court explained in a letter (not specifically addressed to but probably intended for Hummer) that he had escaped because he wasn't insane and did not want to be at Canton Asylum. "Why, I'd be satisfied here," he wrote as he compared himself to the other inmates, "but I don't even get *fits*." He declared an intention to give up moonshine and lead a clean, decent life if he could get out but ended his letter pointedly: "If I am insane why on earth don't I get treatment of some sort."[15]

Hummer wrote an exasperated letter to the commissioner of Indian affairs about the escape, describing how Court had "battered down a re-inforced door, smashed a transom over the employee's office and left through the window of this room." Hummer went on to state that he didn't see any signs of insanity in Court and subsequently sent Commissioner Burke Jerome Court's file and asked for permission to release him. While he made his evaluations and waited for an answer from Burke, Hummer kept Court chained in his room for at least two months.

Appalled at the news of a potential release, Court's home superintendent, W. R. Beyer of Fort Totten, North Dakota, wrote to try and stop it. For his trouble, he received a verbal slap from Hummer, who wrote to the commissioner, "I have the greatest respect for Mr. Beyer's ability as an accountant, but I now find that he possesses much more profound ability, namely the ability to diagnose a case of mental disease at a distance of several hundred miles and not having seen the case since early in July. This surpasses my meager talent so far that I humbly admit that I am ashamed of myself."

In the same sarcastic vein, Hummer wrote that though Court was egotistical, immoral, and potentially violent, he wasn't insane. With self-righteous indignation he asked, "Are we justified in holding this man in chains (for the balance of his life), in an insane asylum, because of this?" He also threw in an innocent question: "Is it possible, do you suppose, that Mr. Beyer is afraid of this man?"

Hummer's concern about holding someone indefinitely is a strong indication that he was merely rationalizing Court's release. Hummer routinely kept many patients for a lifetime because they "might" be difficult for families to handle, "might" get pregnant and have an imbecilic child, or "might" have a relapse after an apparent cessation of symptoms. Either Hummer himself was afraid of Court, or he had just gotten tired of dealing with him.

When he got a copy of Hummer's letter, Beyer immediately fired off a sharp reply to the commissioner that ended, "As far as I know, Dr. Hummer is alone in his opinion as to the mental status of Court. . . . It seems that Dr. Hummer very strongly resents the opinion of any one who does not agree with him."

Beyer then underscored his point with some sarcasm of his own: "If he has cured Court in five months he certainly is entitled to much credit. . . . In view of the questionable miraculous cure of Court, would it not be well to have Dr. Hummer's opinion verified by other experts before Court is released?"

In a testament to Hummer's power as superintendent—or Burke's growing indifference—the commissioner allowed Court to be released, though with the provision that he stay away from Fort Totten. Court honored that provision and immediately began to raise hell at the Sisseton reservation. He got drunk, broke into several houses, beat up a number of fellow Indians, and wound up in jail. Within a month he either escaped or was released. In March 1924 Court thumbed his nose at Hummer by sending him a short postcard that read, "Wishes & regards to all, am in the U.S. Army now."[16]

Hummer had lost that round, though he was probably correct in his judgment that Jerome Court wasn't insane. Characteristically, he had made the assertion for his own convenience or professional purpose. Likewise, he asserted that he kept tubercular patients isolated (he didn't), didn't restrain patients (he did), and gave them better care than they could receive at home (unsupported by the evidence).

He could say whatever suited him, since these assertions were never effectively challenged. Patients and their families sent occasional complaints to the commissioner of Indian affairs, but their voices were stifled as soon as Hummer picked up his pen in reply.

Hummer had hit the fifteen-year mark in his tenure at Canton Asylum and knew the ins and outs of protecting his turf. He was friendly with his inspectors and spent considerable effort entertaining them on their visits. Hummer's temper was nearing legend among his staff, but he was capable of directing charm and affability toward his peers. Hummer was also perfectly ready to render humble mea culpas to his superiors when it suited his purposes. Nothing seriously disturbed Hummer's entrenched position, even as he dragged his feet over improving psychiatric care for his patients or even keeping up their paperwork. Hummer's fiefdom was secure as ever, as he put the first half of the Roaring Twenties behind him.

14. Ripples in the Waters

Dr. Harry R. Hummer had every reason to be enthusiastic about the way things were going at the asylum in 1925. Whether he had initiated the exchange or simply replied to a request for information, Hummer wrote in January or early February to Dr. Emil Kraepelin, who wanted to conduct a study of "general paresis" in "Negroes" and Indians within the United States, Cuba, and Mexico. In his letter, Hummer stated that no other institution in the United States accepted only Indians—information that he surely thought would make Kraepelin anxious to visit Canton Asylum.

General paresis, known more commonly as general paralysis of the insane, occurred in patients with tertiary (late-stage) syphilis. Syphilis spirochetes growing in the body over time attacked various organs, leaving lesions that could manifest as paresis three to fifteen years after the initial infection.[1] Though every syphilitic patient didn't develop it, paresis's symptoms were relentless and horrible. They usually began with forgetfulness and gradual disorientation and incoherence. Patients lost their memories, couldn't define words, or forgot what had happened only moments earlier. At the same time, they began to lose their physical dexterity. Eventually, patients could become incontinent and paralyzed, unable to eat unaided or do more than babble.

Coupled with these physical symptoms were psychological ones. They, too, began innocuously, with perhaps depression and irritability, before moving on to intellectual deterioration, hallucinations, and delusions. Patients could be pitiably frightened, anxious, or restless; the disease's progress was difficult to watch or treat, though patients were often oblivious to their condition toward its end.

Kraepelin described many forms and stages of paresis in his writings, but his most telling words concerned mortality for these unfortunate patients: "The prognosis of the disease is decidedly unfavorable. Death occurs within the vast majority of cases within two years."[2]

General paralysis of the insane was a serious health issue before penicillin began to be used as a treatment for syphilis; it was the seventh leading cause of death in New York State in 1914.[3] This syphilitic syndrome affected perhaps 20 percent of patients in asylums and required lifelong caregiving—no one got well. (Kraepelin's assessment that it proved fatal in two years only meant in its acute stages.) Involvement in researching the disease, especially with someone as eminent as Kraepelin, would be an enormously important and exciting opportunity.

Kraepelin believed that alcohol made syphilis worse and that it might even be the cause of the paresis that sometimes accompanied syphilis. Kraepelin also believed that freed slaves and "the North American Indians, who are well supplied with whiskey in their reservations," were particularly susceptible to both alcohol and general paresis, with North American Indians suffering severely from paresis.[4] All these assumptions were just theory, though, and he had to come to the United States and examine Indians with general paresis to prove any of it.

Dr. William A. White, superintendent at St. Elizabeths, subsequently received a letter from Kraepelin, who had been his professor in Munich. Kraepelin needed help in setting up visits to Canton Asylum, other Indian reservations, and St. Elizabeths, for himself and his colleague Felix Plaut. The two professors planned an eighty-day visit to the United States and wanted to find the largest concentrations of syphilitic Indians and African Americans that they could.

Hummer surely felt validated by the visit: Kraepelin was a giant in the psychiatric world, and Plaut was a highly esteemed serologist. In April 1925, Kraepelin, Plaut, and doctors G. S. Adams and Leo Kanner visited Canton Asylum to conduct Wassermann tests for syphilis on ninety-four patients there.[5] Kanner worked at Yankton State Hospital in South Dakota; he was an Austrian who had been living in Berlin until the previous year and could be expected to help with any language issues the visitors might encounter.

A little more than 9 percent of Canton's patients tested positive for syphilis, but none had general paralysis. Hummer already knew that he had no paralysis cases, but he had neither a laboratory nor the finances to conduct Wassermann tests for syphilis at five dollars per test. (Hummer's resources were so poor that Kanner had to send someone to Yankton for needles and a microscope.) The visit solidified the syphilitic history of his patients, and during the four-day visit, Dr. Kraepelin also examined thirty-seven of the patients. Whether his diagnoses and Hummer's matched is impossible to say for most of the cases.

The doctors examined Canton's medical records and pulled out those for patients with eye problems for further testing. One of these patients was Lizzie Red Owl, whose family had made multiple requests for her release. The doctors found "no signs of intelligence deficiencies" in her and additionally found her "polite and unassuming." Lizzie told them she had been having headaches, unsteadiness, and a stomachache for nearly a year. The examining doctor noted tremors in Lizzie's hands and tongue and signs of Hutchinson teeth, though she had tested negative for syphilis.[6] Hummer had diagnosed her as psychopathic.

Another patient had even fewer problems. Alfred Kennedy spoke English, was polite and animated, did his chores correctly, and had a good memory—"no signs of intelligence deficiencies." He had been hit in the chest prior to admission and subsequently felt weak and unable to work, but he had "no fits or craziness, or hallucinations." Hummer had diagnosed him as psychopathic, as well. Neither Kraepelin nor Plaut commented on these diagnoses in their later publication.

Kraepelin's visit was certainly the high point of scientific inquiry at Canton Asylum, but the visit did nothing to shine a light on Hummer beyond noting his helpfulness. Kraepelin's and Plaut's monograph on their paralysis study, *Paralysestudien Bei Negern Und Indianern*, by simply speaking the truth, instead cast a somewhat unflattering shadow on him.

The doctors noted that Hummer was the only physician at the hospital and thus unable to apply his psychiatric knowledge to any great extent. They also noted that many patients didn't speak English or even each other's languages. The inference, of course, was that with little ability to communicate, Hummer couldn't really aspire to be much more than an administrator. Hummer had only seen about three hundred patients since he took office in 1908, and in the doctors' opinion, it was "a rather stagnant patient picture at Canton." Even more embarrassing, the report told the world that "the complete psychiatric literature consists of one publication from Dr. H. R. Hummer ... published in 1912"—nearly a decade and a half earlier.

When the visit ended, the professors required no further research on Indians at Canton Asylum. They found one subject with paralysis at Yankton and another at the Oregon State Hospital, examined their records, and then requested that the Indian Bureau give them a summary report of other Indians with syphilis. His own lack of a case study for the investigation was disappointing, but Hummer was doomed to further frustration. Two other publications resulted from Kraepelin's visit. One was in the *American Journal of Psychiatry*—coauthored by Yankton's Kanner—and the other in the *British Medical Journal*. Hummer had no hand in either article, so he could not manage to increase his prestige through the visit. Kraepelin's research trip was a lost opportunity that Hummer would never see again.[7]

But life went on. Hummer set aside $12,000 in funds targeted for asylum supplies and maintenance, hoping instead to use the money for items *he* wanted for the facility. Hummer approached Burke with his usual wish list, asking approval for some of the projects because the money came out of his own pocket, so to speak. Unfortunately, Hummer's economies usually came at the expense of his patients—he ran out of money to pay the $27.44 bill for a side of beef that year and had to send it back to the Cudahy Packing Company.

As usual, Hummer's wish list included more buildings so he could accept more patients. He doubtlessly spoke the truth when he claimed that there were patients he couldn't admit because of limited space; a refusal to grant him what he wanted would make only the Interior Department look bad. Among his wants this time were a milking machine, terrazzo flooring in the kitchen and dining room, a new swine house, rugs and draperies for the employees' rooms, and a new rug and better furniture for himself. As savvy as he tried to appear with his savings and economies, Hummer always left out one important factor. He never incorporated the salary for another physician into any of his plans, no matter how many buildings, patients, or other staff he proposed managing.

Members of the Interior Department's subcommittee of the House Appropriations Committee planned a visit to Canton Asylum in July, and this would give Hummer a chance to show his needs to the men who held the purse strings. It was a grand opportunity, and Hummer was eager to take advantage of it.

At the time, Hummer must have believed that 1925 was, indeed, his year. His sense of superiority flourished. Hummer had always resented suggestions by employees and positively prickled at the idea that there might be a better way than his. Even Commissioner Burke couldn't escape his haughty attitude, which surfaced shortly after the Subcommittee on Appropriations made its visit.

Hummer's last inspections had gone well, and he either didn't bother to put his best foot forward this time or played a risky hand at pushing his own agenda. Hummer left one attendant in charge of nearly fifty male patients during the subcommittee's visit and allowed these important subcommittee members to see one of his patients chained and another naked. Commissioner Burke was appalled. He immediately asked the Department of the Interior for another $1,000 to pay an additional attendant's wage, thinking Hummer had only three attendants for nearly one hundred patients. He also spoke to Secretary of the Interior Hubert Work about conditions at the asylum.

Burke wrote to Hummer about his concerns. The commissioner asked Hummer to research his equipment needs and told the superintendent that he would, himself, see about getting additional appropriations for personnel. Burke added that he had discussed the asylum with Work, an expert on mental disease, who had been amazed at Burke's description of the man he had seen in chains. Work made a specific recommendation for a restraining device employed at Yankton's state hospital for the insane and suggested Hummer visit the facility if he wanted to see it in use.

Hummer's reply is a study in condescension and backpedaling. He first told Burke that he had misunderstood the attendant situation. The asylum had only three *male* attendants, but it also had three female attendants and a night watchman who, along with his other duties, attended the males at night. There was no female night watch.

Seven attendants (if you counted the night watchman) made a sufficient ward staff, Hummer felt, because additional staff would only talk and visit among themselves and waste the government money spent on their salaries.

As for the patient in chains and the naked one . . . Hummer told Burke he had *intentionally* left these patients in those conditions, in order to help Burke make a stronger case for additional funding for the institution. Hummer had hoped to "create a lasting impression" on the committee, which "would call up this picture . . . in our coming appropriation." The fact that Hummer told Burke he quickly had a blue denim suit made for the naked patient would seem to imply that the patient had been naked for quite some time, rather than stripped of his usual outfit for Hummer's impression-making purposes.[8] As far as a visit to Yankton went, perhaps Hummer felt outraged to have Kanner's establishment held up to him as a model. He said that he had never learned anything from the state hospital there, except that it had excellent buildings.

Hummer assured Burke that he seldom used chains or any kind of restraint, since he had seen the folly of allowing attendants to use them "at their sweet pleasure" during his time at St. Elizabeths. Newspaper accounts and inspections show that Hummer did use restraints at times, though with what degree of regularity is hard to say.[9]

Hummer didn't seem to take in that Burke had told the most powerful medical man in Hummer's line of supervision—and perhaps in the country—that conditions at the asylum were not up to par. Instead, Hummer mentioned that he had heard Work speak a couple of times at American Medico-Psychological Association meetings he had attended and that it was a shame he couldn't attend them each year, due to finances. It was Hummer's impression, he wrote, that the superintendent of St. Elizabeths *did* receive funding to attend these meetings. After assuring Burke that Canton Asylum was doing fine and that he had managed it well for seventeen years, Hummer closed by saying that as far as the restraints and personnel went, he would be pleased "to sink my wishes into obscurity and to carry out yours, whatever they might be."[10]

Between the subcommittee's visit and this exchange, Burke had sent the Indian Office's medical supervisor, Walter S. Stevens, to inspect the asylum. Stevens agreed with Hummer that the number of person-nel managing patients was adequate and that the two buildings that housed patients were in excellent sanitary condition. The Indian Office might want to consider an additional building, though, to accept the backlog of patients applying to the asylum. What the asylum really needed, said Stevens, was more land on which to graze cattle and to grow feed for hogs.

There were a few problems that Stevens noted. Hummer's iceboxes in the main building and hospital were in such bad condition that odor from the meat permeated the milk and butter, and ice had to be replenished every day to keep the meat itself from spoiling. Canton Asylum had a bad well, too. Stevens recommended replacing the ice-boxes and drilling for a new well and made suggestions to install ter-razzo flooring in the kitchen and dining room and to complete some maintenance on the dairy barn. Finishing his report, Stevens said that "Dr. Hummer is an excellent man for the position of Superintendent."[11]

Hummer may have closed out that episode by the skin of his teeth, but it was a triumph for him, nonetheless. Between the subcommit-tee's and Stevens's visits, he had gained approval for just about every-thing on his wish list with the exception of additional buildings. By the end of the year, he was even able to start negotiating—without much luck—for the additional farmland he so desired.

Hummer was no less successful in blocking patient releases he didn't want to make. Early in December, the San Francisco–based Indian Board of Co-Operation asked Burke to free Peter Kentuck, who had been at the asylum since 1920.[12] They had found three Indian leaders willing to vouch for Kentuck, along with a cousin and aunt who were willing to take him in.

Burke passed on the request to Hummer, who replied to Kentuck's cousin that the patient had homicidal tendencies and his release "was not to be considered." Hummer wrote Burke the next day to say that Kentuck was close to moronic and fought other patients with little prov-ocation. These letters were written on December 20 and 21, 1925, respec-tively, and were at odds with Hummer's medical report to the Hoopa reservation superintendent. Just the previous month, Hummer had said that Kentuck was "quiet and well-behaved. Little trouble. Habits good. Cleanly. Out of door daily, unattended. Assists with work at barn."[13]

Hummer had a history of getting his own way. With relatively powerless people like patients or their families, he could usually dismiss complaints while seemingly responding to their concerns with an authoritative assessment of the patient's conditions and needs. When that was too much trouble, Hummer passed the buck by shifting responsibility to the commissioner's office for decisions he was the only one qualified to make. In Kentuck's case, Hummer carried the day and the young man was not released.

With these successes behind him, Hummer entered 1926 essentially vindicated in his opinions about patients and the need for the asylum projects that he had so continually set before the Indian Office. He enjoyed that refreshing interlude for about six months before he once again enmeshed himself in controversy serious enough to require another investigation.

Hummer had never thought highly of most of his staff. He legitimately found it difficult to hire anyone competent or willing to fill his attendant positions, as they encompassed tasks most rural workers would have found disagreeable or incompatible with former jobs.[14] Few of them stayed in their positions any great length of time, which may have given rise to Hummer's sensitivity about loyalty and dedication. Special inspector T. B. Roberts noted sympathetically that employees in the Indian Service itself "were reluctant to take an assignment there" because of the nature of the work.[15]

For his part, Hummer did little to create a positive atmosphere at the asylum. Roberts had also noted that Hummer didn't have a good word to say about any of his employees and privately made a number of nasty insinuations about their characters that he refused to put into actual charges. The inspector left with an uneasy feeling that he couldn't quite put into words—it was evident that things weren't running smoothly, but he did not feel "competent to say what should be done."

Hummer was not similarly uneasy about what needed to be done. He had definite ideas when it came to his expectations for employees and their willingness to comply with his vision. In Hummer's mind, employees were either loyal and compliant or enemies who needed to be ousted by any means. Ione Landis's experience was not an isolated incident. When confronted by what he termed "disloyal" employees, when his authority was threatened, or when he just didn't like some-one, Hummer's innate pettiness found full scope. In the summer of 1926 he began a campaign against three employees that would have made the behavior of an eighth-grade girls' clique look mature.

Sometime late in spring, the asylum's matron, Lucie Jobin, fell into disfavor with Hummer for an unspecified reason; one document suggests that it was because he wanted a favorite employee, Clara Christopher, to fill Jobin's position. In May 1926 Hummer asked one of the institution's farmers, Herman Van Winkle, if he had had immoral relations with Jobin. Van Winkle replied that he had not, but in June Hummer called Van Winkle into his office and accused him of having immoral relations with both Lucie Jobin and Elizabeth Coleman, another employee.

Hummer asked Van Winkle to turn state's evidence against the two women and resign, with the promise that after he had discharged the two women he would reinstate Van Winkle. Van Winkle refused and suddenly found himself accused of improper conduct with the cook, Mrs. Erna Wahlstrom. Hummer then discharged him. On July 11, Elizabeth Coleman let Van Winkle eat supper at the asylum with her, and Hummer discharged her six days later for "violating positive instructions that she was not to entertain any males while on duty at night."

Perhaps to back himself up, late in July Hummer asked the commissioner of Indian affairs to send an inspector to look into his personnel problems. Medical Director Emil Krulish made a quick visit and offered three particular recommendations: to cover all the radiators so patients couldn't burn themselves, to pay for a subscription for the *Journal of the American Medical Association* and allow Hummer an annual allowance of fifteen dollars for new books on psychiatry, and to abolish the position of matron (Jobin's position) and replace it with that of a trained nurse. A little more ominously, Krulish also made the tentative suggestion that it might be "just as economical and more desirable from the patients' standpoint" to send insane Indians to state asylums closer to their homes.[16]

Hummer replied promptly, saying that he agreed completely with two of Krulish's recommendations. He did want to wait a year to establish the nurse's position and instead to use the money saved to purchase feed for livestock. Krulish's suggestion to replace Jobin with a nurse had little to do with her ability as a matron—he had been regu-larly campaigning to get nurses at the Canton Asylum and the matron's position was the one to replace. What is more indicative of a personal issue between Jobin and Hummer is Hummer's own written statement just five months earlier that he shared a visiting nurse's opinion that "Miss Jobin is a capable and conscientious worker."[17]

Hummer devoted most of his reply to Krulish's report to the sugges-tion that it would be more economical to house patients in state asy-lums. Hummer emphasized the discrimination Indians faced at state institutions, overlooking his own inadequacies in terms of understand-ing his patients' languages and cultures. He also voiced the opinion—shared by a number of psychiatrists—that visits from relatives and friends were harmful to mental patients. Being closer to family and reservations at the more localized state hospitals, therefore, would be a hindrance to recovery rather than a help.

The question of whether visits helped or hurt patients was an impor-tant one, with many psychiatrists weighing in on the side that they impeded progress. Visitors stirred up old memories and associations, disrupted patients' routines, and fueled a desire to return home even if they weren't ready for the transition. Family members seeing the patient at his or her best during the visit were often persuaded to begin the discharge process, against their loved ones' best interests. Even if families agreed a patient wasn't ready to return home, the emotion-ally charged episode often left patients unmanageable or despondent for days. Of course, families who wanted to visit considered it their right and a way of ensuring their loved ones' comfort and safety. A case could be made for either view, depending upon a patient's par-ticular problem and situation. The very real fact remained, however, that even if visitors didn't contribute to setbacks for patients, they were indisputably inconvenient for staff.

The arguments pro and con were immaterial to most patients—visits mattered a great deal to lonely men and women confined in institu-tions. Indian patients at Canton Asylum often expressed acute home-sickness, which a well-timed visit from family might have alleviated. Long distances, language barriers, and poverty prevented many families from coming to Canton, despite its much-touted centralized location.

A dearth of visitors was not unique to Canton Asylum or to Indian patients, however. One contributor wrote in the *Opal* (a mid-nineteenth-century publication at Utica State Lunatic Asylum, written and edited by patients):

A year is gone, and five months more,
My parent, since thy face I saw,
And full twelve months have past me o'er,
Since news from thee I heard or saw
If you had loved me as you ought
A being you had given life,
Some note or message would you not
Have sent to cheer my prison life?[18]

Hummer made the best argument he could against patients' removal to state institutions and then immediately resumed his skirmish with the asylum's personnel. He relieved Jobin of her matron's duties and transferred her to the men's ward, an unprecedented move at Canton Asylum and very rare elsewhere. He then set his spies on Jobin to document every move she made; attendant Robert Ritter made at least twenty-six reports on the former matron's movements in the asylum.

It was a difficult summer in many ways. Hummer had genuine personnel problems, though his inability to delegate supervision or to personally intervene contributed to them. A letter written in 1925 and signed "Susan" (probably Susan Wishecoby) described attendants who mocked patients and got them agitated and uncontrollable before going to Hummer with complaints that they couldn't be managed. She asked Hummer to "please learn them to treat us like human beings not like beast to be teasing all the time."[19] Nothing indicates that Canton's staff had suddenly changed their attitudes or behavior over the course of a year, and 1926 likely saw much of the same misbehavior.

Amid such aggravations, Hummer also faced the imminent departure of his sons into the greater world. Twenty-year-old Harry Jr. was entering his final year at the Naval Academy in Annapolis. Francis, twenty-two, was in his third year at George Washington University, studying medicine. Hummer admitted in a letter that it would be hard to see them leave and that the West would lose its interest for him when his sons remained in the East permanently. At such a reflective time in his life, he undoubtedly considered the two infant children he had buried and what might have been if they had lived.

In May Hummer had sent out bids to drill a new well for which he had recently gained approval. One potential bidder, E. C. Archibald, replied sharply that "you seem to want the world with a fence around it, padlock and extra keys thrown in." After a few more jabs, he told Hummer that it wouldn't surprise him if Hummer didn't get a bid at all, and to look him up when he wanted to be sensible.[20] Later, in July, a severe storm blew down one of the asylum's outbuildings, both an inconvenience and an unexpected financial blow.

The personnel battle continued to intensify. In late August, after he'd had a little time to nurse his grievance and compose his thoughts, Herman Van Winkle wrote an indignant letter to Commissioner Burke about his dismissal. Van Winkle denied the allegations of immorality and lobbed several accusations of his own against Hummer, including Hummer's promise of immunity if he testified against Jobin and Coleman and the superintendent's use of the institution's farm for his own hogs.

By September, Hummer had some new problems. Patient Frank Bear got in a fight and lost an eyeball. Elizabeth Faribault, a female patient, had a baby.[21] Here was another case of Hummer's diagnosis being at odds with his behavior. When Faribault had escaped in 1920, Hummer told the commissioner of Indian affairs that her condition was "comfortable" and that he was willing to let her stay with her family if they would take her. Two days after he informed the commissioner of the escape, he wrote to say that he had already retrieved Faribault; he made no mention whatsoever of meeting with her family. Over the next six years, Hummer refused categorically to release the woman despite the efforts of many individuals working on her behalf. He insisted that she had dementia, delusions, and hallucinations. Suspiciously, however, when Hummer's elderly parents stayed with him, Faribault was the one he tasked with providing their daily care.[22]

In the meantime, Van Winkle's letter had done its job, and Burke sent special inspector T. B. Roberts out to Canton Asylum to investigate. Roberts was not impressed with Lucie Jobin, and he recommended her dismissal because she couldn't give good service. Particularly against her was the fact that she was Indian. Roberts suggested that Jobin be replaced with a white woman, "because white women didn't want to take orders from an Indian."

Roberts instructed Hummer to write a letter clearing up some of Van Winkle's allegations. Hummer actually put in writing, "He tells you truly when he [Van Winkle] says that he was offered immunity if he would give me the facts in reference to other employees."

Then Hummer offered the little spin that so often kept him out of trouble. "The intention," he explained, "was to keep my word and reemploy him after this affair blew over and then, what he did not suspect, to get rid of him at the earliest practicable moment thereafter."[23]

When Burke got hold of this letter in late September, he sent a sharply worded one of his own to Hummer. Burke thought Hummer's ploy a little underhanded, though he apparently believed that Van Winkle "appears to have been the principal offender . . . he was deserving of dismissal." But, said Burke, to have reemployed him and then dismissed him "does not indicate fair dealing and placed the Superintendent in an embarrassing position." He told Hummer to avoid any further embarrassing compromises and to strengthen his weak administration.[24] This letter came on the heels of another from Acting Assistant Commissioner Hauke, stating the Indian Office was looking for a trained nurse for Canton Asylum.

Uncharacteristically, Hummer instead asked for an assistant physician. His history of refusing to back such a position makes the request suspect. Hummer may have gambled that no physician would be interested in coming to Canton Asylum. More importantly, he knew his patient-physician ratio was already superior to that of St. Elizabeths and that his request would not be considered critical. Hummer likely used the request simply to buy time against any change at all. As Hummer had anticipated, Krulish did not agree with him about the need for another physician and continued to push for a trained nurse. However, Krulish immediately ran into at least one of the problems Hummer had undoubtedly expected—no nurse wanted the job for the salary it would pay.

Having successfully moved to thwart or delay any change in staff, Hummer turned his focus back to the attack on his personnel. Jobin had been in the Indian Service since 1901 and undoubtedly knew some of the ins and outs of the system. During her persecution, she made the mistake of advising Herman Van Winkle to demand the vacation that he was due and telling Elizabeth Coleman to ask for reinstatement in the Indian Service. On November 22, 1926, Hummer formally charged Elizabeth's *sister* Mary Coleman (who also worked at the facility) with disloyalty. He accused Lucie Jobin of disloyalty, insubordination, filching of government time, and "conspiracy with two discharged employees."

Special inspector Roberts had written in his report that Hummer was "a peculiar character" and recommended that Dr. Krulish return and make what Roberts considered medical decisions about the asylum's personnel. Burke was dismayed by the continued turmoil, and he wrote to Krulish in December: "Conditions . . . under the superintendency of Dr. H. R. Hummer have been getting serious from the standpoint of employees for more than a year." Burke acknowledged that Hummer had some disloyal employees but added that Hummer's management style undoubtedly contributed to his problems. He asked Krulish to go in, get statements from everyone involved, and make some specific personnel recommendations—even for Hummer.[25]

When Krulish arrived in January 1927, he went through employee records and conducted interviews with nineteen of the institution's twenty-one employees. After a thorough investigation he discovered a molehill instead of Hummer's mountain: Mary Coleman denied being disloyal and Hummer had no proof that she was; Hummer's spy, Robert Ritter, recalled that Jobin sometimes criticized the food served at the institution and once called it "slop"; the cook believed Jobin had criticized Hummer but couldn't remember any particular statement; Clara Christopher believed Jobin was disloyal but could not give any specific statements; and nobody else at the facility thought Jobin was disloyal.

Even Hummer couldn't drum up too much actual evidence, since Mary Coleman's last efficiency report had rated her "Excellent" in every category except "Manners and speech" in which she was rated merely "Good," and in "Loyalty," "Absent." In the "Comments" section, Hummer had written, "This woman is abolurely [*sic*] disloyal to the superintendent since he discharged her sister. She is plotting, with the matron and others, against the superintendent, practically all of her time. . . . She should not remain here."

Jobin had been at the institution since 1919. Her last efficiency report showed her ratings as "Excellent" in all categories except "Openness to suggestion" and "Industry," which were rated "Fair" and "Poor, at present," respectively. She too, earned the biting "None" under "Loyalty." Hummer's comments in Jobin's case were a diatribe against her and ended with a demand that she be removed.

Krulish tried to sort through the ire and accusations flying around the institution and ended up recommending that Coleman remain and that Jobin be transferred to one of the Indian schools.[26] The matron's position had never required nursing skills, but Krulish firmly believed the asylum had a critical need for a registered nurse with special training in an institution for the insane. Now he underscored his recommendation by saying that if it had been carried out in the first place, the trouble at the institution would not have occurred.

Krulish also specified that the institution needed a white nurse but, unlike Roberts, gave no particular reason for specifying "white." He may have had his own racial bias, of course, but he did step in to retain Jobin in the Indian Service. Krulish may have simply felt that the racial bias at the asylum was too strong for an Indian woman to overcome, or perhaps he didn't think any Indian women with the proper training were available.

Krulish certainly didn't seem interested in bolstering Hummer's position and chided the superintendent's management, saying that "he has been trying to manage the institution from a desk instead of by close personal contact. . . . Doctor Hummer has been in charge of this institution for about 17 years, has had but little supervision and has fallen somewhat into a rut in regard to his executive ability. He has evidently not been very regular in making rounds through the hospital."

Regardless of his personal feelings, Hummer knew how to survive in the Indian Service. One tried-and-true method he employed was to graciously accept criticism from a current inspector and then ignore it. Krulish wrote that he went over Hummer's shortcomings and the means of overcoming them very thoroughly with the superintendent and that Hummer "accepted these suggestions very graciously, in good spirit, and promised to put them into effect." Hummer, in fact, told Commissioner Burke that he embraced Krulish's recommendations— Hummer had a policy of *always* telling the commissioners at the Indian Office that he embraced inspection recommendations.

Krulish also spoke to Hummer about the need for a nurse rather than an assistant physician and wrote in his report that Hummer had changed his opinion about the matter. It was a nice concession to Krulish and of little consequence to Hummer, who knew that not many women had the special hospital training Krulish required and that the few who did would not want to work in a South Dakota insane asylum.

Hummer's long experience had paid off in a big way—disfavored employees had been ousted and he still reigned supreme. More importantly, Hummer had once again survived a high-level inspection unscathed, while appearing both repentant and cooperative. However, times were changing, and his next run-in with staff would prove it. When Hummer kicked up his next fuss, he discovered that a lot more had altered in his world than a few innovations in psychiatry and the presence of a medical inspector who didn't completely kowtow to his authority and expertise.

15. The Winds of Change

The mid-1920s, dominated by Prohibition, stock market speculation, and general carousing, were also dominated by new thinking in the Senate and the Interior Department. Reformers' efforts were paying off. Spectacular muckraking articles concerning Oklahoma's tribes and the consortium of judges, guardians, attorneys, bankers, and others who took advantage of their power to legally seize control of the estates of "incompetent" Indians created a sensation in the press and Congress.[1] The House of Representatives ordered an investigation by its Committee on Indian Affairs, which, as always, found little amiss with the administration of Indian property—except in the rich, oil-producing districts.[2]

By this time, Secretary of the Interior Work had become dissatisfied with both partisan and amateurish attempts to investigate Indian affairs. John Collier, increasingly dedicated to helping Indians retain their native cultures and communities, urged Work to use the services of the Institute for Government Research (later called the Brookings Institution), to help with an investigation. Work instead asked the Board of Indian Commissioners to look into the practices of his department's Indian administration.[3] The board found nothing wrong and stoutly defended Commissioner Burke and the superintendent in Oklahoma responsible for the Five Civilized Tribes.

In 1926 Work decided there was too much bias within the Interior Department's usual channels to conduct a proper investigation into the well-being of Indians. He contacted W. F. Willoughby, director of the Institute for Government Research, and asked him to conduct a survey of Indian affairs. The institute sent a nine-member team of experts, headed by Lewis Meriam, to visit Indian reservations, schools, and hospitals.

In February 1928 *The Problem of Indian Administration*, or the Meriam Report as it was popularly called, described government policy toward Indians like no other report before it. Though written in an unemotional, scientific style as opposed to the inflammatory rhetoric of reformers, the report left no doubt that conditions for Indians were miserable, abuses rampant, and mismanagement pervasive.

In a letter that Meriam wrote to W. F. Willoughby from California in 1927, he said, "We are leaving tonight for San Francisco to spend some time in going over the material accumulated by Collier's [American] Indian Defense Association. From what we have been able to learn at the State Department here, and from the Agency, I fear it is true that Collier's organization knows a whole lot more about the Indians of California than does the Government Agency here."[4]

As the Meriam team conducted its survey, Secretary Work also asked engineers Porter Preston (from the Bureau of Reclamation) and C. A. Engle (from the Indian Office) to look at problems with Indian irrigation projects. Issued in June 1928, the *Report of Advisors on Irrigation on Indian Reservations*, more popularly known as the Preston-Engle Report, highlighted the dubious practice of charging irrigation projects to Indian monies. Collier, as a representative of the American Indian Defense Association, later used information from that report to damn the Indian Office once more: while the cost of the projects had been charged to Indians, it was largely white farmers who benefited from them.[5]

Change wafted like a faint perfume—or a creeping stench, depending upon one's viewpoint—through the Interior Department and Indian Office. Burke and Meritt (who had been assistant commissioner since 1913) were increasingly viewed as old school. Though staunchly defended by some, they were just as staunchly attacked by the cohort who wanted to see the entire old school thrown out. Even Hummer, so far away, surrendered to the inevitable and, in April 1927, wrote to Burke positively jumping to secure a head nurse.[6] Actually, Hummer wanted to go on an extended vacation east to see his son graduate from the Naval Academy. He told Burke that if a nurse could be secured by the middle of May, he could leave the asylum in her hands at the end of it.

Hummer had received another quick inspection by the increasingly critical district medical director, Emil Krulish, in early April. Krulish found the asylum in fairly good shape subsequent to his January 1927 investigation concerning the Lucie Jobin brouhaha. The medical director had again urged that the nurse's position be filled, along with the additional positions of a night watchman and fireman. Male patients were housed in two separate buildings, with one attendant to watch over both at night. The attendant also had to inspect the barns and premises and keep up the fires in the two buildings and root cellar. Krulish felt the man was spread rather thin.

Hummer agreed that one attendant was insufficient but explained that he typically locked chronic patients in at night so they wouldn't wander.[7] He tried to arrange for a "fairly intelligent" patient to room with the epileptic patients and help them during the two to three fits they had each night. Hummer ended up by saying he felt it would be a lavish waste of government money to add another employee or two just to reduce the few accidents that occurred due to the staff shortage.

Krulish also wanted to see a couple of new cottages for married employees. A farmer with a wife and five children (Van Winkle) had occupied two rooms before he quit, and other married quarters were almost as cramped. Though a single person had been found for the farmer's position, there was little reason to hope that the asylum had found a permanent solution in him. Hummer asserted that there was no reason to construct additional cottages, since his employees appeared contented with their present quarters. Instead, funds for the construction of cottages could be better used in constructing bed space for additional patients. If anything, Hummer said, that proposed cottage money could go to a separate building for epileptics.

As usual, these minor differences with the Indian Office did little to alter the daily routine of Hummer's life. James Shawano, diagnosed as an imbecile and epileptic, had been in the institution a little over two years before he died of pulmonary tuberculosis in May 1927. When Hummer contacted the young man's reservation superintendent for burial instructions, Superintendent Dawson of Laoana jurisdiction in Wisconsin asked that Shawano's body be sent home to his father. He also asked that James's sister, also an imbecile and epileptic at Canton Asylum, be released at the same time. As usual, Hummer washed his hands of responsibility. He told the commissioner that Annie Shawano was healthy and had nothing in her mental condition that required her residence at the asylum. However, Hummer still couldn't certify that she was "mentally recovered" and therefore didn't have the authority to release her. He was willing to, with Burke's permission, which was granted.[8]

In Shawano's case, Hummer probably did not feel like butting heads with a superintendent (rather than a family member) who was intervening on a patient's behalf, and he was particularly fed up with caring for epileptics. A quiet, cooperative case like Agnes Caldwell was a different matter. Caldwell pleaded to go home to care for her mother, who was old and ill. "I haven't seen my Mother for ten years now," she wrote. Even if she couldn't be released, Caldwell asked, couldn't she just go home for a visit?

Hummer deflected Caldwell's request with the usual excuse that he couldn't release her without proper permission. Caldwell wrote to her sister, Josephine Johnson, for help, and Johnson sent a letter to the commissioner a few months later. She, too, asked if Agnes could come home to help care for their mother but received a reply that it wouldn't be possible. Hummer did consider Caldwell mentally deficient, but he would have been hard-pressed to make a case that she would be difficult to return to family members willing to take her in.[9] Caldwell's mother died late in 1929, leaving Agnes $17.52 as her share of the estate.[10]

Hummer plodded away at his responsibilities: entering into a contract with Universal Film Exchanges, Inc., for weekly moving pictures at the asylum, sending an affidavit in duplicate to the Indian Office stating that a small pig had died and he wanted the animal off his books, and bidding out for a hundred pounds of Prince Albert tobacco at eighty-three cents per pound. He also returned Wilson Honga, described as "a moron, degenerate, and dangerous" by the superintendent who didn't want him back, to his reservation.[11]

Edith A. Wilson arrived as desired on the first of May in 1927, and Hummer was able to leave Canton Asylum in the hands of its first trained nurse. Wilson had studied at St. Elizabeths and seemed quite capable, but Hummer actually relied on his financial clerk, Leon Giles, for updates and assessments while he was gone. It was a well-placed trust, because after clashing with Hummer's favorite employee, Clara Christopher, Wilson got enough of Canton Asylum very quickly and handed in her resignation after only four months at the institution.

During her tenure, however, Giles dutifully informed Hummer that Dr. Herbert R. Edwards had visited in connection with the "Survey on Indian Affairs" going on at the time. Here the clerk and a new nurse were no substitute for Hummer and the personal charm the superintendent used to smooth over his asylum's deficiencies. To Hummer's later embarrassment, Edwards simply reported on what he saw.[12]

It was nevertheless a good summer. Hummer finally purchased 228 acres of additional asylum farmland at $150 an acre—a triumph he had been working toward for years. His social life active, Hummer attended the Grand Commandery of Knights Templar in Spearfish, South Dakota, even though Wilson had resigned by that time. (He often left his financial clerk in charge of the asylum during his absences.) Hummer could report that he had thirty-two applicants waiting for admission—an always-comfortable backlog that underscored the asylum's vital necessity. He had also made a reasonable case for additional funds for the asylum despite the savings he had promised would result from the new acreage. The Indian Office wanted to increase his personnel (adding two nurses and another attendant) and Hummer simply told his superiors that the Indian Office would have to shake loose the funds for their salaries—his budget was based on what had been current expenses.

No new nurses darkened his doorstep that year, and 1927 ended nicely with a public relations opportunity that gave him no trouble and gained him goodwill. A group of Chilocco, Oklahoma, YWCA girls had gathered Christmas presents for Canton Asylum as a service project. The gifts arrived on Christmas Eve, to the delight of his patients, allowing Hummer to distribute largesse without having to pay out of pocket for it. Hummer thanked the girls' coordinator, Mrs. Jose Antone, profusely and asked that the project be made an annual event.

The new year, 1928, dawned in an equally heartwarming manner: in early January Hummer received a promotion of one rate within his classification grade. He also recovered an escaped patient, Charles Hawk. Though he had to request permission to transfer the money from Hawk's individual account to the asylum's general fund, Hummer had the satisfaction of receiving $7.30 from the runaway for expenses related to his recapture and return to the asylum. As a punishment for his misadventure, Hawk was not allowed to attend the moving picture show on January 18. After the attendant left the ward to operate the moving picture machine, Hawk was left alone and committed suicide by hanging himself in his room. The death was reported without further investigation.

Hummer's request for permission to withdraw or disburse funds, though a cumbersome procedure, was typical when it came to anything involving asylum finances. Despite his moral lapse in the matter of feeding his hogs on government swill, Hummer appears to have been scrupulously honest with actual funds, going so far as to send the United States treasurer a check for twenty-five cents that he had collected from Dr. Krulish for a meal at the asylum during one of his inspections. Hummer was also the trustee for patients' Liberty Loan and second Liberty Loan bonds and for any money they received for outside work or selling crafts. His accounting and disbursement of even the smallest sums indicates he did not look to patients' personal funds to meet asylum expenses.

Hummer's financial honesty was never called into question, but his financial decisions were sometimes questioned. Meritt asked Hummer for a detailed statement on the benefits derived from purchasing his additional acreage. The superintendent showed a savings of $2,325.20 in fodder against the $34,170 expended for the land—meaning the investment would take over a decade to pay for itself. The previous May, Meritt had scolded Hummer for offering to return money to the Indian Office while pleading that he was too strapped for cash to install permanent radiator covers to prevent burns to the patients. Now, a year later, Meritt again scolded Hummer for asking to use asylum "savings" to fund an assistant farmer's position while his nurse's position went unfilled. Meritt seems to have caught on to Hummer's tactics and told him to fill the nurse position even if he couldn't get a civil service employee.[13]

Nurse Grace O. Fillius reported to Canton Asylum on September 3, 1928, but probably did not catch Dr. Hummer in the best of moods. The Meriam Report had been handed over to Secretary Work earlier in February, and its ramifications were now trickling out to the inspected facilities. Dr. Edwards, the medical field secretary of the

National Tuberculosis Association, had visited Canton Asylum when Edith Wilson had been in charge for all of a couple of weeks, and neither she nor the financial clerk, Leon Giles, had been able to do much more than show Edwards around.

Edwards had not been favorably impressed to any degree, though he gave a fair account of the facility's importance and scope of service.[14] He found the kitchen and dining room ample, the oven range out of order, kitchen utensils and hot water limited, and the bakery in disorder. Each twenty-two-patient ward had two lavatories, two water closets (not enclosed), one slop sink, and one drinking fountain. The hospital's dining room was in disorder, and its operating room equipment consisted of two lavatories and a slop sink.

In the patients' rooms in the hospital, two patients were sleeping on mattresses placed on the floor. In both buildings, children were housed with adults, and only the violent were segregated into single rooms. Edwards particularly noted that tuberculosis cases were mishandled: patients' dishes weren't sterilized, and no precautions were taken to protect other patients from exposure. Edwards could find no menus on file but saw that on the day he visited, the diet consisted of "a stew of meat and carrots, with more fat and bones than anything else, thin apple sauce, bread, and coffee." The ward dining rooms lacked proper facilities like tables and personnel to supervise the patients, and several patients were eating while seated on the floor.

Edwards found Hummer's records entirely inadequate, saying it was "impossible to obtain a complete picture of a case from the available notes." He specifically advised adding more personnel in the form of a nurse and a subordinate, as well as additional laborers for the farm and dairy. He added that epileptics, children, and patients with tuberculosis needed to be segregated. Edwards ended up by declaring that a system of records "conforming to accepted psychiatric practice in hospitals for the insane" should be installed.

One telling detail was Edwards's table of diagnoses for Canton Asylum's patients:

16 . . . epilepsy

31 . . . dementia praecox

17 . . . imbecility

3 . . . constitutional inferiority

8 . . . idiocy

7 . . . senile dementia

1 . . . paranoia

4 . . . intox. psychoses

3 . . . manic depressive

2 . . . undiagnosed

Nearly half the patients were not insane at all, if one did not buy that epilepsy, idiocy, and the like were actual mental illnesses. It would be safe to say that many of the remaining patients simply couldn't be diagnosed correctly because of cultural and language issues. If they were not diagnosed correctly . . . how many of these men and women *were* insane? Edwards also noted the length of patients' stays: sixty-five had been there longer than five years—an open-ended prison sentence, indeed.

Hummer defended himself by first saying that he was running a mental institution and not a hospital, so he had little justification for installing expensive equipment in his operating room. Hummer contended that he had some equipment that Edwards did not see and patient records that Wilson and Giles hadn't known about. Hummer dismissed the disorderliness and state of disrepair at the asylum as a function of it being a small institution that didn't have dedicated maintenance staff to take care of every little carpentry or painting job that needed to be done. Instead, he used his regular employees for these jobs, and they got around to them when they could.

By that point, of course, the oven range was already repaired. Hummer then explained that he had little furniture and no pictures or other decorations in the wards and dining areas because violent patients used them as weapons. The patients sleeping on the floor were a blind man with a broken hip and a man with hemiplegia, who fell out of bed frequently; they slept on the floor for safety. Though Hummer admitted that he had found the dairy barn and the bakery in disorder himself at times, he always dealt with the conditions promptly and had dismissed a number of employees who had failed to keep up these facilities. He had an excuse for everything: it was a busy season, Miss Wilson hadn't known where the records were kept, and so on.

Hummer summed up his defense by stating that Wilson—who had been at Canton Asylum all of perhaps three weeks before he left for the East Coast—was "hostile." He added, "I am informed that the Doctor and Miss Wilson went to Sioux Falls that night and returned early the next morning, having had 'car trouble.'" Hummer ridiculed Edwards's suggestions for additional personnel and ended up by saying, "It is evident that the institutional care of the insane is a matter that the Doctor has not studied to any great extent."[15]

Actually, Hummer was lucky that Edwards mentioned only what he did. A few months earlier, Hummer had told the commissioner that he had several patients who "plaster the walls of their rooms with urine, feces and food, daily. . . . Our patients frequently stuff anything they can secure down the toilets, blocking them and requiring that they be taken down and opened."[16] It is not likely that these patients stopped doing such things under the direction of Nurse Wilson, so Edwards may have, indeed, considered the difficulties inherent in institutional care of the insane when he filed his report.

The remainder of the year seemed to pass from one exasperating situation to another. Grace Fillius, the new head nurse, wanted a rest period during her twelve-hour day, even though her presence had already caused trouble enough—attendant Amelia Wallace quit when forced to vacate her choice room to make way for Fillius. Luke Stands by Him, a patient since 1916, successfully escaped during the weekly moving picture show. And, perhaps paying more heed to Edwards's recommendation than Hummer thought necessary, the Indian Office had created positions for a total of four nurses.

Hummer was already at work to undermine Fillius, expressing doubts to Krulish about her ability and qualifications. Fillius, forty-one, had graduated from State Hospital #3 in Nevada, Missouri, in 1915, but she had never worked in the Indian Service. However, she had taken a special course in public health nursing and had nursed in the army during World War I . This experience had led to some sort of mental breakdown, and she apparently went to St. Elizabeths for a brief period of treatment in 1918.

Hummer seized on this breakdown a decade earlier as a fatal weakness, but Krulish was determined to give Fillius a chance. In his last inspection of the year, Krulish wrote that he was favorably impressed with the new nurse and specifically added that he didn't think Fillius would get a fair trial until the junior nurses were appointed. Hummer was already finding fault with her, though, and in his December reply to Krulish's report, told the commissioner that he had recently spoken to Fillius about her attitude. On January 21, 1929, Hummer asked for Fillius's removal because of unflattering remarks she had made about him (supposedly) to a female laborer. Two days later, the twenty-six-year-old nurse Doretta L. Koepp arrived and, shortly thereafter, another staff nurse, Mrs. Elsie Behrman. Hummer immediately launched into a rancorous battle that escalated well beyond the matter of incompetent or unwanted nurses.

During all this turmoil, a traveling Indian Office auditor unwittingly stopped at the asylum in February 1929. Hummer telegrammed Commissioner Burke to ask that B. G. Courtright investigate the institution. Assistant Commissioner Meritt replied by the same method, asking what kind of investigation Hummer desired, just as Courtright wrote to Burke about the encounter. Courtright said that Hummer had told him the justification for his request was twofold: to show "his lack of dread of an investigation of the deplorable condition which he said existed at the Asylum" and to have a layman and a stranger give an unbiased report. Courtright had simply told Hummer he was unqualified to look into Canton's affairs.[17]

Meritt agreed that Courtright was not the man to investigate an insane asylum but, by the middle of February, consented to allow an even less qualified committee of Sioux Falls businessmen to do so. Though Meritt made the actual request for these outsiders to conduct an investigation for the Indian Office, circumstances indicate that either Hummer himself lobbied to have them come to the asylum or they lobbied on his behalf. Perhaps satisfied that the committee would both substantiate his claims against Fillius and report favorably on his own behavior when they arrived in March, Hummer wrote to the commissioner at the end of February to say that Fillius's services were unsatisfactory to him and he would like her terminated at the earliest possible moment.

Meanwhile, Hummer had also asked for the removal of a newly hired farmer, Dewey Gilland, because—at another institution—the farmer had once choked a violent patient he and two others were subduing. When Meritt brought up the point that a farmer probably didn't have much to do with patients, Hummer replied that patients were often detailed to help with farm work. Indeed, Hummer said, he was always expecting Gilland to injure one of them. Furthermore, an employee had brought him an empty liquor bottle, found under a coat in the basement, where "I am told Gilland kept his coat. I do not know that this bottle belonged to Gilland, but suspicion points either to him or to Mrs. Fillius, head nurse." Hummer had already written the commissioner that a friend in Sioux Falls (whom Hummer refused to name) had told him that "Fillius could hold a large quantity of liquor."[18]

Hummer's unsubstantiated charges against Fillius may have alarmed Burke, or he may have simply believed that Hummer's additional charges against Gilland indicated the asylum's problems would not be easily resolved. Whatever the reason, Burke took an unprecedented step. He wrote to St. Elizabeths' longtime superintendent, Dr. William White, and asked him to send a staff psychiatrist to Canton to conduct a survey on the physical and professional needs of the institution.

Before that could happen, however, Hummer got the friendly investigation he had craved. In March the committee from Sioux Falls found the asylum's buildings well cared for and nearly all of them immaculately clean. The wards and patients' quarters were also well cared for and clean. Everything about the institution, it seemed, was well cared for and clean, except for the admittedly untidy slaughterhouse. Because of language barriers, the committee couldn't speak to any of the patients but found by their attitude that they were fond of Hummer and the staff. After this visual examination and private interviews with employees, the committee believed the patients were "well treated, housed and cared for."[19]

The exception to all this harmony and cleanliness was Grace O. Fillius, head nurse. Besides lacking the ability to handle subordinates, she was creating strife and dissension by failing to cooperate and trying to assume power outside the scope of her position. The committee was of the unanimous opinion that she would be a difficult person to work with. They stopped just short of suggesting her discharge and instead recommended another, deeper investigation of the matter.

George Pettigrew of that committee wrote personally to Commissioner Burke a day after their visit to the asylum. "We found everything in first class condition," he said. There were no disturbing elements, except one, "a Mrs. G. O. Fillius who pretends to be the head nurse. She has come in and thinks she is the one to run the business of the institution. . . . In other words, she is the only fly in the ointment."

Pettigrew went on to say that he considered Hummer a wonderful superintendent with many fine employees. "It is too bad that a woman of this stamp should be thrust upon them and create the trouble that she is evidently bound to create. You have known me long enough, I think, to know that I would give you a straight tip." Pettigrew signed off, as the grand secretary, on letterhead reflecting the various officers of a South Dakota Masonic lodge.[20]

Burke undoubtedly took this report with a grain of salt. While he waited on the St. Elizabeths physician, Burke dispatched the long-suffering Krulish once more to Canton Asylum. The farmer, Gilland, independently wrote a two-page letter to the commissioner about the problems he had suffered under Hummer. Gilland complained that the superintendent expected him to pick the corn crop that had been neglected the previous fall so that he could get the spring crop in, even though the field was under a foot of water in places. After listing a number of other grievances, Gilland concluded, "If you have a place you can transfer me at once and see fit to do so, I will accept anything you have."[21]

Krulish found that Hummer had lined up a number of statements from an attendant who had seen Fillius and Koepp interacting together in a quite friendly manner. Krulish admonished the employee to pay attention to his own duties and to stop making any further reports, which had little but innuendo and supposition to them. Hummer had assembled a number of personal memos concerning the nurses' work, including a charge that two employees had smelled liquor on Fillius's breath. When Krulish questioned the employees, they both "positively denied the alleged statement of having smelled liquor on Mrs. Fillius' breath." Krulish systematically refuted the bulk of Hummer's charges, not even addressing the superintendent's pure speculation about whether Fillius had lied about various issues or whether she had been drinking.

A week after the Sioux Falls business committee's visit, and in compliance with Krulish's verbal request, Hummer gave Krulish a list of sixteen charges against Fillius and five against Koepp. Krulish spent a good deal of his time investigating the veracity of Hummer's charges, finding that employees Hummer named as witnesses to his charges held their own when they denied them, even in Hummer's presence. Sitting in on Hummer's cross-examination of Nurse Fillius, Krulish said, "He tried court methods to break her down to such an extent that I requested him to change his tactics, but in spite of all she was equal to the occasion and answered him calmly, fiercely, and without showing the least bit of emotion."[22]

Ultimately, Krulish found that Fillius hadn't done much wrong, though she probably had made some unfavorable comments about Hummer and been too friendly with attendants. He was equally convinced that Fillius was trying to work under extremely unfavorable conditions and that her actions were both natural and justified to some extent. At the end of March, Krulish sent his findings to the commissioner with a few biting comments.

Hummer, said Krulish, operated the asylum "without complying with modern standards, as a boarding house for insane Indians, without nurses, insufficient help. . . . The quarters for employees, with the exception of the superintendent who has one of the most desirable homes in my district, have been inadequate." Krulish went on to say that Hummer had not given enough attention to his patients, and "tried to direct the institution from his desk" rather than through any close contact with either patients or employees.

Krulish listed a number of recent problems and stated that it was doubtful whether or not Hummer could really meet the demands of the asylum. Then he got to the heart of the present problem: When the nurses had entered the picture, Hummer was immediately hostile to them. Additionally, a number of employees who had had but the most haphazard supervision came under more control than they were accustomed to having—and didn't always like it. Fillius's natural attempts to impose order and discipline had resulted in some of the turmoil, and Hummer had not backed her at all.

Instead, said Krulish, attendants were being used as "stool pigeons" to spy on the nurses, and were discharged if they wouldn't do so. After detailing a myriad of findings that made Hummer look unprofessional and petty, Krulish concluded that the superintendent and nurse Fillius couldn't work at the same institution. He recommended a change in superintendents, and that Fillius, Koepp, and Gilland be retained.[23]

Krulish visited the asylum again in April, found additional cause for dissatisfaction with Hummer's management, and wrote that it was imperative to change the management of the institution. To emphasize Hummer's incompetence, Krulish included documents written by the recurring thorn in Hummer's side—Dr. Hardin—from twenty years earlier to show that Hummer's mismanagement was of long standing.

By now, Krulish was increasingly impatient with Hummer. He directly addressed Hummer's ploy to get a favorable report from the Sioux Falls committee by saying, "It is also interesting to note that in selecting a citizens' committee to investigate and report upon the management of the asylum not one person was chosen by Dr. Hummer from Canton, but all members serving on this committee are residents of Sioux Falls and social friends of the superintendent."[24]

By this time, Burke was probably impatient with Hummer specifically and exasperated with the rest of the world in general. Over the previous few years, he had had his hands full either waiting out or deflecting investigations into the workings of his office—investigations that were becoming a little too common to be comfortable. He had barely escaped dismissal because of an investigation into his personal conduct in 1923 during the guardianship case of the incompetent (and oil-rich) Jackson Barnett from Oklahoma. Though initiating factors had begun before he became commissioner, Burke allowed the very questionable manipulation of Barnett's estate by a woman who almost forcibly wed the elderly man. In 1925 a subcommittee of the House Committee on Indian Affairs exonerated Burke of maladministration and negligence. A Senate committee investigated him once again for the same issues in 1928 but made no official report.

These close scrapes undoubtedly wearied him of investigations into the affairs of the Indian Office. Though the most recent investigations had uncovered only isolated problems, and the investigation by the Board of Indian Commissioners had been favorable on the whole, the increased scrutiny of his office concerned Burke. Reformers were getting serious, and some of those reformers were in Congress itself—the "sons of the wild jackasses."

Core members of these "jackasses" were westerners and progressive Republicans in the Senate, who sometimes jumped party lines to side with Democrats of like mind on certain issues. William Borah of Idaho, Hiram Johnson of California, George Norris of Nebraska, Burton Wheeler and Thomas Walsh of Montana, Smith Brookhart of Idaho, "Young" Bob La Follette and his father, Robert La Follette, of Wisconsin, and Lynn Frazier of North Dakota were the most prominent members of the group. Walsh had been instrumental in uncovering the Teapot Dome scandal, and Borah had stepped in to oppose the Bursum Bill.

The jackasses got their name when the conservative George H. Moses, himself a colorful and irascible member of the Senate, became so exasperated with them over a tariff battle that he blasted the epitaph during a Washington DC dinner for manufacturers.[25] Though at first insulted, the jackasses eventually embraced the name; they also had no problem showing themselves to be just as stubborn and oppositional as their namesakes.

Boding no good for the old school members of the Indian Office, some of their like-mindedness centered around protecting Indians from at least some of the worst ravages suggested by whites. Concurrent with the investigation by Meriam's team, the jackasses persuaded the Senate Indian Committee to fund a special Indian investigating committee. Members of the committee, often accompanied by the vocal John Collier, traveled throughout Indian Country (including Alaska) holding hearings.

The reports cascaded down—the quietly sensational Meriam Report and stinging the Preston-Engle Report—but Burke's stomach must have churned when he read the inspection that he had ordered for Canton Asylum. Dr. Samuel A. Silk arrived there from St. Elizabeths on March 20, 1929, and spent the next six days reviewing the facility, its administrative procedures, and its personnel. Instead of the typical 5- or 6-page report, or even the dozen or so pages that more rigorous inspections produced, Silk's report was a 108-page litany of disapproval.

He had found a sick, bedridden man with a brain tumor padlocked in a room. He found a ten-year-old boy in a straitjacket, also in a padlocked room. A half-naked girl had slept on a mattress on the floor of the bathroom so she wouldn't annoy others, and an epileptic girl had been shackled to a hot water pipe.

Everywhere, Silk found padlocks, stinking chamber pots overflowing with excreta, and dirt. Patients walked to and from lavatories barefoot and half-clothed, then returned with filthy feet to beds whose linens were changed only once a week. Attendants routinely padlocked patients in rooms or padlocked entire wards for over an hour at a time so they could perform other duties. Often they left unpredictable patients smoking cigarettes in their padlocked rooms.

Like Edwards before him, Silk also found the operating room with nothing more than a surgical table, slop sink, and two washbowls. Even Hummer, who escorted Silk, could not produce overlooked additional equipment. Hummer's much-lauded hydrotherapy apparatus sat unused, and Hummer stored coal in a room meant for hydrotherapy treatment.

"One wonders what Dr. Hummer meant when he stated in several of his annual reports to the Commissioner that the hydrotherapeutic department was functioning satisfactorily," Silk wrote pointedly.

Silk found Hummer's medical records completely inadequate. Hummer conducted no neurological examinations, and psychiatric progress notes were made by uneducated ward attendants. "Most of the information in the records is of a stereotyped and valueless nature," said Silk. "No psychiatrist could get an adequate idea as to the mental condition of a patient from reading such a history."

Silk's other findings were even more damning when he reviewed paperwork for the last five deaths at the institution. One patient died of pulmonary tuberculosis fifteen days after admission, but there was only an attendant's note about it—Hummer had not given the man a physical or mental exam. Charles Hawk had entered the asylum in 1920, but the first physical exam on record was dated 1926. There was no record concerning his suicide, except for a letter from Hummer to the commissioner to report it. Another patient who died of pulmonary tuberculosis worked in the kitchen, according to an attendant note written six months before the patient's death. Her physical deterioration was noted as follows: September 15, 1928, acute coryza (another term for the common cold); October 4, 1928, cough; December 1, 1928, died.

These and the other examples Silk cited were of a pattern, too similar with others in the past to be anomalies: Hummer had written to the commissioner about the patient Elizabeth Faribault early in 1928. The thirty-five-year-old woman awoke and walked to the toilet sometime between six and six-thirty in the morning, returned to her room, and died of no apparent cause. She had been caring for her baby daughter, Winona, just as usual the day before and had shown no signs of illness.[26] Hummer recorded "heart failure" as the cause of death and continued to keep the baby at the asylum.

Silk pointed out many failures in maintenance and supervision, but he particularly focused on the inadequacy of the asylum's personnel. One elderly woman displaying symptoms of Parkinson's disease was responsible for two floors in the main building and two wards in the hospital building, working a shift that began at 6:00 a.m. and lasted until midnight. There was a genuine staff shortage (three attendants had recently quit), which Silk noted, but he also pointed out that even the full complement of attendant personnel—three men and three women during the day and one each at night—would only give the equivalent of four full-time employees during the day.

Hummer never accounted for time off, sickness, holidays, or vacation for his staff and instead refuted the need for additional personnel as though his eight attendants were available twenty-four hours a day. Silk wrote that an analysis of U.S. Veterans Bureau hospitals showed "not less than three-quarters of the maintenance appropriations were spent for salaries." In smaller institutions, added Silk, "this proportion is even larger." Canton Asylum spent only a bit over 50 percent of its appropriation in salaries.

Attendants had so little time for patient care that Silk concluded Canton Asylum acted as little more than a prison for the Indians within it.[27] Attendants often padlocked patients in their rooms or restrained them simply for convenience. Hummer could honestly say he did not give approval for these actions—attendants wishing to restrain a patient simply went to the financial clerk for the various devices (he kept them in the safe) and used them at will.[28] Two patients had been restrained in steel wristlets (one end fastened to the patient's wrist and the other to his bed) for months at a time, and in several instances the keys to the devices had been lost, so that an attendant had to saw through an iron link to free the patient from his bed.

The wards were airless and foul smelling. The attendants would have had to unlock forty-two individual padlocks and remove window blinds each morning to properly ventilate the place, which they patently didn't do. When Silk asked an attendant to open a window guard so he could raise the window, the attendant couldn't reach it without going for a stepladder. Furthermore, when the attendant tried to open the guard, he was surprised to discover that the window blind prevented it—proving to Silk that the windows were almost never opened.

Silk's list of failures went on and on, but the doctor's most damaging points concerned Hummer's management and assessment of the institution. Silk chastised Hummer for classifying all patients with any kind of convulsions as epileptics. When Silk sorted out the various conditions, he found only nine patients with essential epilepsy—far too few to warrant Hummer's separate cottage. Furthermore, Silk thought it unreasonable to expect easily managed, higher-functioning patients to be grouped with violent or "filthy" ones simply because they shared a history of convulsions.

Hummer's record with tubercular patients proved even worse. Hummer "thought" he had eight tubercular patients, but because he did not keep reliable records, conduct examinations, keep temperature charts, or give sputum and X-ray examinations, he couldn't be sure. None were showing clinical symptoms at the time of Silk's visit, but they were distributed throughout the patient population, rather than kept together in isolation. Since Hummer had considered them actively tubercular, this was a failing of the highest order.

Silk found some of the attendants intelligent and helpful, the food palatable and in good quantity, and even some of the rooms clean and neat. In the matter of personnel, he could find no one except the dining room girl, Clara Christopher, who would admit to any difficulties with the head nurse. Silk found that farmer Gilland's work was difficult in the extreme. Even butchering a hog was no insignificant affair, since it was done outdoors under a tree. In bad weather, Gilland and his helper had to immerse their hands in hot water and then expose them to temperatures of twenty-eight or so degrees below zero. Silk recommended constructing a small, enclosed space for this chore.

Silk tried to be fair, pointing out the inadequacy of the buildings and of appropriations for salaries and maintenance. But the fact remained that the patients did not receive psychiatric care of any kind. "They receive the poorest kind of medical attention and custodial care very much below the standard of a modern prison," Silk concluded.

Silk questioned whether the Indian Office even needed a separate institution for insane Indians and came down on the side that it didn't. To bring Canton Asylum up to standard—he said Hummer was practicing patient care in vogue twenty years earlier—would require a per capita outlay that couldn't be justified. Furthermore, said Silk, if the government really intended to eliminate its guardianship over Indians, the need for a separate institution diminished dramatically.

Silk also reminded Commissioner Burke that the secretary of the interior at the time of the institution's creation, C. N. Bliss, had not originally approved of the project, nor had St. Elizabeths' superintendent at the time, Dr. W. W. Godding. Silk then offered a number of practical recommendations in case the facility remained open and submitted his report to Burke through Dr. White on April 13, 1929.[29]

Unlike Burke, Hummer didn't have to worry much about all the congressional activity, and if he was worried about anything Silk discovered, he did not show it. He had never been in the habit of changing his administrative style during, or as a result of, his numerous investigations. Now he continued to immerse himself in minutia. In May he sent a letter to Funk & Wagnall to redeem a coupon for their ten-volume set of *The World's 1,000 Best Poems* and a month later informed the superintendent of the Cherokee Indian Agency that he had dropped his practice of submitting monthly reports.

He discharged Logie Nelson and Dorothy Smith, struggled to retain Lizzie Red Owl and William Harris, whom he did not wish to return to their families even though they were doing very well, and straightened out a problem with the Kellogg Company concerning Bran Flakes and Krumbles. And finally, Grace Fillius—either from desperation or coercion—left Canton in June to transfer to the Indian Service at Large at a lower grade and a lesser salary.

Hummer may have won the round, but he had lost much of his support in the Indian Office. Burke did not defend Hummer after Silk's visit, writing instead to Dr. White at St. Elizabeths that the situation at Canton needed correcting very badly.[30] The recently appointed secretary of the interior, Ray L. Wilbur, agreed. He wanted Hummer replaced, the asylum closed quickly, and the asylum's Indian patients discharged to state hospitals. Wilbur's spirit was willing, but the government's will was weak: the secretary of the interior immediately ran into roadblocks.

Dr. M. C. Guthrie, the Indian Office's medical director, wanted patients from Canton Asylum transferred not to overcrowded state hospitals but to its sister institution, St. Elizabeths. St. Elizabeths' superintendent, Dr. White, couldn't take any patients until he was authorized to do so under federal legislation. He also would need more money for housing, in order to separate the nearly one hundred new patients from white patients. At this point Louis C. Cramton stepped in.

Louis Convers Cramton was a Michigan congressman who served from 1913 to 1931 and acted as a special assistant to the secretary of the interior in 1931 and 1932. He had been impressed enough by Dr. Hummer and Canton Asylum to assist Hummer in gaining his long-sought additional acreage, supposedly in exchange for Hummer's keeping a tight rein on asylum expenses. Cramton inadvertently damned the institution as he defended it during appropriation hearings in 1929.

During debate at the hearings concerning the closure of Canton Asylum, Cramton disparaged Silk's findings by saying, "The Canton Institution is hardly to be called an insane asylum. It is no more doing the class of work that St. Elizabeths is than anything in the world. As a matter of fact, many of those patients are not entirely insane; many of them are defectives rather than insane. We thought it was a very goodlooking plant for those kind of people."[31] He flatly told Commissioner Rhoads that the appropriations committee did not want to close the asylum. If the Interior Department appropriations bill passed, he added, "we will expect that this institution will be continued during 1931."[32]

Cramton hadn't read Silk's report but was convinced it was "unnecessarily harsh" toward Hummer. Cramton based much of his favorable impression on his own visit to the asylum in 1925. Somewhere amid the protests of Cramton and the supportive citizens of Canton, the idea came out that because the asylum had been created by an act of Congress, it could only be closed by a similar act. Whether Wilbur bowed to Cramton's pressure, couldn't see his way to waiting the two to three years White believed he needed for St. Elizabeths to gear up to receive Indian patients, or was convinced that only Congress could close the asylum, he let the matter drop.

Burke was still feeling pressure. Reports pummeled him from all sides, and he finally asserted that Collier and Senator William Bliss Pine of Oklahoma were guilty of subverting the Indians and organizing them against the government. The senate investigating committee promptly invited Burke to appear before it to substantiate his charges. Burke couldn't, or wouldn't, or saw that the tide of political favor had turned against him. Undoubtedly weary of all the battles and allegations, he resigned as commissioner on June 30, 1929.

After a run of bad luck that looked like it would finish his career, Hummer had just been handed the political equivalent of a royal flush. Burke's resignation, Cramton's intervention, and St. Elizabeths' inability to immediately absorb Indian patients hindered any reasonable efforts to act upon the Meriam and Silk Reports. Once again, Canton Asylum dropped through the cracks.

The year ended with a bang as the stock market collapsed and plunged the nation into hard times. The Great Depression spread across the land to swallow the livelihoods of many unfortunates. Hummer, though, still retained a plum position as superintendent of Canton Asylum. No significant action costing taxpayer dollars would be forthcoming from a government whose attention had turned desperately to keeping the country afloat. Canton Asylum—and Hummer—would operate as usual while Dr. Samuel Silk's report gathered dust somewhere in the commissioner's office.

16. The Gale Blows

Having successfully escaped any fallout from the damning reports on his institution, Hummer plodded along with the asylum's business. When someone named William Fett informed Hummer that he was expecting company from out of town and was sure his visitors would enjoy seeing the asylum, Hummer replied, as always, that visiting hours were from one to five, Wednesday and Friday.

In June 1930 the superintendent of Fort Defiance, Arizona, made arrangements for the deceased patient Elizabeth Faribault's child—described as quite intelligent—to go to an orphanage. Hummer concurred with the arrangement and the new commissioner of Indian affairs, Charles Rhoads, approved it. In August four-year-old Winona Faribault finally gained her release from an insane asylum.

Patient Jack Root got into a fight and dislocated a shoulder, and an attendant manhandled Leda Williamson so badly that nurse Lorena Sinning made a lengthy report on the incident. In a horrifying accident, patient Edith Schroder caught both hands in the laundry mangle, and the engineer had to take the machine apart to free her.[1] At Canton Asylum, the days blended into one another as patients did their time under Hummer's indifferent care. Even the land joined their misery: in 1931 the asylum lost its corn and potato crops due to heat and drought.

The superintendent had escaped the consequences of the various investigations that had buried Burke, but he found he could not completely escape Washington's interference. Charles Rhoads was a reform-minded commissioner, and he pushed Hummer to add personnel after an inspection in November 1930 made the need apparent. Hummer sent him an interesting letter in response to this encouragement.

Hummer explained that in 1908, then-commissioner Luepp had told him that he expected the asylum to close in ten years and had directed Hummer not to ask for permanent improvements. (After Luepp's death in 1911, Hummer asked for and received improvements.) Hummer also said that in 1926 he had promised Congressman Cramton, head of the visiting budget committee, that he would keep his expenses to $37,000 a year in exchange for appropriations for the farmland he wanted. Rhoads's push for more staff was in direct opposition to the directives of his predecessors, said Hummer, who had enforced a rigid policy of economy with exhortations to "save and save and then save."[2] Hummer apparently forgot to tell Rhoads about the numerous times he had been chastised for trying to return money to the Indian Office.[3]

Rhoads authorized the salaries for a male and female attendant, but even in the first hard years of the Depression, Canton Asylum couldn't keep its positions filled. Staff bickered and reported on each other, and both nurses and attendants churned through the asylum's employment rolls despite the steady pay its jobs afforded.

Assistant Engineer Vernon E. Ball may not have been a typical employee, but he did represent Hummer's personnel problems. Though married (to the asylum's cook), he was of a rough or coarse enough character that the asylum's female employees were afraid of him. Ball hung around the female ward enough to arouse suspicion, and either the head nurse or Hummer told him to keep away from the female patients there. Ball ignored these instructions and formed an alliance with a patient named Marie Chico, who apparently enjoyed a flirtation, or perhaps a real affair, with him.

Ball enticed Chico to leave the asylum with him in July 1931 and consequently took her to Red Lake, Minnesota, where he had been detailed to pick up a male patient. He then took her to stay with his relatives in Milwaukee. Ball brought Chico back to the asylum after two weeks' absence, promising her he would return to take her out again. His actions were the kind to particularly enrage Hummer: a patient had essentially escaped; an attendant had betrayed his trust; immoral behavior had almost certainly occurred; and the employee didn't even seem to realize he had done much of anything out of the way.[4]

Hummer wrote to the commissioner of Indian affairs asking for an undercover investigator to "work up a case against Mr. Ball," but his own investigation and statements from staff made it unnecessary. Bell admitted to his actions but asked for another chance to prove good. The fact that he was given one is a sure sign that Hummer's personnel situation was desperate. However, Ball returned to the women's ward to continue his pursuit of Chico. Less than a month after the original incident, Nurse Sinning observed Ball stripping to the waist outside Chico's window. He opened his overalls and exposed his penis to Chico, and Sinning went for help. By the time she returned with another female employee, Ball had undressed and was walking, naked, back and forth in front of Chico's window. Presumably Hummer gritted his teeth and fired Ball after such an egregious infraction.[5]

Qualified personnel may not have been readily available, but surprisingly, money was. The asylum's appropriations had been raised to $50,000 for fiscal year 1932, though appropriations for fiscal year 1933 were going to suffer a cut to $40,000. The sum was still more than the $37,000 Hummer had operated on up to Rhoads's intervention, and it probably bought more during the Depression than ordinarily. Hummer did manage to stretch his dollars by ordering penitentiary-made shoes for his patients and again accepting the Chilocco YWCA girls' Christmas presents of games, dolls, teddy bears, picture books, and the like on behalf of asylum patients.

Hummer vigorously pursued the money his paying patients normally gave the asylum, dunning superintendent L. W. Page of Fort Berthold Agency in North Dakota repeatedly until he sent $800 for the care of patient Rose Wash. Hummer didn't have much luck pursuing additional sums from other financially comfortable patients. When Hummer saw that John Gray Blanket had nearly $2,000 in his reservation account, he asked Commissioner Rhoads to authorize payments for the patient's care from it. Rhoads politely told Hummer that the asylum had ample funds for patients' support and that John Gray Blanket's individual funds should be for his personal use.

The Depression didn't just tighten the federal budget, Hummer discovered. It also called into question the need for a separate asylum for Indians. Inspections in 1932 did not so much criticize Hummer's management as they did the state of the asylum itself, with its inadequate buildings, lack of staff, and outdated methods of care.

When he came out to inspect it, Indian school administrator John

H. Holst sarcastically called the asylum "a magnificent political gesture." In a biting condemnation of its usefulness, Holst said that "a heterogeneous number of human derelicts are herded in and practically forgotten." Echoing Edwards's and Silk's complaints, Holst found Hummer's record-keeping appalling, telling Commissioner Rhoads that there was no classification of cases, "no attempt to discover causes or effect cures or mitigate conditions in any scientific way," and ended up calling the institution medieval.

Though Holst found little to like about Canton Asylum, he found Hummer to be genial, optimistic and efficient, and "a man whose enthusiasm for the service has hardly been dampened by twenty-four years of futility and unremitting drudgery."

Bending over backward to be fair, Holst detailed the condition of the buildings and the inadequacy of funds for maintenance and support, along with the staff shortages that contributed largely to the conditions he had found. He made a number of practical recommendations, chief among them that the asylum put in place some sort of eligibility requirements that would help them intelligently select which patients to accept, rather than adhere to the willy-nilly, convenience-based method they were using.[6]

Charles T. Lowndes, a member of the Board of Indian Commissioners, inspected the asylum in November and made his report a month later. He repeated much of Holst's lament but gave his added ominous opinion that the asylum's patients should be transferred to St. Elizabeths. There, they could still be housed in a separate building while enjoying the economies of scale and modern, specialized care that St. Elizabeths' staff could provide.[7]

Lowndes made it clear that he didn't expect any changes until the country's difficult financial times were over, which at the bleak end of 1932 did not seem to be on the horizon anytime soon. Justifiably concerned, though, Hummer told the Canton Chamber of Commerce in January 1933 that he wasn't sure about the future of the asylum unless its members helped him. Hummer asked the chamber members to appeal to their senators and congressmen for an expansion of the facility. Canton's businessmen pledged to act on his recommendation—jobs in Canton were just as precious as they were anywhere else in the jobless country.

Despite the pervasive economic gloom across the country, a growing number of people began to believe that better days were ahead. Franklin Delano Roosevelt had just won the presidential election, and he took office on March 4, 1933. His first hundred days were a whirlwind of activity that began when he called Congress into an emergency session. Between March 8 and June 16, FDR and his supporters created the Civilian Conservation Corps, the Public Works Administration, and the Tennessee Valley Authority, amid a mass of emergency legislation. FDR also instituted his fireside chats during this time, to let the nation know what he was doing to help them as he solidified the New Deal. Urgent to get America back to work, FDR picked, persuaded, and prodded the best people to help him do it, cleaned his political house, and chose his cabinet.

John Collier saw a golden opportunity here, and the race was on to find a new commissioner of Indian affairs to work with whoever would be FDR's new secretary of the interior. The leading contender for the commissioner position was Edgar Meritt, who had built a network of political allies over the years that he had been assistant commissioner. His powerful friends rose to the occasion and pressured FDR to give him the job. The Indian Rights Association wanted to see Rhoads continue as commissioner, while Senators Sam Bratton and Burton Wheeler supported Harry Mitchell from Montana as commissioner and Reuben Perry (Meritt's campaign manager) as his assistant. Collier definitely wanted Meritt out of the race. He was also concerned by candidates for the position who were associated with the previous Republican administrations that had been so disastrous for the Indians.

Collier drew up a list of potential candidates for commissioner, including the former Chicago attorney Harold L. Ickes, Charles de Y. Elkus, Lewis Meriam, Nathan Margold (who had served as legal advisor to the Pueblos), and Senator Joseph O'Mahoney of Wyoming. Collier hastened to make sure his good friend Ickes, in particular, met Roosevelt in time to be considered for the job. Ickes wasn't a national figure, but he had championed the Indian cause for many years and wanted to be commissioner. With the help of Professor Raymond Moley from Columbia University, Collier arranged an interview between Ickes and FDR.[8] Ickes got a surprise when he met with the president: FDR asked him to become secretary of the interior rather than commissioner of Indian affairs. The appointment was a good one from Collier's point of view, but it left the commissioner's position still vacant.

Ickes felt that Collier would be a good candidate for the job, though the latter was reluctant to accept the position. Collier wrote to Lewis Meriam and Nathan Margold; between the three, they agreed that if Roosevelt would consider one of them for the job, the other two would back off and support the decision. Collier also wrote to the governors of the many pueblos and urged them to take part in the selection process. The All Pueblo Council concurred with a resolution addressed to Roosevelt that favored Collier as the new commissioner. The board of directors of the American Indian Defense Association also endorsed Collier, and with Ickes firmly backing him, Collier was presented as the Interior Department's candidate for commissioner of Indian affairs. At the same time, Ickes publicly stated that he would refuse to submit any other candidates for positions requiring Senate confirmation until it had confirmed Collier.

Meritt's friends and Collier's enemies presented powerful opposition to Ickes's proposal, but FDR wasn't ready to back down. He brought Ickes together with Collier's chief obstacle, Senator Joseph Taylor Robinson. Robinson strongly supported his brother-in-law, Meritt, for commissioner of Indian affairs, and FDR gave him a chance to make a case for his candidate. A fully prepared Ickes deftly refuted it, often using Meritt's own words to demonstrate how unsuitable he was for the job in Washington's changed atmosphere. Robinson capitulated and withdrew his support for Meritt under pressure from Roosevelt, and on April 21, 1933, John Collier took office as commissioner of Indian affairs.

Collier was familiar with the Indian Office and how it worked but still needed time to develop a program. Disinclined to sit at a desk in Washington DC, Collier went out west. While at Santa Clara Pueblo in July, he met Severa Tafoya, the wife of an old friend, who begged Collier to help her husband. Cleto Tafoya had worked as a gatekeeper at Tuye Cliff Ruins on the Santa Clara reservation until he began to show signs of a religious mania of some sort. A Catholic, he carried water to his bed and made the sign of the cross over it. Witnesses said he wanted to baptize others and sometimes appeared dazed, as though emerging from a religious fit or spell. In 1930 Tafoya was ordered to

Canton Asylum at the request of Santa Fe officials, where Hummer diagnosed him with dementia praecox, paranoid type.[9]

Tafoya's enemies may have had a hand in his commitment. Native Americans often tried to earn money by selling craftwork to tourists, and unscrupulous non-natives muscled in on the market by setting up "trading posts" that sold cheaper, factory-made goods as authentically handcrafted items. The Maisel Company was the focus of many complaints, which eventually brought the company before the Federal Trade Commission in 1931. Tafoya's wife was a skilled pottery maker who later became well known for her work, and it is very probable that Tafoya was a vocal protester against Maisel's factory-made goods. His convenient committal to an asylum may have resulted from his protests.[10]

Collier had considered his friend Tafoya as one of the brightest of the Pueblo Indians, and he promised Severa he would investigate the matter when he returned from his tour. Not long after his conversation with Tafoya's wife, Collier went back to Washington DC and kept his promise.[11]

That's when the Silk Report landed on his desk. Collier was a fallible man with his share of detractors, but no one disputed his passionate concern for the welfare of America's Indian population. He was shocked by the report. He also read Lowndes's 1932 follow-up report, which showed that little had changed. Collier's shock turned to outrage. "I find that we are conducting an institution so outrageously cruel and injurious that we would deserve to be blown out of the water if we continue it," Collier told Ickes.

Collier did not propose to dally around with the problem for twenty-five years like his predecessors. He immediately spoke to St. Elizabeths' superintendent—perhaps more forcefully than former secretary of the interior Wilber had—because White now agreed to receive Canton Asylum's patients almost immediately. Collier began to look for money to build a separate structure at St. Elizabeths for them and suggested Ickes use funds from the public works program.

Collier declared that Canton should be abolished entirely and its personnel discharged, and he moved to make it happen. After just another few weeks of negotiations, it was settled: if Ickes could free up the money, White would be ready to receive Canton's patients by the first day of 1934. That was exactly what Collier recommended on

August 4, 1933. Out west, Hummer was elected grand commander of the Knights Templar of South Dakota on August 9, and it was possibly the last nice thing that happened to him that year.

Collier moved forward. Before the end of the month, he requested legal advice from the Interior Department's Office of the Solicitor on the issue of transferring patients to St. Elizabeths. Acting Solicitor Charles Fahy advised Collier that the language in the relevant statutes was general enough that it was "quite plain" that the commissioner of Indian affairs had the authority to manage *all* Indian affairs.[12]

An act of 1904 directed that insane Indians in Indian Territory be cared for at Canton, but since Indian Territory no longer existed, the secretary of the interior could provide for insane Indians' care anywhere he wanted. The only question about sending them to St. Elizabeths derived from the fact that they were not citizens of the District of Columbia. However, since the secretary of the interior had authority to transfer the residence of Indians, he could certainly establish their residence in the District of Columbia.

With the legalities settled, Collier sent Dr. Silk back to the institution to make another survey and to classify the patients so they could be properly transferred. He copied Hummer on Silk's letter and directed him to be available to facilitate Silk's visit. The Indian Office made arrangements with the Chicago, Milwaukee, and St. Paul Railroad for an extra train to go to Canton (which specified a breakfast for patients of cereal, eggs, bread and butter, and beverage at sixty cents per capita). It would pick up the ninety patients and twenty-five attendants (some of the latter going to Canton from St. Elizabeths) and accompany them back to Washington DC.

When Silk arrived in Canton on September 6, he found the same dismaying conditions as on his former visit except that the wards were somewhat cleaner. Silk began to examine the asylum's patients and to wade through poorly kept records with little information. The more he learned, the more appalled he became. Hummer could tell him next to nothing about various patients' behaviors or the events that had led to their commitment. In a number of cases where patients were accused of assault within the institution, Hummer didn't know any details of the assaults, even for patients who had been there half a dozen years or more.

During previous inspections, Hummer had been able to rely on his expertise as a psychiatrist to keep any probing medical questions at bay. He could no longer shield his mismanagement and inadequacies under this professional veneer. Silk—St. Elizabeths' clinical director—could run circles around him as a psychiatrist. And he was on the spot with *his* expertise to give a more uncompromising version of Hummer's convenient diagnoses.

Silk discovered that many patients had been sent to the asylum because of problems at a school or agency, such as a fight with a white man or spousal assault. Once at Canton Asylum, they had exhibited normal behavior and often worked at tasks on the farm or in the dairy, kitchen, or various other places, with little or no supervision. They couldn't read or write, however, so Hummer called them mentally deficient and told the Indian Office that there had been "no improvement in their mental condition."

Silk took exception to this policy and asked White, "Should they be judged by the standards of the upper class of cultured white people? Is it fair to keep them at Canton because some minor difficulty landed them there?"

Silk backed up his observations with examples. Emma Amyotte, while residing in Canada in 1923, had had a stroke. Because she was an American Indian, she eventually landed in Canton Asylum on October 15, 1923. The U.S. commissioner of immigration sent Hummer a copy of a letter he had received from Canadian officials. It stated that the medical superintendent at the Ponoka Hospital (where Amyotte had been treated) reported on the ninth of October that she was in excellent physical health. Additionally, she had been "very well mentally for the past three month, and in his opinion it will not be necessary to have her committed to any institution." Hummer ignored the letter and kept her at the institution, going on now for ten years.

Patient William Deroin, a blind paraplegic suffering from syphilis, entered Canton Asylum in 1931. Hummer tentatively diagnosed him with a syphilitic condition (locomotor ataxia) but didn't perform either a blood or spinal fluid test to confirm it. Deroin had received treatment for syphilis at the hospital where he stayed before his transfer, but at the asylum Hummer did nothing for him. Silk wrote that the patient "just spends his time lying helpless in bed. He is frequently left alone on the ward unattended, the ward being locked from the outside with a padlock. . . . Mr. Deroin does not show any mental symptoms."

Hummer had a quick defense for Silk's contention that many of his patients showed few signs of any active mental disease or other striking abnormalities. He not only agreed, he further admitted that many of these patients could take care of themselves, "especially on an Indian reservation," where they would presumably be somewhat protected.

However, even if the patients were not insane, they were still mentally deficient, said Hummer, and "should only be discharged after they were sterilized." Since he didn't have the means to sterilize them, Hummer felt there was nothing left for him to do but keep them in the asylum.

Hummer performed no sputum tests on suspected tubercular patients, and Silk observed three with active coughs and loss of weight that would point to such a diagnosis. Highly contagious if they indeed had tuberculosis, the three mingled freely with other patients. Silk also pointed out another matter that was minor in itself but showcased Hummer's poor management. The hospital had a refrigerating plant for keeping food, said Silk, but no ice. When a patient ran a fever, the nurse had to run to Dr. Hummer's home "and beg a few ice cubes from Mrs. Hummer."

Patients were still padlocked in their rooms all too frequently, and Silk described how a male attendant with one month's experience locked a number of patients in their room, then locked the entire ward, so he could go eat his meals. One day during Silk's visit, a nurse and a male attendant—the only caretakers on duty—both went to lunch at the same time and locked all the wards from the outside. Certain patients were additionally locked in their rooms so they wouldn't fight.

Hummer never allowed patients to go home on trial visits, though these kinds of furloughs had been accepted by other superintendents for many years. Hummer also admitted that though he discharged about ten patients a year, nine of the ten were usually discharged through death. Since many of his patients had chronic illness or were elderly, this statistic is not as damning as it seems at face value. Many other institutions shared in that situation, since asylums were becoming custodial institutions for chronic patients, rather than hospitals where acute cases of insanity might recover.

Though little could excuse the medical negligence he saw, Silk noted in fairness that Hummer faced some insurmountable hardships in managing the institution, mainly due to the unsuitable buildings he had to use. Per capita costs would have to be extraordinarily high to give patients even adequate care, said Silk. He pointed out that there was general agreement in the field that no institution with fewer than five hundred patients could operate economically.[13]

Collier may have given Canton Asylum a political death sentence, but Silk's second report was the medical nail in the asylum's coffin. However, rumors about the purpose of Silk's visit had already circulated in town and its leaders were ready and waiting to take action. They launched an aggressive counteroffensive within a day of Silk's arrival at the asylum, pulling their state politicians into the fray as point men.

Collier was the fourth person to recommend closing Canton Asylum (Secretery of the interior Ray Wilbur had recommended its closure after the first Silk report, while Holst and Lowndes had felt the same way after their inspections in 1932) and the sixth person to recommend Hummer's dismissal. Charles L. Davis had recommended it in 1909, Dr. Joseph Murphy concurred in 1910, someone else of influence in the Indian Office recommended that Hummer be replaced in 1915 in the aftermath of the Landis investigation, Dr. Emil Krulish recommended a change in superintendents in 1929, and Secretary Wilbur had wanted Hummer replaced as well. But . . . Hummer was still superintendent of Canton Asylum. He must have been confident that this was just one more round in a battle that resumed every few years.

The fight began with a flurry of telegrams on September 8, 1933. Canton attorney Claude A. Bennett wired Ickes that the asylum had been created by an act of Congress and could be closed only through another act of Congress. Congressman Fred H. Hildebrandt sent a telegram to Ickes to relay that the citizens of Canton were protesting the closure because it would deprive them of a $40,000 annual payroll. Senator W. J. Bulow sent Collier a telegram asking him to postpone his decision until he met with Canton citizens. Senator Peter Norbeck asked for a stay of ten days to present facts against a closure.

Collier informed Silk of the telegrams a day after he received them. He told Silk he would allow the ten-day delay Senator Norbeck had requested, noting that at least that amount of time would pass before the transfer could begin, anyway.

Bennett had followed his telegram with a long letter detailing the reasons the asylum should stay open—in Canton—and included his prediction that the Republicans who had voted for FDR would be angered by such a move as closure of the institution. Ickes replied to Bennett and Norbeck, stating calmly that the numerous reports on the matter pointed to the fact that the physical structure of the asylum itself was a large part of the problem. He made it plain that it would be cost-prohibitive to bring the institution up to acceptable standards.

Hummer asked Collier to visit the asylum, but Collier replied that he could not really say when he could come. "Since measures are now under way for the transfer of the Canton patients to St. Elizabeth's Hospital, Washington, DC, and the closing of the Canton Asylum in the reasonably near future is contemplated, it is not thought that a visit there now is feasible," Collier replied. Both the secretary and the commissioner had made their positions clear.[14]

With a delegation from Canton on its way to Washington, Silk had an extra ten days to study conditions at the asylum. Of the ninety patients he examined, Silk believed only twenty-five to thirty were actually insane. About twenty showed no signs of *any* mental trouble, another twenty were mildly affected and could live on a reservation or with relatives with just a little supervision, and twenty to twenty-five patients were mentally deficient—without psychosis—and needed to live in a home for the feebleminded rather than in an insane asylum.

The extended stay was awkward for Silk as persona non grata and the town's unwanted center of attention. Newspaper articles both discussed and denounced the closure while Silk patiently waited out the uproar and went ahead with his arrangements to transfer patients. He became particularly involved with the cases of Logan Lovejoy and Reuben Taylor at Collier's request and discharged them to their relatives. Meanwhile, Collier met with the South Dakota delegation, refused to keep Canton Asylum open, and telegraphed Silk to get ready to move patients on September 25.

On September 23, Silk was served an injunction issued by Justice James D. Elliot of the U.S. District Court in Sioux Falls. The injunction restrained him from removing patients from Canton Asylum. The court order included restraints against John Collier, Harry Hummer, and their agents and employees.

Hummer's defensive mechanism against the Indian Office had been a time-tested combination of acting passive-aggressively on any problem, standing on his expertise as a psychiatrist, and bending the truth to his advantage. In this instance, Hummer performed his first maneuver admirably by wiring Collier about the injunction as though it had come as a complete surprise to him.

G. J. Moen, head of the Canton Chamber of Commerce and a guardian for patient Albert Blaine Jr., had engineered the injunction. Silk believed that Hummer both knew about it and had likely aided Moen in obtaining it. Silk wrote a letter to Dr. White that same day, saying, "This is of course all the work of D. Hummer—he was in Sioux Falls all day yesterday and only this morning I heard him give the name of the patient Albert Blaine to someone over the phone."[15]

A court date was set for a month later, October 23, so Silk and the seven attendants who had just arrived to escort the patients received permission to leave South Dakota and return to St. Elizabeths. The situation was certainly on Silk's mind, for he fired off another letter to Dr. White on the twenty-fourth, reiterating that the injunction had been completed with Hummer's knowledge.

Obviously irate, Silk offered White a plan to close the institution another way: simply have Collier transfer Hummer somewhere else in the Indian Service and replace him with another field service physician. Since only about ten cases at the asylum had been committed via insanity hearings before a court, Silk felt the replacement physician could simply return the other patients to their reservations. Silk ended his letter by telling White that he had just received a phone call ordering him to be at the U.S. attorney's office in Sioux Falls the next morning.

Silk, who had expected to be in Canton only a few days, wrote in exasperation, "I am quite fed up with Canton, Dr. Hummer, the Indians and everything else that goes with it." He was out of clean clothes and had nothing warm to wear but was willing to stick it out a little longer if needed. "I fear that Dr. Hummer and his friends are not going to give up this battle so easily," he finished bleakly.

Hummer had rarely encountered anyone in the Indian Service who had actually become angry over his affairs, but the current commissioner was quite angry at Moen's trickery and knew about Hummer's role in it. Collier sent Moen a sharp note as a matter of public record. He called Moen out for asking for a ten-day delay: "You asked and received an excessive courtesy, more than was due you," said Collier, and told him that he had abused that courtesy.[16]

Collier's ire may have stung Moen a bit, but the latter had still gained a solid victory for the asylum. The *Sioux Valley News* crowed triumphantly, describing the legal battle as it might a prize fight:

FIRST ROUND: Collier darted from his corner in a surprise attack...

SECOND ROUND: ... his opponent countered by securing a ten-day stay, stopping Collier in his tracks.

THIRD ROUND: Moen parried with a trip to Washington and ... jabbed in another five-day stay which busted up Collier's plan of attack and left him wide open and unguarded.

FOURTH ROUND: Moen slipped in a haymaker to the jaw in the form of a federal court injunction which tied Collier's hands, sent him rocking on his heels and left him gasping for breath.[17]

As supporters vigorously kept up their attack, opponents of the asylum also began to move. Helen Groth, who had been so surprised to discover that she was insane after collapsing from overwork, wrote to J. E. Hoover, director of the Division of Investigation in the Department of Justice, to detail her experience with Dr. Hummer:

After all that had transpired, I was nearly paralyzed with fright and refused to go the Asylum at Canton where Hummer was to examine me. Finally Hummer came into the court house at Canton where he questioned me for ½ hour or so, insulted my mother who was with me, thumbing his nose at her and asking if she would rather go back to her home in Missouri or with me, where I was going for about six months "hospitalization." His entire manner was one of burly brutality, insolence and co-operation with the doctor who had advised my unsuspecting husband to take me there.

Groth finished her letter with the exhortation, "Move them [the patients] to Washington where intelligent people are interested in science and progress."[18]

Others who had been misused by Hummer jumped in. G. W. Karlson wrote to Silk about his own experience: "On June 30, 1932 Dr. Hummer acting as a member of the Lincoln County Insanity Board and F. J. Cooper Judge of said County had me taken from my place of business, staged a fake examination on my mentality and had me removed to the State Hospital for the Insane [at Yankton]."

Karlson explicitly blamed Hummer for the episode. After being released from the hospital, Karlson tried to find records concerning the complaint against him without success. He initiated a petition to the governor to have his name cleared but quickly found himself once more before Hummer and Cooper. That same night, he was back in the state hospital.

Thirty-three responsible men from Canton signed a petition to the governor stating that Karlson was not insane, but Karlson told Silk that nothing happened until "Judge Cooper in later part of March was arrested for taking the Widows pension fund. The Superintendent became alarmed and let me go."

Karlson was bitter about his treatment and offered his services to Silk. He had heard that Hummer wanted a trial and felt that "in the interests of humanity, Doctor H. R. Hummer should be restrained for all time to come from ever again to give a professional opinion of the mentality of any Red, White, or Black person."[19]

Despite the efforts of people like Groth and Karlson, by the end of September all appeared well at Canton Asylum once more. Silk and the attendants from St. Elizabeths were gone, the Canton delegation had returned from Washington, and the town's delaying tactics and injunction had proven effective. The Canton Chamber of Commerce even upped the ante by writing directly to FDR, appealing to him to stop Collier from closing the asylum. All three hundred chamber members agreed that Dr. Silk's report was false.

Hummer even felt comfortable writing to an agent at C. M. Youman's Lumber Company in Canton that the commissioner of Indian affairs had informed a delegation from Canton that if the asylum didn't close, he was prepared to obtain $250,000 for the asylum from the Public Works Fund. (Hummer was replying to a letter from the agent, which referenced an eight-point letter of Collier's, now unavailable, but probably written to the chamber of commerce.)

Hummer reiterated the idea that the asylum could be closed only by an act of Congress, saying that the Indian Office had endeavored to close the institution four years earlier and couldn't, because of that provision. Hummer ended his letter by charging the Indian Office with trying to "railroad the patients to St. Elizabeths while Congress is not in session." He stated that he welcomed a congressional investigation into the Indian Office and that "there are certain facts in my possession that would embarrass them to a very great degree."

Hummer's letter to the lumberman made its way to Senator Henrik Shipstead, who forwarded it to Collier. Collier immediately made it plain to Shipstead that he had said the opposite: that there were already facilities that could care for the Indians in the best possible way without new expenditures and that he wasn't seeking funds to reconstruct the asylum.[20]

Silk's second report was already in Collier's hands, though, and it was disturbing on any number of levels. One condition that Silk underscored was the dubiousness of Hummer's diagnoses: Silk believed that about twenty patients were actually sane. Agnes Caldwell, admitted as "rather fussy, discontented, irritable, refuses to work at times, limited mentality," had been characterized by Hummer himself ever since as "usually quiet and well behaved . . . no mannerisms, correctly oriented, memory fair, education limited, judgment undeveloped, no delusions or hallucinations but is over-sexed. Mentally she is deficient." Based on this assessment, Caldwell had been confined at Canton Asylum for the past sixteen years. Others that Silk specifically mentioned were kept at the asylum based on even flimsier observations.

Hummer may have fallen into a little indulgent daydreaming about the $250,000 he thought his asylum might receive from the commissioner, but he was positively unbalanced if he thought he would remain in charge to spend it. A week after giving his hopeful prognosis to the lumberman, Hummer received a communication that brought him down to earth with a thud.

In a terse letter, Collier informed Hummer that various inspections—with supporting detail—showed that he had permitted "an incredibly bad condition to exist and continue" at the asylum. Collier made it plain that these conditions existed outside and beyond any that could be attributed to old buildings or lack of funds. The commissioner spelled it out: Hummer had allowed attendants to lock Indians in rooms without attendants to rescue them in case of fire, had chained them to beds and water pipes, and had neglected their cleanliness and health in the most fundamental ways. Furthermore, he had kept sane patients in the asylum. Collier accused Hummer of misfeasance and malfeasance "of an extreme character" and gave him five days to refute the charges.[21]

This is where Collier made it plain that Hummer was out of his league when it came to an all-out scrap with the government. As a reformer, Collier had been in many such battles over the years and was in dead earnest with this one. If Hummer and his cohorts thought they could breathe easy until the injunction hearing on October 23, they now found they were badly mistaken. Hummer may have drummed up some favorable publicity for himself in Canton, but Collier had used the power of publicity many times in his own fights with the government. Now he and Ickes launched a counterattack at a national level.

On October 14, 1933, the Department of the Interior issued a press release detailing the most sensational of the asylum's shortcomings. Even as Interior Secretary Ickes released information about Hummer's imminent dismissal, he included facts about Silk's investigation, the dreadful conditions at Canton Asylum, and the town of Canton's efforts to delay the transfer of the Indian patients to St. Elizabeths.

The release gave everyone involved on the Canton side a public black eye and made it next to impossible for any politician to defend keeping the asylum open. Suddenly, Senator Norbeck was asking Collier only to let Hummer retire without prejudice; any further assistance would have had the senator defending the asylum against headlines that screamed "Sane Indians in Asylum" and "Canton Asylum Conditions 'Sickening', Director Says: Indians 'Chained to Pipes.'"[22]

"Lies!" Hummer shouted back to the headlines. He sputtered that the charges were all "politics" and that he was considering asking for what had to be the worst possible thing he could think of: a congressional investigation. Hummer's rebuttal came a day after headlines across the nation spilled out the Interior Department's charges. A day after that, Ickes acted on the charges Collier had made and dismissed Hummer from government service.

Others still fought for the asylum. Six thousand Indians from around the country met at the Rosebud Reservation (South Dakota) on October 14–15 to elect a committee to gather signatures for a petition to the federal court. Led by William J. Bordeaux, the group hoped to obtain thirty thousand Indian signatures to act as a powerful voice against the asylum's closure.[23] Activists could not secure the required signatures, and Clement Valandra, a member of the Board of Advisors, Rosebud Sioux Council, publicly refuted Bordeaux's authority as any kind of committee member acting on behalf of the Sioux Council. Naming the real members of the Board of Advisors to the Rosebud Sioux Council, Valandra said, "We, the committee, have decided not to take part in this scrap."[24]

Economic benefit to the city aside, some Indians had legitimate reasons for wanting the asylum to remain in Canton. Washington DC represented a tremendous financial and logistical challenge to family visits because of its great distance from the homes of most patients. Though many patients never received visits (Silk noted that only three patients had visitors during his three-week stay), those who did would almost assuredly find them curtailed if family members had to take on the expense of a train ticket to the East Coast. Another concern was the difference in climate between South Dakota and the District of Columbia. Though the district's climate was milder and more beneficial to patients in ill health, the atmosphere was more humid and oppressive than South Dakota's. Finally, many Indians experienced with the horrors of the boarding school system could not feel comfortable seeing helpless patients shipped east, where they knew so many helpless children had died of tuberculosis and been mistreated.

Despite these concerns, Collier and Ickes made it clear that the problems at Canton Asylum could not be resolved by merely retrofitting it with better buildings. Ickes wrote to Representative Fred H. Hildebrandt in explanation: "If the Canton Asylum were to be maintained, a large new investment in plant would be necessary. The facilities and means for the treatment of the patients would still be greatly inferior to those now accessible at St. Elizabeths Hospital."

Ickes pointedly stated that the asylum had been a mistake from the beginning and that the mistake should have been remedied years early. He then continued, "The treatment of the patients at the Canton Asylum is not merely inadequate; it is excessively and indefensibly inadequate. The fault lies in part with personnel, but in part it is a deficiency of plant which could only be remedied by a large new investment. That investment is not justified either from the standpoint of government economy or of Indian need."[25]

Dr. L. L. Culp, special physician in the Indian Service at Large, was told to report immediately to Canton Asylum to assume administrative duties there. Driving home Hummer's utter defeat was a second notification: James W. Balmer, superintendent of the Pipestone School in Minnesota, was detailed to proceed to Canton immediately to give Hummer a receipt for all funds and property under his charge and to turn him out. No matter what happened at the injunction hearing, the asylum was effectively closed. More importantly, Hummer was no longer a force at the institution he had ruled for twenty-five years.

It was a cleanup operation after that. Hummer sputtered and fumed and immediately retained E. C. Mahoney, a Sioux Falls attorney. The former superintendent demanded a hearing concerning the charges against him, but the matter was already closed. Ickes and Collier stood firm. The federal government filed a brief to dismiss Moen's injunction suit against the removal of Indian patients, and federal district judge James D. Elliot overturned the injunction without demur. And finally, a White House executive order stated that "the functions of the Canton Asylum [are] to be transferred to St. Elizabeths Hospital, and that the Canton Asylum be abolished."[26]

Hummer accepted his defeat and moved to Sioux Falls in November. He promptly opened an office "for the treatment of mental and nervous diseases" in the Citizens National Bank & Trust Company building.[27]

On Wednesday, December 20, 1933, a doctor from the Indian Service and three attendants from Washington arrived in Canton on the 9:30 a.m. passenger train. They called Dr. Culp and told him to start making arrangements to remove the Indian patients. At 6:00 p.m. they began to help patients board the train, and by 7:00 p.m. sixty-nine patients and fourteen attendants from Canton were ready to go. At least a hundred Canton residents gathered to watch the death of "the only institution of its kind in the world."[28]

Epilogue

Sixty-nine patients from Canton Asylum were admitted to St. Elizabeths on December 22, 1933, and two others who had been too ill to travel were admitted six days later.[1] Only nine of the patients had any kind of court records that showed a legal commitment. Seventeen Canton patients were released as sane, including the unfortunate Edith Schroder, Peter Kentuck, Emma Amyotte, and Agnes Caldwell. One of the sane seventeen, Rosa Bite, died at the age of thirty-four of advanced pulmonary tuberculosis a day before she would have been free.

Dr. Culp sent Collier a plot of Canton Asylum's cemetery, along with names, ages, dates of death, and tribal designation, and told the commissioner that he had marked the graves and erected a "substantial wire fence with iron posts" around the plot.[2] He recommended either erecting permanent markers or exhuming the bodies and sending the remains to homes or home reservations. There were 121 graves, with one holding both a mother and her two-month-old baby. Neither markers nor exhumation were forthcoming.

The asylum was largely abandoned for several years, though in 1934 South Dakota governor Tom Berry signed a lease with the federal government permitting the property's use as a penitentiary. The lease was not long, and a farmer then leased the land for approximately ten years. According to local witnesses, he used the main building as a granary and kept hogs in the asylum basement. In 1946 the federal government deeded the land (to be used only for public purposes or revert to the federal government) and the asylum's buildings to the city of Canton. Several buildings were sold to the Canton Hospital Association and to the Augustana Academy Association. A dormitory, Hofstad Hall, was built with granite and slate from the razed main asylum building. Hummer's prized cottage was moved to Newton Hills State Park, South Dakota, in 2006, where it can be rented by the public.

Citizens in Canton and Inwood voted in 1947 to establish a joint community hospital at the site, and after remodeling, the old hospital reopened in May 1949 as the Canton-Inwood Memorial Hospital. In 2008 Sanford Health purchased the hospital, clinics, and assisted living center, which became the Sanford Canton-Inwood Medical Center and Sanford Health Hiawatha Heights Living Center.

The city also developed a municipal golf course (Hiawatha Golf Course) around the cemetery, which fell into neglect. Only a single grave marker between the fourth and fifth holes stated the names of those buried there, and golfers sometimes hit balls off the graves. Finally they instituted a rule that if a ball landed on a grave, the player could take a free drop and play the shot outside the cemetery.

In 1988 the late Harold Iron Shield, a member of the Lakota Nation's Yankton tribe, initiated memorial services for the dead at the cemetery. The ceremony became an annual event, during which golfers stopped play. Iron Shield, also a member of the Native American Reburial Restoration Committee, pursued recognition of the cemetery as a national historical site. The Canton Asylum for American Indians Cemetery was added to the National Register of Historical Places (#98000074) in 1998.

Cleto Tafoya, whose commitment had sparked the asylum's closure, was released from St. Elizabeths six months later, on June 1, 1934. He returned to Santa Clara Pueblo and by 1935 was the secretary of its election board and a signer of the pueblo's constitution.[3] He became governor of Santa Clara Pueblo and later (1947) worked as a chef at Los Alamos National Laboratory in New Mexico.[4] Tafoya must have been pleased when Secretary of the Interior Ickes later stepped in on the battle that had probably landed Tafoya in Canton Asylum. Ickes asked in the late 1930s for a ruling that only *handmade* Indian crafts could be sold in national parks.[5]

Dr. Harry Reid Hummer landed on his feet after his defeat at Canton Asylum. He and his wife initially lived in an apartment after moving to Sioux Falls but bought a home on North Euclid Street in 1935, where they remained until Hummer died. He was elected secretary of the Seventh District Medical Society in 1936 and, beginning in 1947, served five years as a staff consultant at the Sioux Falls Veterans Hospital. He retired in 1954 and died on August 28, 1957, at the age of seventy-eight after an unspecified illness of several months. He was survived by his sons, Francis, a doctor, and Harry Jr., a retired rear admiral who received a Legion of Merit in 1943 for his service while commanding the destroyer USS *McLanahan* during World War II; by his wife of fifty-six years, Norena; and by a sister, brother, and four grandchildren. He was interred in the Congressional Cemetery in Washington DC on September 1, 1957, and Norena Hummer joined him on October 8, 1962.

Afterthoughts

Some readers may say that the history of the Canton Asylum for Insane Indians is a Native American story, which only a Native American should tell. I disagree, believing instead that it is a societal story that reveals much about the culture and time in which it occurred. In addition to Native Americans, government employees, policy makers, educators, medical personnel, reformers, caregivers, politicians, and others were involved in Canton's story. A qualified person with an interest in any of these areas would be able to shed an interesting—and perhaps entirely different—light on the Native American/U.S./South Dakotan/medical/political history that occurred there. My own special interest lay in the time period and in medical history, particularly the study of insanity; my graduate thesis concerned insane asylums in Appalachia and was a long study on the evolution of care for the insane.

Few people would be qualified in every respect to write about Canton Asylum. I have never worked in an insane asylum, though coincidentally enough my parents met and fell in love at the Chicago State Hospital, the former Cook County Insane Asylum, in the late 1940s. I worked in a nursing home just as I turned eighteen, and found it a job that has continued to enlighten me long afterward. I was untrained, fearful, young, and out of my comfort zone when I showed up for work that first day. Bedridden or disoriented "old people" were almost as foreign to me as a teenager as insane patients would have been to staff in a remote part of the West. Here I have to admit to a less than laudable affinity with Canton Asylum's staff: I worked in that nursing home simply because it was the only job available and the day shift included a free meal. Most asylum attendants probably worked for the same selfish reasons rather than from any call to higher purpose.

My experience at the nursing home gave me insight into Canton's situation in a way few other jobs could have done. A number of my elderly patients were strong and violent, and I remember being afraid to approach anyone who had resolutely decided not to cooperate with me. I was fortunate in that I had the option of calling in more experienced staff for assistance. Though we were all stretched thin with far too much work, most of us could drop our own immediate tasks and help one another through difficulties. I am not convinced that staff at Canton Asylum ever had the same option, or had it very often. And of course, their patients were not confined merely to the elderly and (theoretically) infirm but included strong young men and women. Not all my patients were difficult, of course. I met residents who were personable and verbal enough to express *their* side of life in an institution, and I felt great sadness for their diminished boundaries and autonomy. This eye-opening experience as a youth has given me empathy for *all* of Canton Asylum's inhabitants.

Historians are charged not only with digging out information on their topic but also with evaluating, analyzing, and reconstructing the past through that information. Like many others who have been interested in Canton Asylum, I initially approached my examination with several preconceived ideas and plenty of judgment and blame. As I examined the records, researched the time period, and got a better feel for what the country was like at the turn of the twentieth century and through the early 1930s, my opinions changed. I began to see how complicated Canton Asylum was, how little even doctors knew about insanity or how to treat it, and how largely government policy lay at the heart of the situation.

I found many reasons why the Canton Asylum for Insane Indians failed so miserably. The asylum was never given enough money to run efficiently and well. Staff were untrained and largely uneducated until nurses came onto the scene late in in the asylum's existence. The Indian Office didn't support continuing education for Dr. Hummer or allow him to attend conferences where he might have stayed in touch with current psychiatric methods or found inspiration in his peers.

No provision was ever made for patient interpreters or cultural representatives. But these reasons are merely practical ones and the list is incomplete at that.

The overarching problem was that Indians had no political voice, and this underlying issue led to the real reason for Canton Asylum's failure. The federal government's assimilation mentality had dismissed Indian culture and concerns so completely that its solution to the problem of their (possible) insanity was unworkable. Until and unless the asylum could accommodate Native American languages, customs, worldviews, and culture, it was able to offer only the barest medical assistance to its patients. Under Hummer's care it scarcely offered that, and the institution continued to exist as it did because no one with enough power to rectify the situation cared enough to do so.

It is true that John Collier and Harold Ickes (probably) could not have closed the facility quite so quickly if they had arrived on the scene before reformers laid the groundwork necessary to make their point of view less radical. However, the idea that the country before 1933 was not ready to help Indian mental patients does not ring true as a reason for the asylum's continued existence and relentless decline.

Collier, Ickes, and numerous others helped lay the policy-changing groundwork that finally closed Canton Asylum, but it is unlikely that any of these reformers would have stood by in a position of power at any period and not intervened in the best way they could. And early on, one person in power, Commissioner of Indian Affairs Francis Luepp, did take appropriate action. He saw the inherent inadequacy of asking a layperson like Oscar Gifford to administer what was essentially a medical facility and replaced the asylum's nonmedical superintendent with a physician. He rode out a storm of protest and political intervention to enforce what he knew made sense. After that, no one stepped up to the responsibility and challenge of keeping the Canton Asylum for Insane Indians on track with its mission.

Despite claims to the contrary, there were numerous inspections by conscientious people who pointed out failures and made commonsense recommendations—including getting rid of Superintendent Hummer—that could have gotten the facility back on track or ended its existence. Supervisor Charles Davis recommended Hummer's dismissal as early as 1909, and Dr. Joseph Murphy's follow-up investigation in 1910 suggested that Hummer ought to resign because of the strength of negative feeling against him in the community. An indignant writer in the Indian Office (possibly Meritt) suggested in the aftermath of Dr. L. F. Michael's investigation into Ione Landis's charges that Hummer be suspended and Michael take temporary charge of the facility. Dr. Emil Krulish recommended a change in superintendents in 1929, as did Secretary of the Interior Ray Wilbur after Dr. Samuel Silk submitted his report. Nothing happened, though.

Throughout their tenures, both asylum superintendents pleaded for additional monies, which would have allowed them to run the institution—albeit according to their own lights and through their pet projects—more humanely, hygienically, and efficiently. The Indian Office (and Congress) repeatedly denied many of their reasonable requests. Chairman of the House Appropriations Committee Louis C. Cramton's eagerness to deny Indian children more than twenty cents a day for food clearly shows where the government's interests did *not* lie. When it came to the country's Indian population, there was never enough money even for basics like nutritious food, good health care, and social support. Indians were unimportant to most government officials in positions of power and authority.

Racism, misguided humanitarianism, muddled eugenic thought, and plain old politics had played a role in creating Canton Asylum. Indifference is what sustained it. Even worse, a complete failure to incorporate Native American cultural practices into its medical care guaranteed that the asylum would not help patients who needed to rely on a supportive network of trusted personnel and traditional practices to get well.

Some improvements in federal care have been made since that time. The Navajo surgeon Dr. Lori Arviso Alvord saw the difference it made to patients when a hospital occasionally allowed a medicine man to perform a ceremony at a patient's bedside. Some Indian Health Service clinics and hospitals later built kivas (holy ceremonial rooms) within their facilities, and Alvord adds that the National Institutes of Mental Health has even funded training for medicine men. Indian Health Service training now includes information about how to interact appropriately with patients; among other things, it advises medical staff to give body tissues such as toenails, scalp hair, and placental material back to patients so that they can be disposed of in a traditional way. The Department of Veterans Affairs supports Native American and Alaskan Native traditional practitioners and allows patients coordinating through its Chaplain Service to participate in such things as purification and sweat lodge ceremonies, formal healing ceremonies, talking circles, and vision quests. What might have happened at Canton Asylum if even the smallest concessions had been made to Native American sensibilities?

Many people of the time would not have recognized their cultural indifference, but today's observers often remark on both that and the heartlessness of the Canton Asylum experience. This heartlessness must also be brought into perspective.

At the time of Canton Asylum's operation, mentally ill people who did not recover quickly usually did not recover at all. Patients who missed timely intervention and a quick cure were almost always doomed to abandonment in an asylum. Insanity wasn't understood at all well during most of Canton Asylum's existence, as medical men tried to hammer out whether excessive studying, masturbation, epilepsy, internal lesions, faulty genetics, emotional experiences, and the like caused or contributed to insanity. Prevailing attitudes that considered an Anglo-based culture superior to others hurt *any* non-Anglo person accused of insanity, not just Native Americans. Though ill-advised and arrogant when considered through today's lens, the desire to uplift "inferior" cultures through education and assimilation was considered an enlightened view at the time.

Alienists had few medicines or methods to treat mental illness effectively, and after the first hopeful flush of asylum building, they lacked the time to divert and encourage patients into wellness through recreation and occupational therapy. Large institutions didn't have the opportunity to delve into psychoanalysis with patients when that practice began to show promise.

Later, up-and-coming psychiatrists wanted to move away from a hospital setting into private or clinical practice where they had a chance to work with acute and more generally curable cases. They gave asylums the leftovers—mainly elderly and chronic patients who couldn't be cured. Asylums across the country turned into warehouses rather than sanctuaries where patients could recover. The Canton Asylum experience—including abuse and neglect—was duplicated in greater or lesser degrees in many places.

Is any blame appropriate, then? Oscar Gifford, Canton's first superintendent, is certainly guilty of biting off more than he could chew. As a politician, he failed to analyze the exact content of his spoils before he accepted them. Gifford seems to have been an old-school frontiersman, comfortable with top-down, paternalistic Indian policy that always assumed educated whites knew what was better for native people than they did. Gifford was incompetent and out of his milieu running an insane asylum but didn't appear to bear any noteworthy prejudice or animosity toward his charges. With the proper background, he might have done a better job running Canton Asylum. But he didn't have the proper background, probably discovered the truth after a year or two, and yet chose to remain as the asylum's superintendent. That was clearly his weakness, his decision, and his mistake.

Dr. Harry Hummer is much more of a puzzle. Certainly, no one in a modern workplace would have wanted him as an employer. However, Hummer's era routinely installed and countenanced workplace tyrants. When unions gathered strength in the 1920s—organized in large part to protect workers from shockingly callous and dangerous working conditions—employers responded with calculated violence to destroy anything that threatened their power. The horrific Triangle Shirtwaist Factory fire in 1911 killed 146 people because managers locked the factory's doors to keep employees from taking unauthorized breaks or pilfering goods. Draconian methods of supervision were almost the norm. Superintendent Hummer's opportunities to indulge his pettiness and egotism reflect his time period almost as much as they do his flawed personality.

Several factors seem to have fed into Hummer's character. He had an immense desire to be respected and honored and found the perfect medium to satisfy these traits in the medical field. Moreover, he could feel assured of his superiority in an insane asylum, where "defectives" could not possibly rise to his level—unlike patients in a mere hospital might have. St. Elizabeths was a prestigious workplace, while the civil service gave him security. Because it catered to the military and was run somewhat along military lines, St. Elizabeths also provided an atmosphere of top-down authority along with the standards of behavior and ceremony Hummer enjoyed.

Even considering what he left behind, Hummer's move to South Dakota is quite understandable. Running his own facility was a step up for him despite Canton Asylum's comparative smallness. It *was* the only asylum of its kind in the world. And being in charge suited Hummer's personality. He may have gone west with the idea that he would put in his time, make a mark for himself as a superintendent, publish findings on whatever fieldwork he thought he could perform, and then return to the East with an improved chance for advancement.

Hummer was educated, ambitious, and obviously could be charming and gracious. At times he seemed to understand the difficulties his employees faced and worked hard to provide amenities that made their lives easier. Hummer was also intolerant of those he didn't consider his social equals, exacting to a fault, arrogant, egotistical, and highly strung—none of which made him guilty of running a bad asylum. Beyond that, he cared deeply about his reputation and demanded respect for his position and skills. How was it that he could allow an asylum with which he was so closely affiliated to fall into such discredit and disrepair? What made him stay in a situation that seemed to promise little but stress and aggravation?

Sheer perversity cannot be the entire answer, even if he had compelling reasons to "prove" himself either to his family or to former colleagues at St. Elizabeths. Instead, he probably felt certain during his first few years that he could make a huge difference in care at the asylum and that there was much he could study and contribute to his field. His paper at the 1912 Medico-Psychological Association conference proved he could get noticed for where he worked and what he did. That taste of fame beyond his workplace walls may have been the psychological carrot that inspired him for many years.

Hummer may also have been reluctant to leave the asylum under a cloud. Inspections that found fault with his facility made him dig in his heels all the harder, trying to deflect blame anywhere but toward himself. He would have felt disgraced to have left with a poor inspection held up as the reason for his departure.

Hummer still cut an admirable figure in his new community in terms of education and patronage. He obviously knew important people in Washington, returned there often for visits, and probably found himself much respected among his peers. Hummer grew comfortable. He eventually cultivated social ties with area organizations and compatible new colleagues. His sons were growing up in the West and likely enjoyed the life there. Hummer found a niche as an administrator who didn't have to bother much with medicine, ensconcing himself comfortably in his office with only necessary forays into patient affairs. He was well paid and had next to no competition in any area of his life. Hummer was a big fish in a small pond, a position many others have found attractive and desirable.

Though Harry Reid Hummer has often been held up as the epitome of indifference, mismanagement, and egotism, many in his own day and age would not have especially censured him. To be sure, inspectors sometimes thought he was a bad fit for the job, but they found little wrong with his morals and character. His bad temper was nearly legendary, and his views concerning employee loyalty and other management issues are almost ridiculous in retrospect. However, the West had room for strong-willed or larger-than-life characters, and in his early years, Hummer's actual administration of Canton Asylum was not always far removed from what his peers were doing.

Hummer was not the only superintendent who allowed restraints. His views concerning the sterilization of "defectives" were fairly mainstream, as evidenced by the many states that passed sterilization laws during his tenure at Canton Asylum. Also, mental institutions across the country—not just Canton Asylum—were turning into chronic care facilities whose patients had little hope of recovery.

Hummer could also point out that he had repeatedly requested more buildings and other necessary equipment over the years. Whether he was right or wrong in lumping all patients with seizures into one category, Hummer undeniably tried to get a separate building for those he called his epileptic patients. He gave time and attention to his livestock, tenaciously pursued moving picture equipment that he thought would bring his patients and staff pleasure, and tried over and over to acquire an amusement hall, chapel, and other amenities for the asylum. Even disapproving inspectors granted that the asylum's buildings and personnel left much to be desired. It would be fair to say that the odds were stacked against Hummer to some extent, since these two factors were ultimately beyond his control.

Not every deficiency at the asylum was Hummer's fault, nor were all failures in patient care. Records show that he promptly dismissed anyone on staff that he found engaged in immoral or egregious behavior. Though he could be faulted for the extent to which he tried to make employees behave exactly as he liked, Hummer seems to have acted quickly when abuse or other misconduct caught his attention. However, none of these observations implies that Hummer was not also *himself* guilty of neglect, abuse, and dereliction of duty.

Hummer had power and choice, and in that lies his blame. At no time did this well-educated psychiatric specialist ever seem to take a stand for his asylum, though he had almost absolute authority to admit or refuse patients. He allowed the asylum to fill with unfortunates who were not insane, to the detriment of the many he was charged with helping. Callous to the extreme, Hummer did not seem to consider for a moment how a person who was not insane would feel in a chaotic asylum, especially children. Worse, his files almost always held a backlog of applicants; Hummer could have afforded to choose patients who were actually insane rather than feebleminded, elderly, or merely troublesome or "immoral."

Hummer complained about epileptics and others who took up too much staff attention, yet Hummer is the one who allowed them in. Indian Office personnel showed time and again that they considered Hummer their expert on insanity—he could have made them follow his agenda. He could have made Canton Asylum a place *only* for the insane. Additionally, Hummer's discussion with Dr. Silk shows clearly that he did realize some patients weren't insane. But he overrode the demands of their sanity with a desire to keep them from reproducing. Hummer's alliance with eugenics took precedence over his responsibilities as a psychiatrist.

Hummer may have fallen into his era's mind-set that the dominant Anglo culture was superior to native ones, but he chose not to familiarize himself at all with his patients' cultures. That was a medical failing of the first magnitude if he honored his role as a physician of mental health. Hummer could have developed culturally appropriate ways of treating their insanity or of helping them to at least feel more comfortable in the asylum. Even nonpsychiatrists like Gifford and Turner did not dismiss their patients' desires to enjoy traditional pastimes like dancing and craft making.

The asylum operated under the boarding school model—which used interpreters—yet no records show that Hummer ever requested interpreters' services or made a case for needing them. Surely the Indian Office could have found someone to send Hummer on occasion, if he had only asked. Hummer could have hired someone temporarily to help him communicate with patients, or he could have used the money he tried to return to the government for such an expense. What a difference this might have made to frightened people who were figuratively in solitary confinement due to language barriers.

Hummer deliberately shut himself off from patient care. He may well have believed that he would be faulted if the institution's paperwork was not completed. But he took no real steps to alleviate the situation. Indeed, he actually took steps to *keep* the status quo by refusing to hire trained nurses or another physician until they were forced upon him. He deliberately ignored good advice on how to run a better facility and instead scrambled to circumvent "interference" so he could run the asylum his own way. By choosing paperwork over patients, Hummer defaulted from physician to administrator. Ironically, reports show that Gifford had made hospital rounds just as frequently, or more so, than Hummer.

Because he would not supervise his staff properly, Hummer took part in every shortcoming and failing that occurred and was partner to his staff's abuse, neglect, and cruelty. *Anyone* walking through the building could see the chains, locked rooms, and filth at Canton Asylum just as easily as Dr. Silk had. Hummer saw it, overlooked it, and allowed these conditions to continue. His cruelty was renewed every morning as he allowed patients to live in conditions that he knew were inhumane.

That Hummer *allowed* these conditions seems borne out by two particular facts: he never changed his management focus despite numerous calls from inspectors and higher-ups to do so, and he constantly emphasized unnecessary frugality. Both factors worked against patient welfare, and Hummer was very consistent in these areas. While the

Indian Office may never have funded the asylum the way it should have, it was Hummer who decided to pinch pennies and try to return money targeted for patient care. Hummer himself was the obstacle to the asylum receiving more staff; he fought the acquisition of more attendants and nurses every time the issue arose. He seems to have deliberately abandoned his responsibility toward those who could not help themselves. Yet, as the asylum's only physician, he was also his patients' only hope. He let them down in an inexcusable way.

Those who are familiar with Canton Asylum's story believe that locals are also partly to blame for prolonging the misery suffered by its patients. Those who benefited from the fruits of the asylum in terms of its reliable wages, labor contracts, and so on obviously wanted to keep it open. In this, they would be similar to any of today's workers who want their industries supported despite adverse conditions, safety issues, or the availability of newer technology. Jobs and money are jobs and money. The question with Canton Asylum is whether citizens were guilty of anything other than normal self-interest.

It would probably be safe to say that few of Canton's citizens had specific knowledge of patient mistreatment. How many of us today feel any need to tour a hospital or nursing home to ascertain that the patients there are properly cared for? The same would have held true for Canton's citizens. The Indian Service regularly inspected the facility, while neighbors, friends, or even family members worked there. Surely, everything was fine.

The institution was open to the public during its twice-weekly visiting hours, and plenty of tourists and locals did go there. Newspapers regularly wrote glowing reviews of the asylum's wonderful facilities and staff and generally painted a very positive picture of life inside. The two assistant physicians who had worked there were resolved to hinder the institution whenever they could, but only once or twice did their disapproval become public enough to catch the attention of area citizens. Even then, counterarguments or explanations managed to quell any misgivings that might have been generated.

The greater focus should be on the staff—who *were* at the asylum every day and *were* in a position to see how the patients were treated. There a different pattern emerges. Some attendants were simply ignorant and didn't know what to expect from an insane patient. They may not have thought that insane people even felt the same sensations as sane ones. Staff were never trained, and consequently they tried to deal with their work in any manner that made sense to them given their individual backgrounds. They had little understanding of psychiatric conditions, probably had a poor idea of what any given patient was capable of doing, and didn't know how to manage patients who weren't docile or didn't understand English. Impatience or frustration would result, with each staff member's personality coming out in the way he or she expressed it. In an era that accepted much harsher disciplinary measures than society does today, striking or confining patients likely seemed commonsense rather than abusive.

Other attendants were bullies and predators, or just a step shy: they teased or mocked patients, laughed at their mishaps, or preyed on them sexually. Many were dismissed as quickly as their misbehavior was uncovered, but that is not to say that some situations didn't exist far too long before that happened. These attendants deserve full condemnation.

Most attendants probably fell into a third category: ordinary people with their own frailties and faults who were trying to do their best. Much of asylum work *everywhere* was laborious and thankless. A woman who fought you as you dressed her might urinate in her chair less than an hour later, necessitating another strenuous change of clothing. Some patients wandered, got into mischief, fought with other patients, or became agitated, restless, and possibly destructive. Through it all, one attendant in charge of perhaps twenty or thirty patients would be required to make beds, scrub floors, feed helpless patients, give others baths, change bandages, and on and on. At mealtime, many attendants chose to lock patients in their rooms and go eat; if they didn't, they would forego an important chance to sit down and rest during their ten- or twelve-hour day. Their real error lay in eating together, rather than in shifts that would have made all the locking-up unnecessary.

Some patients fought with or assaulted attendants, wouldn't follow directions, or otherwise impeded the schedule and rhythm of the day. Unless the windows were open and a breeze blowing, the air inside the building would be close and pungent from bodies that were washed only once a week unless accidents of a foul nature required bathing more frequently. It would have been noisy, too, with calls and shouts from patients, unintelligible mutterings, petitions for water, food, release, and so on. Staff who broke up one too many fights or were themselves the targets of violence, perhaps discovered feces in unexpected places, or found themselves overwhelmed with too much work might have easily turned to locks and restraints to keep patients at bay until they could complete their tasks.

Caretaking is a stressful occupation. Being on call day and night is wearing. Living in quarters composed of one or two rooms is dispiriting. Canton Asylum's staff reacted to their situation just as one might expect humans who were not particularly dedicated to a profession to act. Some attendants abused their positions of power, some took out their stress and frustration on helpless patients, some looked down on the "defectives" they cared for . . . and some attendants were kind and selfless, as described in a few patients' letters. Fortunately, there were always a few employees who raised the alarm or made complaints that triggered investigations.

Ultimately, there are no excuses for Canton Asylum. The Interior Department could have done better, the commissioners of Indian affairs could have done better, its superintendents could have done better, and the staff could have come up higher. Those who were especially charged with looking after the interests of federal wards failed to do so. Ultimately, however, Dr. Harry R. Hummer deserves the greatest blame. He asked for buildings and livestock rather than personnel and mental health programs. He holed himself up in an office rather than venture out to take care of his patients. He looked the other way at terrible conditions others saw at a glance and spent his energies thwarting all attempts to rein him in. These were choices, not temperament.

Children confined in such a place had to be horrified and frightened. Helpless men and women locked in their rooms, shackled to bedposts, or left neglected in their beds had to be miserable. Just as appalling is the issue of patients' sanity. If Dr. Silk's findings in 1929 held true throughout the asylum's life, the vast majority of patients there had not been insane. That means they were aware of their surroundings, could feel the injustice of their imprisonment, and suffered longer and felt deeper despair than patients less aware of their situations.

Abandoned, ignored, lonely, and despairing, they might well cry out across the years, "Remember us."

ACKNOWLEDGMENTS

No one writes or researches in a vacuum, and I want to thank all who have written about the Canton Asylum for Insane Indians before me. Historians in many areas related to this story previously laid the groundwork for my own research, and I have necessarily used their great strengths in presenting information and analyzing my subject matter. Archivists whose dedication to preserving the documents that make the past come alive have my heartfelt thanks and gratitude.

Determined and expressive people have tried to keep the facility and its victims alive in memory, and I commend their efforts. One particular group continues to advance the asylum's history and make it part of a public conversation: the Keepers of the Canton Native Asylum Story. Since 2012, these dedicated native and non-native volunteers have come together to work toward education, reconciliation, and restoration; the City of Canton, South Dakota, passed a resolution in 2014 to approve them as a city task force.

There are many individuals who have played an important role in helping me write this book. My editor, Matthew Bokovoy, has been extraordinarily patient and understanding—a pleasure to work with. I want to especially thank Amanda Mecke for helping me early on to pull together my thoughts and initial narrative for this piece of history. As soon as we connected, Maureen Jais-Mick at St. Elizabeths shared my enthusiasm for the Canton Asylum story; besides her encouragement, she sent me a great deal of information and assisted me with valuable contacts. Dr. Jogues Prandoni spent his own valuable time researching photos and sharing some of his favorite aspects of St. Elizabeths' history, for which I am greatly indebted. These two professionals from

St. Elizabeths epitomize the generosity available in the researcher and historian community. Anne Dilenschneider of the Keepers of the Canton Native Asylum Story has given me an extraordinary amount of her time and has graciously shared her contacts within that group; her efforts have greatly enhanced my understanding of Canton Asylum's history. I also appreciate the time, attention, and information other Keepers have personally given me: Bud Johnson, Ross Lothrop, Jerry Fogg, Susan Jennys, David Jennys, and Julie Kellogg. I cannot thank them enough for their kindness and willingness to share. I was also delighted to meet Manfred Hill, who shared his boyhood memories of visiting the asylum to play with the employees' children and of that final, dramatic day when it closed. I particularly appreciate all the family members who have listened and empathized with my joy, frustration, hope, discouragement, and the gamut of emotions in between as I spent time learning about this particular aspect of America's past. I must also give special thanks to three faithful friends who sustained and encouraged me over a very long time: Valery Garrett, who helped me see this story with a historian's eye; Adelaida Lucena-Lower, who read, re-read, and commented astutely on every version put in her hands; and Michael Williams, nitpicker extraordinaire, whose keen eye and insightful comments kept me on track. My longtime friend and fellow writer Diane Bertrand has been a faithful encourager for many years, as well as an insightful critique partner. May all writers have such wonderful people in their lives.

Patients Treated at Canton Asylum

Officially, there is no complete list of Canton patients with dates of admission, psychiatric notes, health notes, discharge or death dates, and so on. Information about patients has been gathered from many sources, which do include some admission cards and other official forms. However, other information—sometimes even the bare names of patients—has been culled from written correspondence between the asylum superintendents and the Indian Office, census records, newspapers, letters, and reports from other sources. One list of names, for instance, came from a journal voucher within a "Report of Deposit Funds to the Credit of the United States," which listed small amounts of money spent for individual patient needs in February, 1927. For some patients, the only source that acknowledges their stay at the asylum is Dr. L. L. Culp's letter detailing the cemetery arrangement that the asylum's two superintendents had kept (see appendix B).

The Indian Service itself did not know how many patients had come through Canton Asylum. At the time of Dr. Kraepelin's visit in 1925, Hummer *estimated* about 300 patients had been in the institution; at the time of Dr. Silk's visit in 1929, a little over 350. I have found 384 separate names (including babies), though a few of them may very well refer to the same person. "Colonel" is a nickname and cannot be tied to any particular patient, even though his true name is probably recorded; some patients known by both native and Anglo names may possibly appear twice. There are also a few discrepancies in the data (such as admission or death dates), which may have resulted from typos or carelessness in transcribing data during the operation of the asylum. An asterisk (*) following a patient's name indicates a discrepancy in two or more records. Patients are listed alphabetically by last name under three categories: Male Admissions, Female Admissions, and Other Admissions. "Other Admissions" have not been included in the total.

Male Admissions

Patient name: William Abdulhena (Shoshone)
Date of admission: Unknown, but involved in a fight with Frank Bear in 1926
Diagnosis: Unknown

Patient name: Albert Allison (Pima)
Date of admission: June 25, 1927
Diagnosis: Unknown
Notes: Thirty-nine in 1910; died on May 16, 1928

Patient name: Antone (Papago)
Date of admission: July 29, 1905
Diagnosis: Chronic dementia, revised to dementia praecox, hebephrenia
Notes: Died on April 4, 1912, age forty-two, of pulmonary TB

Patient name: John Arrow (this may be John Brings-the-Arrow)
Date of admission: Unknown
Diagnosis: Unknown
Notes: Mentioned in an employee letter in 1914

Patient name: Wilbur Baldwin
Date of admission: June 29, 1926 (received from Immigration Service)
Diagnosis: Insane prisoner
Notes: Held at asylum until he could be deported to Canada

Patient name: George Battise or Beautiste (Winnebago)
Date of admission: July 18, 1903 (committed from Wittenberg)
Diagnosis: Epilepsy, grand mal
Notes: Died on May 30, 1909, age seventeen

Patient name: Frank Bear (Navajo)
Date of admission: February 14, 1924
Diagnosis: Psychosis, lethargic encephalitis
Notes: Transferred to St. Elizabeths, age thirty; died on January 16, 1938

Patient name: Pugay Beel (Northern Navajo)
Date of admission: February 16, 1931
Diagnosis: Unknown
Notes: Died on September 12, 1931, age fifty-one

Patient name: Big Day (Crow)
Date of admission: June 1, 1905
Diagnosis: Paresis
Notes: Died on July 3, 1905, age forty-five

Patient name: Big John (Navajo)
Date of admission: Unknown
Diagnosis: Unknown
Notes: Died on August 25, 1920, age thirty-eight

Patient name: Joseph Bigmane* (Sioux)
Date of admission: May 6 or 12, 1906 (committed from Standing Rock ND)
Diagnosis: Epilepsy, grand mal, revised to epileptic psychosis, deteriorating
Notes: Died on May 20, 1916, age thirty

Patient name: Tujo Thlani Bitzili (Navajo)
Date of admission: August 13, 1919
Diagnosis: Unknown
Notes: Discharged on January 14, 1920

Patient name: Sam Black Buffalo (Sioux)
Date of admission: November 9, 1905
Diagnosis: Mutism
Notes: Discharged January 24, 1908

Patient name: James Black Bull (Sioux)
Date of admission: July 23, 1923 (committed from Rosebud)
Diagnosis: Unknown
Notes: Died on February 6, 1926, age forty

Patient name: James or Simon Blackeye (Chippewa)
Date of admission: February 23, 1920 (committed from Red Lake Agency)
Diagnosis: Epileptic, limited mentality
Notes: Admitted at age nineteen; within nine months suffered 313 recorded convulsions; died on May 4, 1922, age twenty

Patient name: Albert Blaine (Sioux)
Date of admission: May 1, 1928 (committed from Yankton)
Diagnosis: Imbecility, revised to mental deficiency, probably without psychosis
Notes: Transferred to St. Elizabeths; died from a fall in January 1942

Patient name: Andrew Bray Blair (Sioux)
Date of admission: Unknown
Diagnosis: Unknown
Notes: Died on August 4, 1921, age sixteen

Patient name: Tome Bole
Date of admission: Unknown
Diagnosis: Unknown

Patient name: Jule (Papa) Brien (Kickapoo)
Date of admission: February 3, 1911 (committed from Topeka State Hospital)
Diagnosis: Alcoholic, pseudo-paresis
Notes: Died on February 5, 1918

Patient name: Robert Brings Plenty (Sioux)
Date of admission: January 17, 1903
Diagnosis: Chronic epileptic dementia
Notes: Transferred from St. Elizabeths; died on May 20, 1903, age twenty-one

Patient name: John Brings-the-Arrow (Sioux)
Date of admission: October 21, 1903 (committed from Cheyenne River Agency)
Diagnosis: Chronic melancholia, intoxication psychosis and alcoholic dementia
Notes: Died on January 23, 1915

Patient name: Charles Brown* (Winnebago)
Date of admission: Unknown (committed from Wittenberg Indian School)
Diagnosis: Acute melancholia
Notes: Died on November 2, 1907, age sixty or sixty-three, after Gifford withheld treatment for biliary calculi

Patient name: John Brown (Sioux)
Date of admission: March 9, 1909
Diagnosis: Paranoid, dementia praecox
Notes: Admitted at age forty-two; only one exam on record in over twenty years; released as sane at asylum's closing

Patient name: Amos Brown Ears (Sioux)
Date of admission: January 15, 1913 (committed from Pine Ridge)
Diagnosis: Hemiplegia with epilepsy
Notes: Died on May 1, 1921, age thirty-one

Patient name: Joseph Louis Bruce (Chippewa)
Date of admission: July 5, 1908 (committed from Turtle Mountain Agency)
Diagnosis: Acute melancholia
Notes: Admitted at age twenty-five; admitted from county jail, Glasgow, Montana; discharged on December 17, 1908

Patient name: John Burrs
Date of admission: Unknown
Diagnosis: Unknown
Notes: Listed in 1910 asylum census

Patient name: Joseph Carpenter (Sioux)
Date of admission: November 7, 1914
Diagnosis: Dementia praecox
Notes: Transferred to St. Elizabeths

Patient name: Philip Carson (Osage)
Date of admission: October 1, 1918 (committed from Pawhuska OK)
Diagnosis: In a letter, said he was not a fool, insane, or drunken fighter, so may have been committed due to an alcohol incident
Notes: Wrote to Indian Department in 1918 to say he would join the Army on January 1, 1919

Patient name: Kee Catron (Navajo)
Date of admission: April 13, 1922
Diagnosis: Imbecile, revised to dementia praecox
Notes: Admitted at age seventeen; transferred to St. Elizabeths

Patient name: Albert or Alfred or Ben Chapman (Sioux)
Date of admission: October 3, 1928 (committed from Yankton)
Diagnosis: Epileptic, imbecility

Patient name: Joseph Charbonneau or Charbonreau (Chippewa)
Date of admission: November 11, 1921 (committed from Ft. Totten)
Diagnosis: Atactic disturbances years earlier, hallucinated, became senile
Notes: Died of a stroke on January 29, 1923

Patient name: Frederick Charging Eagle (Sioux)
Date of admission: Unknown
Diagnosis: Unknown
Notes: Died on September 1, 1918, age forty-three

Patient name: Charlie (Andy Navajo Mountain Shukgie) (Navajo)
Date of admission: October 30, 1928 (committed from Western Navajo Agency)
Diagnosis: Dementia praecox
Notes: Transferred to St. Elizabeths at age thirty-six; died on March 24, 1934

Patient name: Thomas Chasing Bear (Sioux)
Date of admission: August 28, 1913 (committed from Standing Rock)
Diagnosis: Unknown
Notes: Died on February 2, 1915, age thirty-one

Patient name: Francisco Chico* (Papago)
Date of admission: April 23, 1923 (committed from Sells Agency)
Diagnosis: Manic
Notes: Died on April 17 (or May 9), 1927, age fifty-one

Patient name: James Chief Crow (Piegan)
Date of admission: June 19, 1906
Diagnosis: Epileptic dementia
Notes: Died on October 24, 1908, age twenty-eight

Patient name: Charles Clafflin (Menominee)
Date of admission: January 28, 1909
Diagnosis: Senile dementia, revised to senile psychosis, dementing
Notes: Admitted at age seventy-eight; died on February 28, 1914

Patient name: Peter Clafin or Clafflin (Menominee)
Date of admission: November 8, 1917
Diagnosis: Imbecility
Notes: Seventy-eight in 1909; released from Canton Asylum and returned to
Keshena Indian Agency at asylum's closing

Patient name: David Cloud Shield (Sioux)
Date of admission: Unknown
Diagnosis: Epilepsy, imbecility

Patient name: John Coal-of-Fire (Arapahoe)
Date of admission: March 27, 1918 (committed from Cantonment Indian School)
Diagnosis: Unknown
Notes: Died on June 17, 1919, age thirty-two

Patient name: Fred Collins (Ute)
Date of admission: January 3, 1916
Diagnosis: Unknown
Notes: Died on May 30, 1919, age twenty-one

Patient name: Colonel (a nickname with no other identifier)
Date of admission: Unknown
Diagnosis: Had a fit, according to patient James Herman

Patient name: Conley, Herbert (W. Navajo)
Date of admission: Unknown
Diagnosis: Unknown
Notes: Died on March 17, 1933, age twenty-five

Patient name: Richard Cottonwood
Date of admission: March 9, 1919 (committed from Standing Rock Agency)
Diagnosis: Unknown
Notes: Died of anasarca on April 30, 1920

Patient name: Jerome Court (Sioux)
Date of admission: July 12, 1923
Diagnosis: Violent, possibly syphilitic
Notes: Escaped and joined U.S. Army in March 1924

Patient name: John Charles Cox (Omaha)
Date of admission: July 14, 1923
Diagnosis: Dementia praecox
Notes: Mentioned as a recipient of funds in a February 1927 journal voucher

Patient name: Charley Creeping, Tah-poot-sah (Paiute)
Date of admission: June 5, 1916 (committed from Nevada School)
Diagnosis: Paraplegia, imbecility, revised to mental deficiency, without psychosis
Notes: Transferred to St. Elizabeths at age fifty-six; died on October 23, 1949

Patient name: Crooked Eyes (Sioux)
Date of admission: December 14, 1925
Diagnosis: Unknown
Notes: Admitted around age sixty; discharged April 10, 1926

Patient name: Alfred Crow Feather or One Feather
Date of admission: October 19, 1907 (committed from Cheyenne River Agency)
Diagnosis: Unknown, but had auditory hallucinations
Notes: Discharged in July 1909 after escaping July 1, 1909

Patient name: James Crow Lightning (Sioux)
Date of admission: (committed from Santee NE)
Diagnosis: Unknown
Notes: Died on May 8, 1921, age sixty-one

Patient name: Guy Crow Neck (Cheyenne)
Date of admission: April 15, 1919
Diagnosis: Unknown
Notes: Died of epileptic convulsion on July 26, 1920, age nineteen

Patient name: Danaghonginiwa (Moqui)
Date of admission: July 29, 1905
Diagnosis: Acute mania
Notes: Spoke no English; died on March 27, 1916, age forty-one

Patient name: Andrew Dancer (Sioux)
Date of admission: Unknown (committed from Yankton)
Diagnosis: Unknown
Notes: Died on November 21, 1918, age twenty-four

Patient name: Dasgol (Apache)
Date of admission: November 18, 1906 (committed from San Carlos)
Diagnosis: Toxic insanity
Notes: Admitted at age nineteen; released April 14, 1908, on furlough

Patient name: George Davis (Creek)
Date of admission: February 28, 1921
Diagnosis: Unknown
Notes: Discharged on July 20, 1925

Patient name: Willie Dayea* (Navajo)
Date of admission: March 13, 1922, and April 13, 1922
Diagnosis: Constitutional psychopathic inferiority
Notes: Admitted at age twenty-three; diagnosed as not insane at asylum's closing; taken to St. Elizabeths and returned to his home on January 21, 1934

Patient name: Amos Deere (Shawnee)
Date of admission: February 8, 1908
Diagnosis: Manic-depressive, amentia
Notes: Admitted at age thirty-two; died of peritonitis on July 11, 1914, age thirty-eight

Patient name: William Deroin (Sac & Fox)
Date of admission: October 15, 1931
Diagnosis: Syphilis, taboretic symptoms, psychosis
Notes: Transferred to St. Elizabeths

Patient name: Dirt (Northern Navajo)
Date of admission: February 16, 1931
Diagnosis: Unknown
Notes: No other name known; admitted with Pugay Beel

Patient name: Philip Doctor (Catkaptecena) (Yanktonai Sioux)
Date of admission: Unknown
Diagnosis: Unknown
Notes: Over ninety years old in 1905; medicine man; died on June 19, 1906

Patient name: Kee D. J. Dodge (Navajo)
Date of admission: April 13, 1922
Diagnosis: Suffering from gonorrhea

Patient name: Charles Ducharme or Ducheine (Sioux)
Date of admission: November 14, 1907 (committed from Cheyenne River Agency)
Diagnosis: Acute alcoholic insanity
Notes: Returned home to Cheyenne River Agency SD on January 20, 1908

Patient name: Edward O. C. Dupois
Date of admission: November 10, 1926 (committed from Pawnee Indian Agency)
Diagnosis: Epilepsy
Notes: Admitted at age twenty-three; Hummer recommended discharge on March 16, 1929

Patient name: Louis Eagle Bear (Sioux)
Date of admission: August 2, 1926 (committed from Pine Ridge)
Diagnosis: Epilepsy
Notes: Mentioned as a recipient in a February 1927 journal voucher

Patient name: John Enos (Pima)
Date of admission: July 3, 1928 (committed from Phoenix)
Diagnosis: Dementia praecox, paranoid
Notes: Transferred to St. Elizabeths

Patient name: Richard Fairbanks (Chippewa)
Date of admission: August 5, 1920 (committed from Leech Lake Agency)
Diagnosis: Idiocy, demented (idiocy with psychosis)
Notes: Described as an "insane child" (age fourteen in 1927); transferred to St. Elizabeths at age twenty-one; died on March 10, 1935

Patient name: James Fishtrap (Chippewa)
Date of admission: May 14, 1930
Diagnosis: Idiocy with psychosis, revised to without psychosis
Notes: Transferred to St. Elizabeths

Patient name: Thomas Floodwood
Date of admission: May 13, 1923 (Chippewa)
Diagnosis: Unknown
Notes: Died on September 26, 1923, age sixty-two

Patient name: Pisquoponoke or Pisquopomoke Fredericks (Menominee)
Date of admission: Unknown
Diagnosis: Unknown
Notes: Mentioned in fiscal year 1926 and in 1930

Patient name: Lloyd C. Freeman
Date of admission: Unknown (committed from Union Agency Indian Territory)
Diagnosis: Alcoholic dementia
Notes: An escape on September 8, 1907, is mentioned

Patient name: Henry Frenier (Sioux)
Date of admission: May 15, 1923 (committed from Cheyenne River)
Diagnosis: Idiocy, epilepsy
Notes: Frenier was twelve in 1927; died on August 1, 1928

Patient name: Willie George (Paiute)
Date of admission: November 15, 1917 (committed from Walker River Reservation)
Diagnosis: Unknown
Notes: Died on November 18, 1919, age twenty-four

Patient name: Baptiste Gingras (Flathead)
Date of admission: December 26, 1906
Diagnosis: Sexual neurasthenia
Notes: Died on December 19, 1909, age nineteen

Patient name: William Goforth (Choctaw)
Date of admission: December 3, 1907 (Union Agency)
Diagnosis: Traumatic dementia, revised to traumatic psychosis, deteriorating
Notes: Admitted at age forty-seven; died on September 17, 1910

Patient name: Peter Thompson Good Boy (Sioux)
Date of admission: May 3, 1916
Diagnosis: Constitutional inferiority (meaning obsessions, compulsions, etc.)
Notes: Admitted from St. Elizabeths; released in 1918

Patient name: Oliver Grass Rope (Sioux)
Date of admission: May 17, 1916 (committed from Lower Brule)
Diagnosis: Unknown
Notes: Died on May 24, 1918

Patient name: Anson Graves (Chippewa)
Date of admission: October 10, 1918 (committed from Red Lake)
Diagnosis: Epileptic
Notes: Died on February 12, 1926

Patient name: John Gray Blanket (Sioux)
Date of admission: February 5, 1917
Diagnosis: Epileptic psychosis, syphilis
Notes: Transferred to St. Elizabeths

Patient name: Louis Green* (Sioux)
Date of admission: August 5, 1909 (Pine Ridge Agency)
Diagnosis: Epileptic psychosis, dementing
Notes: Died on March 20, 1910, age forty-two; shown as twenty-two in 1909

Patient name: Peter Greenwood (Brule Sioux)
Date of admission: Unknown
Diagnosis: Syphilitic dementia
Notes: Died on September 22, 1903, age forty-two

Patient name: Ira Gristeau (Menominee)
Date of admission: Unknown
Diagnosis: Unknown
Notes: Died on March 24, 1920, age fourteen

Patient name: Charley Guerio or Guerno
Date of admission: Unknown
Diagnosis: Dipsomania
Notes: *Sioux Valley News* article, July 20, 1906, said he had been cured and accompanied Dr. Turner on his trip to New Mexico and Arizona (and presumably dropped off at his home)

Patient name: John Hall (Pima)
Date of admission: November 10, 1905
Diagnosis: Chronic dementia, revised to dementia praecox, hebephrenia
Notes: Died of diabetes complications on May 25, 1914, age thirty-four

Patient name: William Harris (Cherokee)
Date of admission: September 10, 1928
Diagnosis: Dementia praecox
Notes: According to a note on the June 15, 1929, Report of Attendance, patient was "about recovered"; discharged June 28, 1930

Patient name: Stephen Harrison (Sac & Fox)
Date of admission: June 17, 1910
Diagnosis: Dementia praecox, hebephrenic
Notes: Died on September 29, 1930

Patient name: Mark or Marcus Hart, Missee-way-guh-noo (Ojibwe)
Date of admission: Unknown
Diagnosis: Alcoholic psychosis, deteriorated
Notes: Transferred to St. Elizabeths

Patient name: Robert Harwood (Blackfeet)
Date of admission: Unknown
Diagnosis: Unknown

Patient name: James Hathorn (Navajo)
Date of admission: March 14, 1904
Diagnosis: Diplegia spastica infantalis, revised to congenital imbecility
Notes: Patient was age twelve in the 1910 asylum census; died on November 26, 1919

Patient name: Charles Hawk (Sioux)
Date of admission: December 7, 1920

Diagnosis: Unknown
Notes: Silk notes that his first physical was performed on January 7, 1926; died as a result of suicide by hanging on January 18, 1929

Patient name: Silas Hawk (Sac & Fox)
Date of admission: August 4, 1905
Diagnosis: Congenital imbecility
Notes: Died on May 12, 1910, age twenty-four

Patient name: Jacob Hayes
Date of admission: Unknown (committed from Pima Boarding School)
Diagnosis: Senile dementia
Notes: Died on October 14, 1907, age sixty-five

Patient name: Robert Hayes (Chippewa)
Date of admission: November 4, 1920 (committed from Turtle Mountain Agency)
Diagnosis: Imbecility
Notes: Hayes was age sixteen in 1927; released in 1933

Patient name: Edward Hedges (Sioux)
Date of admission: December 31, 1902 (committed from Santee Agency)
Diagnosis: Acute melancholia, revised to manic-depressive insanity
Notes: Hedges was the asylum's first patient; his wife began divorce proceedings while he was in the asylum in 1909; died on March 18, 1920, age fifty-one

Patient name: George Harry Henry (Chippewa)
Date of admission: December 7, 1916 (committed from Turtle Mountain Agency)
Diagnosis: Unknown
Notes: Died of pulmonary and intestinal TB on June 3, 1923

Patient name: James Henry (Creek)
Date of admission: August 31, 1923
Diagnosis: Unknown
Notes: Transferred from Norman State Hospital

Patient name: James Herman (Sioux)
Date of admission: February 28, 1914
Diagnosis: Unknown, but committed by the Gregory County (SD) Insanity Commission as mentally unsound and suffering from the excessive use of alcohol
Notes: Declared "sane" by chief medical supervisor Dr. Robert Newberne April 28, 1920, and stricken from Canton Asylum's list of patients

Patient name: Wilson Honga
Date of admission: Unknown (committed from Truxton)
Diagnosis: Moron
Notes: Returned to reservation in May 1927

Patient name: Hon-sah-sah-kah (Osage)
Date of admission: Unknown
Diagnosis: Congenital epileptic idiocy
Notes: October 23, 1905, age twenty-three

Patient name: Abraham Hopkins (Sioux)
Date of admission: March 27, 1929 (committed from Sisseton Agency)
Diagnosis: Not insane, apparently normal
Notes: Silk mentions Hopkins in 1933 as one of nine patients committed through the courts; discharged to Sisseton December 28, 1933

Patient name: John Howling Horse (Sioux)
Date of admission: May 31, 1919
Diagnosis: Unknown
Notes: TB and streptococcic infection; died on May 17, 1923

Patient name: Howling Wolfe (Arickaree)
Date of admission: June 9, 1910 (committed from Ft. Berthold School ND)
Diagnosis: Diagnosis reserved
Notes: Listed in the June 28, 1910, asylum census; died on March 30, 1911, age fifty-nine

Patient name: Herbert Iron (Arapahoe)
Date of admission: August 6, 1908 (committed from Shoshone School)
Diagnosis: Hemiplegia, epileptic dementia, revised to epileptic psychosis, deteriorating
Notes: Admitted at age thirty; died on May 18, 1919, age forty-one

Patient name: Robert Jackson (Shoshone)
Date of admission: September 4, 1932 (Ft. Washakie WY)
Diagnosis: Psychosis, cerebral arteriosclerosis
Notes: Transferred to St. Elizabeths, age seventy-one; died on January 3, 1939

Patient name: Amos Jaundron
Date of admission: Unknown
Diagnosis: Epilepsy, grand mal

Patient name: Rowley Johnson* (Klamath)
Date of admission: December 4, 1919
Diagnosis: Epileptic insanity
Notes: Hummer recommended discharge to Johnson's mother on August 4, 1920, when he was dying; discharged on April 11, 1920

Patient name: Joseph Jordan (Chippewa)
Date of admission: March 28, 1903 (committed from White Earth)

Diagnosis: Alcoholic dementia
Notes: Died on March 1, 1916

Patient name: Benito Juan (Papago)
Date of admission: April 23, 1923
Diagnosis: Unknown
Notes: Died on March 21, 1926, age thirty-three

Patient name: Alex Kennedy (Chippewa)
Date of admission: September 7, 1917 (committed from Standing Rock Agency)
Diagnosis: Unknown
Notes: Died on February 15, 1921, age sixty-four

Patient name: Alfred Kennedy (Sioux)
Date of admission: January or November 1, 1923
Diagnosis: Psychopathic
Notes: Discharged on February 15, 1926

Patient name: Peter Kentuck* (Hoopa)
Date of admission: December 15, 1920 or December 12, 1920
Diagnosis: Psychopathic inferiority, revised to imbecility
Notes: Released as sane at asylum's closing

Patient name: Keosoht or Ke-O-Soht (Potawatomi)
Date of admission: May 22, 1922
Diagnosis: Unknown
Notes: Reported as an escapee on May 1, 1926; died on December 31, 1927

Patient name: Moses Keynote or Kenote (Menominee)
Date of admission: Unknown
Diagnosis: Hysteric angina pectoris
Notes: Discharged as cured on May 5, 1905

Patient name: Simon Kirk (Sioux)
Date of admission: October 9, 1931 (committed from Sisseton)
Diagnosis: Dementia praecox
Notes: Transferred to St. Elizabeths at age twenty-two

Patient name: William LaClaire (Sioux)
Date of admission: July 14, 1927 (committed from Yankton)
Diagnosis: Dementia, senile
Notes: Died on September 22, 1930

Patient name: Charles LaComte (Chippewa)
Date of admission: Unknown
Diagnosis: Multiple sclerosis

Patient name: John LaDeaux or LaDue (Sioux)
Date of admission: Unknown
Diagnosis: Acute melancholia
Notes: Discharged as cured on May 5, 1905

Patient name: Joseph Langer
Date of admission: Unknown (committed from Devils Lake Reservation [ND])
Diagnosis: Congenital imbecility
Notes: Escaped three times

Patient name: Earl Leve Leve (Walapai, Hualapi Tribe)
Date of admission: May 2, 1919
Diagnosis: Epileptic psychosis, TB
Notes: Transferred to St. Elizabeths

Patient name: Alfred Littlewind (Sioux)
Date of admission: August 31, 1917 (committed from Ft. Totten)
Diagnosis: Unknown
Notes: Listed in 1921 asylum census; died on January 7, 1923

Patient name: Charles Lodgeskin (Sioux)
Date of admission: Unknown
Diagnosis: Demented, revised to idiocy

Patient name: Thomas Lone War (Sioux)
Date of admission: April 28, 1908 (Pine Ridge Agency)
Diagnosis: Epileptic dementia
Notes: Admitted at age fifty-one; died on December 24, 1909 of croupous pneumonia, age fifty-two

Patient name: Logan Lovejoy (Winnebago)
Date of admission: October 15, 1931
Diagnosis: Epilepsy
Notes: Collier asked Dr. Silk to look into his case; discharged on September 22, 1933

Patient name: Anselmo Lucas (Papago)
Date of admission: October 14, 1921 (committed from Sells Agency)
Diagnosis: Dementia praecox
Notes: Died on December 19, 1926, age forty

Patient name: Miguel Macy
Date of admission: Unknown
Diagnosis: Chronic melancholia

Patient name: Peter Mahkimetas (Menominee)
Date of admission: Unknown
Diagnosis: Unknown
Notes: Mahkimetas was twenty-one in 1933

Patient name: Earl F. Mahkimetass (Menominee)
Date of admission: April 11, 1917
Diagnosis: Imbecility
Notes: Had trachoma in 1923, mentioned as being of school age in a report that year; said to be fourteen in 1927; released at asylum's closing, age twenty-one

Patient name: George Marlow or Marlowe (Sioux)
Date of admission: January 14, 1905
Diagnosis: Congenital imbecility, revised to dementia praecox, hebephrenia
Notes: Twenty-three in 1909; transferred to St. Elizabeths

Patient name: Joseph D. Marshall* (Sioux)
Date of admission: January 17, 1903 (Rosebud Agency)
Diagnosis: Chronic epileptic dementia, revised to epileptic psychosis
Notes: Transferred from St. Elizabeths; died on November 17, 1919, age twenty-five; shown as thirty in 1909

Patient name: John Martin (Chippewa)
Date of admission: March 4, 1933 (committed from Lac du Flambeau)
Diagnosis: Psychosis
Notes: Transferred to St. Elizabeths

Patient name: John Masten
Date of admission: Unknown (committed from Hoopa Valley Agency)
Diagnosis: Unknown
Notes: Masten is noted in a list of patients from June 30, 1921; died on April 4, 1922, age thirty

Patient name: Miguel Maxcy (Mesa Grande)
Date of admission: January 17, 1903
Diagnosis: Chronic melancholia
Notes: Transferred from St. Elizabeths; discharged in December 1906

Patient name: Watt McCarter* (Cherokee)
Date of admission: September 27, 1920; telegram to Hummer requests admittance September 23, 1933
Diagnosis: Dementia praecox
Notes: Request for admittance said insanity as a result of influenza; transferred to St. Elizabeths

Patient name: Willie McCarthy (Osage)
Date of admission: November 30, 1906
Diagnosis: Hemiplegia with epilepsy, revised to epileptic psychosis
Notes: Age twenty at admittance; listed in June 28, 1910, asylum census; mentioned as deceased in a 1924 letter

Patient name: James McCloskey or McClusky (Sioux)
Date of admission: Unknown (committed from Rosebud Reservation)
Diagnosis: Imbecility, high-grade
Notes: Discharged as cured on May 5, 1905

Patient name: Frank McEwin (Cherokee, Five Civilized Tribes)
Date of admission: December 24, 1918
Diagnosis: Harmless imbecile

Patient name: Joe McEwin (Cherokee)
Date of admission: April 7, 1918
Diagnosis: Psychosis, brain disease, revised to imbecility
Notes: Transferred to St. Elizabeths

Patient name: Ernest McGinty* (Washoe)
Date of admission: October 13, 1924, also July 30, 1924 (committed from Carson School)
Diagnosis: Epilepsy, imbecility
Notes: Admitted at age twelve; died on December 2, 1930

Patient name: Abraham Meacham (Makah)
Date of admission: September 7, 1920 (Neah Bay Agency)
Diagnosis: Unknown
Notes: Discharged June 6, 1922, but readmitted August 7, 1922; died on November 7, 1922, age sixty-two (from Dr. Culp's cemetery list)

Patient name: Juan Mendoza (Papago)
Date of admission: June 3, 1916
Diagnosis: Psychosis, imbecility, revised to dementia praecox
Notes: Transferred to St. Elizabeths

Patient name: Harry Miller (Paiute)
Date of admission: November 11, 1916 (committed from Walker River)
Diagnosis: Unknown
Notes: Died on April 20, 1919, age sixteen

Patient name: Apolonio Miranda (Papago)
Date of admission: Unknown

Diagnosis: Unknown
Notes: Died on January 14, 1919, age fifty-four

Patient name: Willie J. S. Mitchell (Potawatomi)
Date of admission: October 18, 1921
Diagnosis: Dementia praecox
Notes: Transferred to St. Elizabeths

Patient name: Oscar Moccasin Top
Date of admission: February 18, 1921 (committed from Pine Ridge Agency)
Diagnosis: Unknown
Notes: Mentioned in 1924 asylum census

Patient name: James Monroe (Chippewa)
Date of admission: August 27, 1923 (committed from Red Lake)
Diagnosis: Epilepsy
Notes: Died on May 10, 1929

Patient name: Jose Augustine Montoya (Pueblo)
Date of admission: July 14, 1928
Diagnosis: Psychosis, schizophrenia, imbecile, revised to dementia praecox
Notes: Transferred to St. Elizabeths

Patient name: Aloysius Moore* (Sioux)
Date of admission: May 13, 1917
Diagnosis: Unknown
Notes: Listed in the June 30, 1921, asylum census; died on May 12, 1923, age twenty-nine (death also listed as May 7)

Patient name: Moxey (Mesa Grande)
Date of admission: Unknown
Diagnosis: Unknown
Notes: Mentioned as an escapee in 1906; this is very likely Miguel Maxcy

Patient name: Nadesoode (Apache)
Date of admission: Unknown (committed from San Carlos)
Diagnosis: Chronic dementia
Notes: Died of consumption on February 8, 1908, age sixty-three

Patient name: Ne-bow-o-sah (Potawatomi)
Date of admission: February 6, 1913
Diagnosis: Unknown
Notes: Died on December 18, 1914, age fifty

Patient name: Logie Nelson (Pima)
Date of admission: June 25, 1927

Diagnosis: Constitutional inferiority
Notes: Age sixteen when admitted; discharged on July 21, 1929

Patient name: Spot Omudis (Chippewa)
Date of admission: June 30, 1905 (committed from White Earth)
Diagnosis: Imbecility, demented, epileptic, kleptomaniac
Notes: Said to be eighteen years old in a 1909 report; died on June 1, 1920, age thirty

Patient name: Alfred One-Feather or Crow-Feather
Date of admission: Unknown
Diagnosis: Chronic melancholia
Notes: Escaped October 19, 1907, and July 1, 1909; officially discharged to agency in July 1909

Patient name: Allen Owl (Cherokee)
Date of admission: September 22, 1917
Diagnosis: Unknown
Notes: Owl was allowed to work for a farmer while at the asylum; discharged October 26, 1920

Patient name: George Pappan (Pawnee)
Date of admission: April 16, 1930
Diagnosis: Dementia praecox
Notes: Transferred to St. Elizabeths, age twenty-seven

Patient name: Peter Pecot (Sioux?)
Date of admission: Unknown
Diagnosis: Unknown
Notes: Silk mentions Pecot in 1933

Patient name: Peo (Umatilla)
Date of admission: January 1905
Diagnosis: Senile or arterio sclerotic dementia, revised to senile psychosis, dementing
Notes: Former chief; apparently discharged and escorted home by Hummer on February 21, 1912

Patient name: Peter Picotte
Date of admission: Unknown
Diagnosis: Senile dementia
Notes: Transferred to St. Elizabeths

Patient name: Fidel Podillia (Pueblo)
Date of admission: September 29, 1918

Diagnosis: Unknown
Notes: Discharged October 4, 1921

Patient name: John Rave (Winnebago)
Date of admission: Unknown
Diagnosis: Unknown

Patient name: Red Cloud (Sioux)
Date of admission: April 10, 1907 (committed from Pine Ridge)
Diagnosis: Chronic dementia, revised to dementia praecox, hebephrenic
Notes: Died on December 7, 1910, age fifty-eight

Patient name: Red Crow (Sioux)
Date of admission: February 5, 1922 (committed from Crow Creek Agency)
Diagnosis: Unknown
Notes: Died on April 8, 1922, age eighty-four

Patient name: Benjamin Red Rock (Sioux)
Date of admission: February 18, 1921 (Pine Ridge Agency)
Diagnosis: Unknown
Notes: Listed in the June 1921 and June 1924 asylum censuses and in a 1927 journal voucher

Patient name: George Red Rock (Sioux)
Date of admission: Unknown
Diagnosis: Unknown
Notes: Mentioned February 28, 1927

Patient name: Amos Ree (Sioux)
Date of admission: January 21, 1921 (committed from Yankton Agency)
Diagnosis: Epileptic psychosis
Notes: Mentioned February 28, 1927

Patient name: Alfred Richard (Sioux)
Date of admission: May 10, 1931 (committed from Pine Ridge)
Diagnosis: Alcohol incident
Notes: Brought to the asylum from jail; discharged by Silk on December 26, 1933

Patient name: Alfred Richards (Chippewa)
Date of admission: October 31, 1921
Diagnosis: Idiocy
Notes: Age sixteen in 1927; transferred to St. Elizabeths

Patient name: Arthur Richards (Sioux)
Date of admission: Unknown
Diagnosis: Unknown

Patient name: **George Roberts (Pima)**
Date of admission: July 14, 1928
Diagnosis: Dementia praecox
Notes: Admitted at age thirty-four

Patient name: **Henry Roberts (Chippewa)**
Date of admission: August 27, 1923 (committed from Red Lake)
Diagnosis: Epileptic psychosis
Notes: Admitted at age fourteen; mentioned in Silk Report, 1929

Patient name: **James Romero (Sioux)**
Date of admission: January 31, 1920 (committed from Pine Ridge Agency)
Diagnosis: Unknown
Notes: Escaped February 9, 1920; listed in the June 1924 asylum census; died on March 14, 1925

Patient name: **Jack Root (Chippewa)**
Date of admission: Unknown (committed from Lac du Flambeau)
Diagnosis: Unknown
Notes: Dislocated shoulder in 1930; died October 27, 1933, age eighty-two

Patient name: **David or Davis Roubideaux or Rubidoux (Sioux)**
Date of admission: September 5, 1903
Diagnosis: Chronic epileptic dementia, revised to idiocy with epilepsy
Notes: Died of epileptic convulsion on September 14, 1920

Patient name: **Thomas Ruby (Pima)**
Date of admission: Unknown
Diagnosis: Dementia praecox
Notes: Discharged 1930

Patient name: **John Sandborn (Gros Ventre)**
Date of admission: Unknown (committed from Ft. Belknap)
Diagnosis: Unknown
Notes: Escaped in 1918 and remained at large

Patient name: **Sam Scabby Robe* (Blackfeet)**
Date of admission: May 2, 1919
Diagnosis: Epileptic, hallucinated
Notes: Transferred to Montana State Hospital on December 31, 1921, where he died on February 5, 1922, of exhaustion of paresis; Kraepelin's report says he died November 5, 1922

Patient name: **Robert Scott Jr. (Paiute)**
Date of admission: January 23, 1920 (committed from Walker River Agency)

Diagnosis: Unknown
Notes: Referred to as a "boy"; died of epileptic convulsion on October 21, 1923

Patient name: Frank Shanahan (Chippewa)
Date of admission: Unknown, but a patient by 1906
Diagnosis: Delusional melancholia
Notes: Shanahan triggered an investigation of the asylum after impregnating Lizzie Vipont

Patient name: James Shawano (Chippewa)
Date of admission: May 30, 1925 (committed from Union Indian Agency OK)
Diagnosis: Imbecility, epilepsy
Notes: Died of pulmonary TB on May 4, 1927

Patient name: Richard Sheppard (Chippewa)
Date of admission: November 3, 1906
Diagnosis: Chronic dementia, dementia praecox, catatonic
Notes: Discharged to state asylum in Vinita OK on March 3, 1922

Patient name: Steve Simons (Cherokee)
Date of admission: Unknown
Diagnosis: Unknown
Notes: Died on October 8, 1917, age forty-five

Patient name: Frank Smith (Winnebago)
Date of admission: December 29, 1909
Diagnosis: Imbecility
Notes: Fractured arm while helping unload hay in 1910; died on May 18, 1914, of exhaustion from general paralysis of the insane

Patient name: Matt Smith (Chemehueve)
Date of admission: September 30, 1918 (committed from Colorado River Agency)
Diagnosis: Paranoia, auditory hallucinations; Kraepelin noted dementia praecox
Notes: Died on November 28, 1928, age fifty-one

Patient name: Paul Spry Bear (Sioux)
Date of admission: February 1, 1924 (committed from Yankton)
Diagnosis: Unknown
Notes: Listed as "very old"; died of cerebral hemorrhage on April 4, 1924

Patient name: Luke Stands-By-Him (Sioux)
Date of admission: January 20, 1916
Diagnosis: Dementia praecox
Notes: Transferred to St. Elizabeths, age forty-four

Patient name: Frank Starr* (Chippewa)
Date of admission: February 22, 1907 (Leech Lake)
Diagnosis: Imbecility, high-grade, revised to dementia praecox, hebephrenic
Notes: Died on April 28, 1913, age thirty-one; age given as twenty in 1909 report

Patient name: Dneas Stoely (Flathead)
Date of admission: Unknown
Diagnosis: Unknown

Patient name: Jacob Sweet Medicine (Cheyenne)
Date of admission: September 26, 1920 (Tongue River Agency)
Diagnosis: Dementia praecox
Notes: Transferred to St. Elizabeths, age thirty-nine

Patient name: Adam Swift Horse
Date of admission: July 4, 1923 (committed from Cheyenne River Agency)
Diagnosis: Unknown

Patient name: Cleto (Jose) Tafoya (Pueblo)
Date of admission: November 13, 1930
Diagnosis: Dementia praecox, paranoid type, dazed religious spells
Notes: John Collier's investigation of Tafoya's case led to the asylum's closing; transferred to St. Elizabeths

Patient name: Fred or George Tatsup (Bannock)
Date of admission: January 30, 1905
Diagnosis: Galloping paresis, revised to syphilitic paresis
Notes: Died on February 6, 1905, age forty-five

Patient name: Joseph Taylor (Joe Big Bear) (Chippewa)
Date of admission: April 20, 1910 (committed from White Earth Agency)
Diagnosis: Congenital imbecility
Notes: Died of pulmonary and intestinal TB on September 18, 1913, age twenty-four; weighed ninety pounds at death

Patient name: Reuben Taylor (Sioux)
Date of admission: Unknown
Diagnosis: Feebleminded
Notes: Age eighteen in 1933 and discharged by Silk to South Dakota State School for the Feeble Minded

Patient name: Leonard Thomas (Papago)
Date of admission: June 4, 1931 (committed from Sells Agency)
Diagnosis: Dementia praecox, alcoholic
Notes: Transferred to St. Elizabeths

Patient name: John Thompson (Winnebago)
Date of admission: Unknown
Diagnosis: Unknown

Patient name: Peter Thompson
Date of admission: February 14, 1929 (committed from Red Lake)
Diagnosis: Feebleminded, tubercular
Notes: Died on February 21, 1929

Patient name: Robert Thompson (Quapaw)
Date of admission: October 30, 1907
Diagnosis: Hemiplegia, chronic epileptic dementia, revised to epileptic psychosis
Notes: Admitted at age thirty; discharged September 26, 1923; had "considerable interests" in lead and zinc mines

Patient name: Three Striker (Osage)
Date of admission: March 1906
Diagnosis: Senile dementia
Notes: Discharged March 27, 1913

Patient name: Toby or Koz-he-la (Apache)
Date of admission: Unknown
Diagnosis: Chronic dementia, spastic spinal paralysis
Notes: Died on March 6, 1906, age thirty-five

Patient name: Toistoto or To-is-to-to (Northern Navajo)
Date of admission: Unknown (committed from San Juan School)
Diagnosis: Spastic spinal paralysis, revised to chronic dementia
Notes: Died of consumption on May 17, 1908, age thirty-two

Patient name: Bob "Lo" Tom (Paiute)
Date of admission: July 6, 1905 (committed from Walker Indian School)
Diagnosis: Chronic dementia, paranoid, intoxication psychosis, alcoholic
Notes: Subject of Gifford's pursuit in newspaper story; died on November 20, 1912

Patient name: Trucha (Apache)
Date of admission: Unknown
Diagnosis: Unknown
Notes: November 17, 1905, age forty-six

Patient name: Hosteen Tso (Navajo)
Date of admission: February 16, 1931
Diagnosis: Syphilitic dementia
Notes: Admitted at age eighteen; spoke no English; released as sane at asylum's closing

Patient name: **William Tucker**
Date of admission: 1904
Diagnosis: Circular insanity
Notes: Discharged November 5, 1906 to Meshena w i

Patient name: **Peter Turpin (Chippewa)**
Date of admission: March 11, 1905 (committed from White Earth)
Diagnosis: Imbecility, spastic diplegia
Notes: Age sixteen in 1909; transferred to St. Elizabeths

Patient name: **James or John Two Crows (Gros Ventre)**
Date of admission: March 6, 1909
Diagnosis: Imbecility, epileptic, deteriorating psychosis
Notes: Age sixteen in 1909

Patient name: **Two Teeth**
Date of admission: March 2, 1921 (committed from Crow Creek Agency)
Diagnosis: Dementia, senile
Notes: Married to Mrs. Two Teeth; age seventy-nine on July 16, 1930

Patient name: **Baby (Frank) Vipont (Paiute, Chippewa)**
Date of admission: November 8, 1906
Diagnosis: Imbecility, bastard
Notes: Named Frank Shanahan; sent to children's home in Sioux Falls, September 19, 1907; died on December 16, 1907

Patient name: **Fidel Virgil (Jicarilla Apache)**
Date of admission: May 29, 1932 (committed from Dulce n v)
Diagnosis: Epilepsy, idiocy
Notes: Transferred to St. Elizabeths, age fifteen or sixteen; died July 6, 1935

Patient name: **Walker**
Date of admission: Unknown
Diagnosis: Unknown
Notes: Mentioned as being "old" and mistreated by an attendant in 1915

Patient name: **Walkkas or Wah-kas (Potawatomi)**
Date of admission: April 17, 1912 (committed from Jackson County k s)
Diagnosis: Unknown
Notes: Admitted at age seventy-five; died on January 21, 1917, age seventy-nine

Patient name: **Edward Wauketch (Menominee)**
Date of admission: April 11, 1917 (committed from Keshena)
Diagnosis: Epileptic psychosis
Notes: Died from epileptic convulsion on June 29, 1929

Patient name: Seymour Wauketch (Menominee)
Date of admission: November 8, 1917 (committed from Keshena Agency)
Diagnosis: Unknown
Notes: Died on May 27, 1926, age seventy-one

Patient name: Joe Wellwin
Date of admission: Unknown
Diagnosis: Unknown
Notes: Mentioned on February 28, 1927

Patient name: Elmer Whitehorse (Sioux)
Date of admission: Unknown
Diagnosis: Unknown

Patient name: Navajo Willie
Date of admission: April 13, 1922 (committed from Navajo Indian Agency)
Diagnosis: Unknown

Patient name: Charley Willow, also Guerio
Date of admission: January 30, 1908 (committed from Albuquerque School NM)
Diagnosis: Chronic alcoholic insanity
Notes: Admitted at age thirty-five; discharged January 26, 1909

Patient name: Herbert Wilson (Pima, Southern Pueblos)
Date of admission: July 14, 1928
Diagnosis: Unknown

Patient name: Robert Winans (Arickara)
Date of admission: April 7, 1926
Diagnosis: Intoxication psychosis
Notes: Released as sane at asylum's closing

Patient name: Arch Wolf (Cherokee)
Date of admission: January 17, 1903
Diagnosis: Chronic melancholia, dementia praecox, paranoid
Notes: Transferred from St. Elizabeths; died of diabetes and pulmonary TB
on July 2, 1912, age thirty-eight

Patient name: Joe Wolfe* (Cherokee)
Date of admission: December 21, 1924, and December 21, 1922
Diagnosis: Idiocy ("patient was born insane")
Notes: Transferred to St. Elizabeths

Patient name: Roy Wolfe (Cherokee)
Date of admission: January 18, 1923 (committed from Cherokee Orphan Training School OK)

Diagnosis: Epileptic, imbecility
Notes: Died on March 28, 1928, age eighteen

Patient name: John Woodruff (mulatto or Sioux-mulatto)
Date of admission: January 17, 1903
Diagnosis: Chronic melancholia
Notes: Transferred from St. Elizabeths; died May 15, 1909, age fifty-one

Patient name: Hoskee Yazzie (Navajo)
Date of admission: May 25, 1930 (committed from Leupp Agency AZ)
Diagnosis: Idiocy
Notes: Admitted at age thirteen (?); transferred to St. Elizabeths, age sixteen; died March 11, 1936

Patient name: Yells-at-Night (Piegan)
Date of admission: July 28, 1906
Diagnosis: Cortical epilepsy
Notes: Died November 21, 1908, age thirty-three; diagnosed with TB

Patient name: Nakai Yezza (Navajo); records also show the name reversed
Date of admission: September 18, 1907
Diagnosis: Amentia, revised to imbecility, reputed sorcerer
Notes: Reported as escaped in October 1907 and July 1922; age thirty when admitted

Patient name: Peter Young Bird (Gros Ventre)
Date of admission: May 21, 1927
Diagnosis: Dementia praecox
Notes: Transferred to St. Elizabeths, age twenty-seven

Patient name: David Zephyr or Zephier (Sioux)
Date of admission: Unknown
Diagnosis: Senile dementia
Notes: Discharged by Silk in September 1933

Patient name: Alex Zimmerman* (Cheyenne)
Date of admission: April 13, 1919
Diagnosis: Hemiplegia
Notes: Mentioned as "discharged" on September 17, 1924, but probably read-mitted; died on June 1, 1928

Female Admissions

Patient name: Vivian Ambrose (Colville)
Date of admission: October 18, 1923 (committed from Spokane Agency)

Diagnosis: Encephalitis, lethargic; dementia, organic
Notes: Died of exhaustion following TB on September 8, 1931

Patient name: Christine Amour (Menominee)
Date of admission: November 8, 1917 (committed from Keshina)
Diagnosis: Epileptic
Notes: Died on May 5, 1928

Patient name: Emma Amyotte (Chippewa)
Date of admission: October 15, 1923
Diagnosis: Mental deficiency, imbecility
Notes: Released as sane at asylum's closing

Patient name: Milsie Antone (Papago)
Date of admission: March 18, 1926
Diagnosis: Dementia praecox
Notes: Age fifteen in April 1927

Patient name: Tchee Asal (Southern Navajo)
Date of admission: July 18, 1906
Diagnosis: Toxic insanity
Notes: Died on February 11, 1909, age twenty-nine

Patient name: Joanna Augusta (Papago)
Date of admission: July 9, 1920 (committed from Sells Agency)
Diagnosis: Senile psychosis, revised to dementia praecox
Notes: Transferred to St. Elizabeths, age sixty-eight; died on July 24, 1935

Patient name: Mary Bah (Western Navajo)
Date of admission: October 30, 1928
Diagnosis: Dementia praecox
Notes: Age eighteen in 1929; died on August 22, 1930, age twenty

Patient name: Priscilla Benally (Navajo)
Date of admission: Unknown (committed from Shiprock Agency)
Diagnosis: Dementia praecox
Notes: Transferred to St. Elizabeths in 1933

Patient name: Rosa Bite (Blackfeet)
Date of admission: August 14, 1919
Diagnosis: Idiocy, revised to imbecility
Notes: Died of pulmonary TB before release as sane at asylum's closing; died on December 19, 1933

Patient name: Maggie Black Cat (Sioux)
Date of admission: May 17, 1903

Diagnosis: Dementia praecox, feebleminded; revised to manic-depressive psychosis
Notes: Transferred to St. Elizabeths, age fifty-five

Patient name: Black Medicine (Gros Ventre)
Date of admission: Unknown
Diagnosis: Unknown
Notes: Listed in June 30, 1921, asylum census

Patient name: A. B. Blair
Date of admission: Unknown
Diagnosis: Unknown
Notes: Died on August 6, 1921

Patient name: Maggie Blanchard (Chippewa)
Date of admission: January 30, 1916
Diagnosis: Dementia praecox
Notes: Transferred to St. Elizabeths, age thirty

Patient name: Blue Sky (Chippewa)
Date of admission: March 9, 1903
Diagnosis: Dementia, arteriosclerotic or senile
Notes: Discharged September 1908 and later readmitted; died on June 18, 1914, age sixty-eight

Patient name: Mary G. Buck (Southern Ute)
Date of admission: September 9, 1918
Diagnosis: Unknown
Notes: Died of starvation and constipation on December 14, 1918, age twenty-seven

Patient name: Susan Bull (Choctaw)
Date of admission: June 20, 1907 (committed from Ardmore OK)
Diagnosis: Acute melancholia
Notes: Discharged April 14, 1908

Patient name: Minnie Bunker
Date of admission: Unknown
Diagnosis: Acute mania

Patient name: Baby Burch (Southern Ute)
Date of admission: March 9 or 10, 1913
Diagnosis: Unknown
Notes: Daughter of Susan Burch

Patient name: Jane Burch (Mrs. James Allen) (Southern Ute)
Date of admission: October 3, 1912
Diagnosis: Unknown
Notes: Died on March 1, 1916, age thirty-five

Patient name: Susan Burch (Southern Ute)
Date of admission: October 3, 1912
Diagnosis: Pregnant upon arrival
Notes: Delivered child on March 9, 1913; died on August 16, 1913

Patient name: Lillian Burns (Laguna)
Date of admission: June 25, 1912
Diagnosis: Violent, manic-depressive
Notes: Age twenty-three; discharged on April 22, 1913

Patient name: Agnes Caldwell (Menominee)
Date of admission: November 8, 1917
Diagnosis: Feebleminded with weakness for sex, revised to imbecility
Notes: Released from Canton Asylum and returned to Keshena Indian Agency
at asylum's closing

Patient name: Delores Caldwell (baby of Agnes) (Menominee)
Date of admission: May 26, 1921
Diagnosis: Unknown
Notes: Died on October 31, 1921, age five months

Patient name: Kate Canoe (Thibeau) (Winnebago)
Date of admission: April 21, 1919
Diagnosis: Dementia praecox with Froelich's syndrome, catatonic; revised to
undifferentiated psychosis
Notes: Transferred to St. Elizabeths

Patient name: Janet Carrier
Date of admission: May 1, 1933 (committed from Ft. Peck MT)
Diagnosis: Reputed epilepsy, no fits here; no mental disease, not insane
Notes: Age eighteen when admitted; no note on release

Patient name: Juanita Casildo (Pueblo)
Date of admission: Unknown (committed from Albuquerque School)
Diagnosis: Toxic insanity
Notes: Died on June 22, 1908, age forty

Patient name: Lillian Chavez (Pueblo)
Date of admission: September 25, 1913
Diagnosis: Manic-depressive psychosis, revised to dementia praecox

Notes: Father took her home on May 25, 1914, when she was eighteen; readmitted on January 22, 1923; transferred to St. Elizabeths at age thirty-seven

Patient name: Chee* (Southern Navajo)
Date of admission: March 1906 or November 18, 1906
Diagnosis: Chronic dementia, revised to dementia praecox; hebephrenic
Notes: Died on May 4, 1911, age thirty-seven

Patient name: Nancy Chewie (Cherokee)
Date of admission: December 26, 1917 (committed from Ft. Yuma)
Diagnosis: Pellagra
Notes: Critically ill upon arrival; died on February 7, 1918, age twenty-three

Patient name: Marie Chico (Papago)
Date of admission: May 15, 1922
Diagnosis: Dementia praecox
Notes: Admitted at age twenty-five; transferred to St. Elizabeths

Patient name: Ruth Chief on Top (Arikara)
Date of admission: August 13, 1916 (committed from Ft. Berthold)
Diagnosis: Unknown
Notes: Died on May 11, 1918, age twenty-five

Patient name: Kittie Chu-e-rah-rah-he-kah (Pawnee)
Date of admission: January 1903
Diagnosis: Chronic mania
Notes: Transferred from St. Elizabeths; died on January 1, 1905, age seventy-two

Patient name: Caroline Collins (Cheyenne)
Date of admission: April 4, 1932
Diagnosis: Unknown

Patient name: Cecile Comes-at-night (Piegan)
Date of admission: Unknown
Diagnosis: Unknown
Notes: Died on August 9, 1919, age twenty-five

Patient name: Lucy Crane (Seminole)
Date of admission: April 17, 1910
Diagnosis: Hypochondriacal melancholia
Notes: Died on April 27, 1915

Patient name: Dasia or Pidajoltaha (Apache)
Date of admission: April 22, 1908 (committed from San Carlos)
Diagnosis: Hemiplegia, cortical epilepsy
Notes: Died on May 20, 1916, age twenty-nine

Patient name: Madeline Dauphinais (Chippewa)
Date of admission: July 23, 1913
Diagnosis: Senile, manic-depressive; revised to senile psychosis
Notes: Transferred to St. Elizabeths at age seventy-nine; died on July 12, 1934

Patient name: Eliza L. Davis (Cherokee)
Date of admission: June 18, 1907
Diagnosis: Chronic dementia, revised to dementia praecox; paranoid
Notes: About sixty-eight in June 1917; discharged on March 3, 1922, to the state asylum in Vinita OK

Patient name: Josephine DeCoteau (Chippewa)
Date of admission: Unknown, but was in asylum by 1921 (committed from Turtle Mountain Agency)
Diagnosis: Unknown
Notes: Born in 1905; died on April 5, 1923, age eighteen

Patient name: Margaret DeCoteau (Sioux)
Date of admission: August 7, 1916 (committed from Sisseton Agency)
Diagnosis: Epileptic
Notes: Died on October 13, 1924

Patient name: Drag Toes (West Navajo)
Date of admission: January 21, 1920
Diagnosis: Spastic diplegia, imbecility
Notes: Mother of Zonna Yazza; died on February 21, 1932, age seventy-two

Patient name: Emily Eldridge (Blackfeet)
Date of admission: September 3, 1909
Diagnosis: Dementia praecox
Notes: Listed as a "Care and Maintenance" patient in fiscal year 1927

Patient name: E-nas-pah (Northern Navajo)
Date of admission: April 5, 1909
Diagnosis: Manic-depressive, tubercular (she was pregnant when admitted)
Notes: At the asylum, had a premature female child in 1909; died on September 30, 1909, age twenty-six

Patient name: Ruth E-nas-pah (Navajo)
Date of admission: August 1909
Diagnosis: Tubercular meningitis
Notes: Baby of E-nas-pah; died on October 14, 1909, age two months; mother and daughter are buried in the same grave

Patient name: Meda Ensign (Shoshone)
Date of admission: March 22, 1913
Diagnosis: Psychosis, idiocy; had trachoma in 1923
Notes: Transferred to St. Elizabeths at age forty-four; died on October 11, 1935

Patient name: Frances Espinoza (Pueblo)
Date of admission: June 23, 1923
Diagnosis: Paranoia, revised to dementia praecox, paranoid type
Notes: Transferred to St. Elizabeths at age forty-three

Patient name: Juanita Espinoza (Pueblo)
Date of admission: June 23, 1923
Diagnosis: Senile, dementia praecox
Notes: Mother to Frances; transferred to St. Elizabeths at age seventy-three

Patient name: E-we-jar or E-we-gar (Bannock)
Date of admission: January 30, 1905 (committed from Rossfork ID)
Diagnosis: Kleptomania, revised to arterio-sclerotic dementia
Notes: Died on October 4, 1910, age forty-five

Patient name: Mary Fairchild (Klamath)
Date of admission: Unknown
Diagnosis: Syphilitic dementia
Notes: Died on April 29, 1907, age fifty-eight

Patient name: Elizabeth Faribault (Sioux)
Date of admission: May 29, 1915
Diagnosis: Intoxication psychosis; diagnosed by Dr. Emil Kraepelin as dementia praecox
Notes: Escaped in 1920 but was returned to asylum; died on March 2, 1928

Patient name: Winona Faribault (Sioux and Navajo)
Date of admission: Born to Elizabeth on September 28, 1926
Diagnosis: Imbecile
Notes: Stayed at Canton Asylum four years; released to Episcopal Orphanage/ Good Shepard Mission in Ft. Defiance AZ on July 24, 1930

Patient name: Stella Fast Horse (Sioux)
Date of admission: July 30, 1923
Diagnosis: Dementia praecox, catatonic symptoms; revised to manic-depressive
Notes: Transferred to St. Elizabeths; became pregnant by another patient in 1937

Patient name: Susie Fish (Sioux)
Date of admission: Unknown
Diagnosis: Unknown

Patient name: Mary Mann Fisher (Winnebago)
Date of admission: June 16, 1917
Diagnosis: Dementia praecox
Notes: Discharged on December 28, 1918

Patient name: Pisquoponoke Fredericka (Menominee)
Date of admission: January 30, 1918
Diagnosis: Epileptic psychosis
Notes: Listed as a recipient in a February 1927 journal voucher

Patient name: Lizzie Giroux (Sioux)
Date of admission: February 2, 1903
Diagnosis: Congenital imbecility, ataxic aphasia
Notes: Admitted at age twelve; discharged May 16, 1908, at age seventeen

Patient name: Lucy or Lillian Gladstone (Flathead)
Date of admission: March 4, 1911
Diagnosis: Chronic depression, probably hysteria
Notes: Discharged on September 5, 1911

Patient name: Gonda say quay* (Chippewa)
Date of admission: July 12, 1918
Diagnosis: Demented, senile psychosis
Notes: Transferred to St. Elizabeths at age seventy-six; age seventy-nine in 1929

Patient name: Frances Goodbear (Winnebago)
Date of admission: February 28, 1932
Diagnosis: Dementia praecox
Notes: Transferred to St. Elizabeths

Patient name: Gertrude Gould (Navajo)
Date of admission: August 12, 1932
Diagnosis: Dementia praecox and Parkinson's
Notes: Transferred to St. Elizabeths

Patient name: Emma Gregory (Creek)
Date of admission: August 4, 1905
Diagnosis: Terminal dementia, revised to dementia praecox; paranoid
Notes: Died on March 12, 1912, age forty-six

Patient name: Maggie Hale or O-zowsh-quah (Potawatomi)
Date of admission: February 22, 1908
Diagnosis: Climacteric insanity, intoxication psychosis
Notes: Transferred to St. Elizabeths, though Hummer offered to let her go home in March 1909

Patient name: Lulu L. Vincent Hall (Jicarilla Apache)
Date of admission: May 29, 1932
Diagnosis: Admitted with chronic melancholia, revised to dementia praecox
Notes: Transferred to St Elizabeths at age thirty

Patient name: Jessie Hallock* (Caddo)
Date of admission: January 29, 1903 (committed from Kiowa Agency)
Diagnosis: Congenital imbecility, high-grade
Notes: Died on June 8, 1923, age twenty-one; listed as twenty-five in 1909 report

Patient name: May Harris (Winnebago)
Date of admission: Unknown
Diagnosis: Died of epilepsy
Notes: Listed as a "girl"; died on February 28, 1918

Patient name: Mellum Harris (Winnebago)
Date of admission: April 26, 1911 (committed from Klamath Agency)
Diagnosis: Senile dementia
Notes: Age around fifty-five but looked seventy; died on August 23, 1912

Patient name: Olnya Houla
Date of admission: Unknown
Diagnosis: Unknown

Patient name: Cynthia or Cynia Houle (Cree)
Date of admission: June 22, 1911
Diagnosis: Manic-depressive
Notes: Mentioned in 1927; died on January 17, 1932, age sixty-nine

Patient name: Ollie House* (Shoshone)
Date of admission: Unknown
Diagnosis: Senile dementia
Notes: Died on February 11, 1909, age sixty-nine, according to L. L. Culp's cemetery listing; patient's death is mentioned in a 1907 investigation as occurring at 2:00 a.m. on July 19, 1904

Patient name: Nellie Hurley (Pima)
Date of admission: November 21, 1922

Diagnosis: Dementia praecox
Notes: Transferred to St. Elizabeths at age thirty-one

Patient name: Mary Ignatio (Papago)
Date of admission: March 14, 1921 (committed from Ft. Yuma School)
Diagnosis: Dementia praecox, catatonic
Notes: Transferred to St. Elizabeths at age thirty-five

Patient name: Grace Jim (Paiute)
Date of admission: February 28, 1929
Diagnosis: Psychosis, feebleminded; revised as epilepsy with deterioration
Notes: Transferred to St. Elizabeths

Patient name: Edith Kaloneheskie or Kalonehuskie, Kalonuheskie (Cherokee)
Date of admission: December 21, 1922 (committed from Cherokee Agency NC)
Diagnosis: Imbecility
Notes: Age eighteen in 1927; transferred to St. Elizabeths at age twenty-five; died on January 26, 1937

Patient name: Nellie Kampeska
Date of admission: September 12, 1917
Diagnosis: Constitutional psychopath, hysterical, nymphomania
Notes: Discharged on July 24, 1919

Patient name: Kay-ge-gay-aush-oak or Kay-ge-gay-aush-eak* (Martha Smith) (Chippewa)
Date of admission: December 1908 (also listed as May 5, 1903)
Diagnosis: Dementing psychosis with epilepsy
Notes: Seventeen in 1909; her neglect led to an investigation; died on March 12, 1913, age twenty-one

Patient name: Kaygwaydahsegaik (Chippewa)
Date of admission: December 20, 1908 (committed from Leech Lake)
Diagnosis: Senile dementia
Notes: Admitted at age sixty-eight; died on October 14, 1910, age seventy-one

Patient name: Kay-she-ah-bow or Kay-she-ah-bo* (Maggie Francis) (Chippewa)
Date of admission: May 21, 1903 (committed from White Earth)
Diagnosis: Senile dementia
Notes: Age 101 in June 28, 1910, asylum census; died on June 22, 1912, age 95

Patient name: Kayso (Menominee)
Date of admission: April 6, 1920 (committed from Keshena Agency)
Diagnosis: Unknown
Notes: Died of a series of epileptic fits on March 23, 1923, age fifty-nine

Patient name: No Walk Kiger* (Paiute)
Date of admission: June 5, 1916 (committed from Reno Agency)
Diagnosis: Paraplegia
Notes: Age sixty-two in 1929; died on July 2, 1929 (also listed as June 29, 1929)

Patient name: Sadie LaMere (Winnebago)
Date of admission: June 7, 1922
Diagnosis: Unknown
Notes: Died of status epilepticus on January 31, 1926

Patient name: Mary Le Beaux
Date of admission: Unknown
Diagnosis: Acute melancholia
Notes: Died of consumption on December 17, 1905

Patient name: Minne LeCount or LaCount (Chickasaw)
Date of admission: Unknown
Diagnosis: Chronic dementia
Notes: Died on July 5, 1906, age thirty-four

Patient name: Leona LeLakes or LaLakes (Klamath)
Date of admission: August 7, 1920
Diagnosis: Unknown
Notes: Died of tubercular meningitis on August 6, 1928

Patient name: Long Time Owl Woman (Blackfeet)
Date of admission: Unknown
Diagnosis: Epileptic dementia
Notes: Died on August 25, 1908, age thirty-four

Patient name: Maria or Marie Lupe* (Pueblo)
Date of admission: May 31, 1905
Diagnosis: Hemiplegia with epilepsy, syphilitic; revised to epilepsy with idiocy
Notes: Nineteen in 1909; died on October 27, 1916

Patient name: Maud Magpie (Cheyenne)
Date of admission: February 18, 1918 (committed from Tongue River Agency)
Diagnosis: Epileptic
Notes: Died on April 22, 1920, age forty-one

Patient name: Magwon (Chippewa)
Date of admission: June 30, 1905 (committed from Leech Lake)
Diagnosis: Senile dementia
Notes: Eighty-four in 1910 asylum census; died on March 23, 1912

Patient name: Mahjegeshig (Chippewa)
Date of admission: May 2, 1917 (committed from White Earth)
Diagnosis: Senile, demented
Notes: Died on July 15, 1920

Patient name: May-go-wun-a-be-quay* (Chippewa)
Date of admission: Unknown
Diagnosis: Senile dementia, revised to senile psychosis
Notes: Eighty-seven in 1910 asylum census; died on March 23, 1912, age eighty-seven

Patient name: Louisa Porter McIntosh (Cherokee)
Date of admission: April 21, 1905
Diagnosis: Chronic dementia, revised to dementia praecox, paranoid
Notes: Died on April 10, 1915, age sixty

Patient name: Adele Montriel (Chippewa)
Date of admission: Unknown (committed from Turtle Mountain Agency)
Diagnosis: Manic-depressive
Notes: Discharged on December 15, 1915, but listed in June 30, 1921, and June 30, 1924, asylum censuses

Patient name: Amelia Moss (Caddo)
Date of admission: May 31, 1922 (committed from Kiowa Agency)
Diagnosis: Idiocy with epilepsy, revised to mental deficiency
Notes: Age six when admitted; transferred to St. Elizabeths

Patient name: Magdelene Nacjewiske or Nachewiske (Menominee)
Date of admission: Unknown
Diagnosis: Unknown
Notes: Discharged on April 7, 1919

Patient name: Nesba (Navajo)
Date of admission: February 14, 1924
Diagnosis: Paraplegic, imbecile, revised to idiocy
Notes: Transferred to St. Elizabeths

Patient name: Maggie Nicholson (Gros Ventre)
Date of admission: August 4, 1917
Diagnosis: Dementia praecox
Notes: Transferred to St. Elizabeths at age forty-nine

Patient name: Oche-chago-oke-zhig-oke* (Chippewa)
Date of admission: July 17, 1906, or August 1908
Diagnosis: Periodic insanity, revised to manic-depressive
Notes: Discharged on March 23, 1910

Patient name: Victoria Martinez Ortiz (Pueblo)
Date of admission: September 4, 1922
Diagnosis: Manic-depressive
Notes: Listed as discharged on November 21, 1924, and admitted on July 26, 1926; died on October 20, 1929, of carcinoma of the pylorus

Patient name: Marie Pancho (Papago)
Date of admission: December 11, 1920 (committed from Sells Indian School)
Diagnosis: Unknown
Notes: Died on October 14, 1923, age forty-three

Patient name: Marie Parker (Chippewa)
Date of admission: April 5, 1919
Diagnosis: Unknown
Notes: Discharged on November 6, 1921

Patient name: Sophia Pecore (Menominee)
Date of admission: September 14, 1919, and January 11, 1921 (committed from Keshena Agency)
Diagnosis: Unknown
Notes: Discharged on September 23, 1920, but readmitted

Patient name: Josephine Pejihutaskana (Sioux)
Date of admission: Unknown
Diagnosis: Unknown
Notes: Died on September 25, 1921, age thirty-three

Patient name: Mary Pierre (Flathead)
Date of admission: January 1917
Diagnosis: Unknown
Notes: Died on May 16, 1917, age seventy-six

Patient name: Celina Pilon (Chippewa)
Date of admission: November 25, 1911 (committed from Rapid City Indian School)
Diagnosis: Unknown
Notes: Died on October 11, 1922, age thirty-five

Patient name: Poke ah doo ah (Comanche)
Date of admission: Unknown
Diagnosis: Unknown
Notes: Died on December 22, 1920, age seventy-two

Patient name: Louisa Porlier (Menominee)
Date of admission: August 7, 1909 (committed from Keshena)

Diagnosis: Alcoholic psychosis
Notes: Died on December 22, 1928

Patient name: Isabella Porter (Chippewa)
Date of admission: August 15, 1906 or 1908
Diagnosis: Congenital imbecility, amentia
Notes: Suffered a miscarriage on March 20, 1910; discharged September 8, 1910, at age twenty-two

Patient name: Pretty Nest (Crow)
Date of admission: January 14, 1919
Diagnosis: Unknown; lost her reason when her daughter died in a train wreck
Notes: Died of stomach cancer on March 31, 1921

Patient name: Mabel Red Hair
Date of admission: Unknown
Diagnosis: Nymphomania

Patient name: Lizzie Red Owl (Sioux)
Date of admission: March 30, 1922
Diagnosis: Dementia praecox, paranoid form; Kraepelin examined her and found "no signs of intelligence deficiencies"
Notes: Hummer denied her release in letter dated December 4, 1929; released by Silk

Patient name: Lucy Reed (Creek)
Date of admission: Unknown
Diagnosis: Epileptic dementia
Notes: Died on April 19, 1907, age twenty-two

Patient name: Josephine Rider (Cherokee)
Date of admission: October 13, 1905
Diagnosis: Circular insanity
Notes: Furloughed on February 18, 1907; readmitted on April 20, 1907; furloughed again on April 6, 1909

Patient name: Sylvia Ridley (Choctaw)
Date of admission: Unknown
Diagnosis: Neurasthenia
Notes: Died on June 12, 1905, age thirty-four

Patient name: Bessie Rising Fire (Cheyenne)
Date of admission: January 12, 1933 (committed from Tongue River Agency)
Diagnosis: Psychosis, cerebral arteriosclerosis, revised to senile psychosis

Notes: Transferred to St. Elizabeths, age seventy-six or seventy-seven; died on June 29, 1938

Patient name: Melinda Robinson (Sioux)
Date of admission: August 17, 1929 (committed from Rosebud)
Diagnosis: Violent and delirious, advanced pulmonary TB; tentatively diagnosed infection-exhausted psychosis
Notes: Dr. Hummer believed she would die within a few days of admittance

Patient name: Ida Roubideaux (Sioux)
Date of admission: June 28, 1929 (committed from Rosebud)
Diagnosis: Unknown
Notes: Discharged by Silk in September 1933 to hospital in Rosebud Agency

Patient name: Edith Schroder (Chippewa)
Date of admission: November 17, 1924
Diagnosis: Diagnosed feebleminded; "immoral, used liquor, neglected infants, bad temper" on medical certificate
Notes: Admitted at age twenty-nine; lost her right hand in laundry mangle at asylum in 1930; released as sane at asylum's closing, age thirty-eight

Patient name: Sallie Seabolt (Cherokee)
Date of admission: September 29, 1917
Diagnosis: Unknown
Notes: Died on July 9, 1922, age forty-six

Patient name: Susie Sharp Fish (Sioux)
Date of admission: June 28, 1929 (committed from Rosebud)
Diagnosis: Epilepsy

Patient name: Annie Shawano (Chippewa)
Date of admission: April 16, 1926
Diagnosis: Epilepsy, imbecility
Notes: Sister of James Shawano; discharged at time of brother's death in May 1927

Patient name: Minnie Sheayounena (Hopi or Moqui)
Date of admission: October 5, 1907
Diagnosis: Congenital imbecility, revised to dementia praecox, catatonic symptoms
Notes: Age seventeen when committed; transferred to St. Elizabeths

Patient name: Catherine Sheshequeam (Menominee)
Date of admission: September 10, 1914 (committed from Keshena Agency)
Diagnosis: Unknown

Notes: Died on November 29, 1922, of tubercular pneumonia; had $700 at time of death

Patient name: Alice Short (Bannock)
Date of admission: June 1, 1905 (Ft. Hall Agency)
Diagnosis: Dementia, syphilis, revised to general paralysis of the insane
Notes: Died on April 17, 1909, age thirty-four, of exhaustion from general paresis of the insane

Patient name: Sarah Shortwoman (Cheyenne)
Date of admission: February 17, 1933 (committed from Cheyenne Agency)
Diagnosis: Senile psychosis
Notes: Transferred to St. Elizabeths, age eighty-six; died on February 21, 1936

Patient name: Sits in it (Sioux)
Date of admission: Unknown
Diagnosis: Unknown
Notes: Died on January 22, 1921, age seventy-five

Patient name: Agnes Sloan (Puyallup)
Date of admission: March 24, 1909
Diagnosis: Epileptic idiocy
Notes: Age sixteen when committed; died on February 14, 1910, age seventeen, of exhaustion following TB of the bones

Patient name: Dorothy Smith (Chippewa)
Date of admission: October 9, 1928 (committed from Lac du Flambeau)
Diagnosis: Manic-depressive
Notes: Discharged on August 7, 1929

Patient name: Annie Smoke (Paiute)
Date of admission: December 31, 1918 (committed from Warm Springs OR)
Diagnosis: Dementia praecox, paranoid
Notes: Transferred to St. Elizabeths, age fifty-one

Patient name: Maggie Snow (Chippewa)
Date of admission: May 20, 1916
Diagnosis: Weak-minded
Notes: Admitted around age thirty; died on July 7, 1929

Patient name: Ebe Snowboy (Sioux)
Date of admission: February 4, 1926
Diagnosis: Dementia, encephalitis
Notes: Died on August 9, 1928, age fifty-eight

Patient name: Kittie Spicer (Peacock) (Wyandotte)
Date of admission: April 27, 1908 (committed from Seneca School)
Diagnosis: Epilepsy with dementia
Notes: Admitted at age twenty; transferred to St. Elizabeths

Patient name: Nellie Spotted Elk (Cheyenne)
Date of admission: January 12, 1933 (committed from Tongue River)
Diagnosis: Psychosis with epilepsy
Notes: Transferred to St. Elizabeths, age twenty

Patient name: Edith Standingbear (Sioux)
Date of admission: Unknown
Diagnosis: Sporadic cretinism
Notes: Died on May 13, 1905, age seventeen

Patient name: Mary Stubbs (Chippewa)
Date of admission: Admitted sometime between July 1925 and October 1928
Diagnosis: Unknown
Notes: Died on October 26, 1928

Patient name: Sweetgrass Woman (Mandan)
Date of admission: May 19, 1923 (committed from Ft. Berthold)
Diagnosis: Senility

Patient name: Lu Lu Taylor (Chippewa)
Date of admission: Before 1905 and on June 17, 1910 (committed from Leech Lake)
Diagnosis: Epilepsy, grand mal, revised to epileptic psychosis
Notes: Admitted at age thirty-five (?); returned home sometime in 1905, but listed
in June 28, 1910, and June 30, 1921, asylum censuses; died on September 13, 1923

Patient name: Sophie or Sophia Three Stars (Sioux)
Date of admission: August 25, 1922
Diagnosis: Dementia praecox
Notes: Transferred to St. Elizabeths, age forty

Patient name: Ida Todd
Date of admission: Unknown
Diagnosis: Epilepsy, petit mal
Notes: Nearly fourteen years old when furloughed to go to school (Flandreau)
in 1908

Patient name: Trucha (Jicarilla Apache)
Date of admission: Unknown
Diagnosis: Chronic dementia

Patient name: Mabel Tsinnijinni (Navaho)
Date of admission: February 8, 1931 (committed from Leupp Agency)
Diagnosis: Psychosis, idiocy, epilepsy
Notes: Age ten when committed to Canton Asylum; transferred to St. Elizabeths, age twelve; died on October 5, 1934

Patient name: Emma Twin
Date of admission: May 15, 1919 (committed from Standing Rock Agency)
Diagnosis: Unknown
Notes: Died suddenly on May 21, 1920

Patient name: Mrs. Two Teeth*
Date of admission: August 22, 1919 (committed from Crow Creek Agency)
Diagnosis: Unknown
Notes: Died of uremic coma, chronic nephritis on January 1, 1925 (also listed as January 7, 1922), age sixty-nine

Patient name: Lizzie Vipont (Paiute)
Date of admission: July 6, 1905
Diagnosis: Chronic epileptic dementia, hysteria
Notes: Died on April 17, 1917, age forty-one

Patient name: Wah-bis-ay-she-quay or Wah-be-she-she-quay (Chippewa)
Date of admission: June 23, 1907 (committed from Leech Lake)
Diagnosis: Congenital imbecility
Notes: Listed in June 30, 1924, asylum census and as recipient in February 1927 journal voucher

Patient name: Emily Waite (Chickasaw)
Date of admission: March 30, 1906
Diagnosis: Delusional melancholia, revised to paranoia
Notes: Found dead in bed on August 3, 1929

Patient name: Mary Walking Day
Date of admission: April 18, 1918 (committed from Winnebago Agency)
Diagnosis: Manic-depressive insanity
Notes: Discharged on May 16, 1918

Patient name: Rose Wash (Arickara)
Date of admission: June 30, 1906
Diagnosis: Organic dementia, hemiplegia
Notes: Transferred to St. Elizabeths

Patient name: Nannie Washington (Caddo)
Date of admission: December 21, 1907 (committed from Kiowa Agency)

Diagnosis: Traumatic epileptic dementia with epilepsy
Notes: Admitted at age twenty; died on February 25, 1919

Patient name: Mary Wauketch (Menominee)
Date of admission: January 30, 1918
Diagnosis: Dementia praecox
Notes: Transferred to St. Elizabeths

Patient name: Josephine Wells (Chippewa)
Date of admission: January 10, 1905
Diagnosis: Chronic epileptic dementia
Notes: Died on June 27, 1921, age thirty-six

Patient name: Lucy Cline Wells
Date of admission: June 22, 1922 (committed from Omaha Indian Agency)
Diagnosis: Unknown
Notes: Died on September 29, 1922

Patient name: Amy Whiteboy (?)
Date of admission: Unknown (committed from Crow Creek Reservation)
Diagnosis: Unknown

Patient name: Leda Williamson (Crow)
Date of admission: February 3, 1929
Diagnosis: Psychosis, epilepsy
Notes: Admitted at age twenty-eight; transferred to St. Elizabeths

Patient name: Susan Wishecoby (Menominee)
Date of admission: November 8, 1917
Diagnosis: Epilepsy
Notes: Discharged on September 14, 1925

Patient name: Mrs. Womak (Osage)
Date of admission: April 24, 1906
Diagnosis: Senile mania
Notes: Age eighty-eight in June 28, 1910, asylum census; died on June 22, 1912

Patient name: Ollie Yarlott (Crow)
Date of admission: September 14, 1930
Diagnosis: Dementia praecox
Notes: Had ten children, the youngest was eight; transferred to St. Elizabeths, age fifty

Patient name: Zonna Yazza (Navajo)
Date of admission: April 29, 1919 (committed from Southern Navajo Agency, Ft. Defiance)

Diagnosis: Epileptic
Notes: Age eighteen in 1927; transferred to St. Elizabeths, age twenty-five; died on March 15, 1974

Other Admissions

Dr. Hummer noted on January 18, 1921, that he had admitted a "very old, feeble blind woman" from Crow Creek Indian Agency and did not have her name yet.

Patient name: Atsoni (Navajo)
Date of admission: Unknown
Diagnosis: Unknown

Patient Name: Dan
Affidavits by employees Jesse Watkins and Joab N. Johnson in November 1909 reference a patient named "Dan"; could possibly refer to Danaghonginiwa

Patient name: Francisco
Date of admission: October 14, 1921
Diagnosis: Unknown

Patient name: Bi-co-dy Hosteen (Navajo)
Date of admission: Unknown
Diagnosis: Intoxication psychosis, alcoholic

Patient name: Jimmie
Date of admission: Unknown
Diagnosis: Unknown
Note: During the Perry/Allen investigation, an attendant mentioned someone named "Jimmie" who weighed fifty pounds

Patient name: Lufkins (Chippewa)
Date of admission: Unknown
Diagnosis: Unknown

Patient name: Pasue
Date of admission: Unknown
Diagnosis: Unknown
Notes: Died on May 20, 1916

APPENDIX B

Patients Interred in Canton Asylum Cemetery

This listing is taken from a report from Dr. L. L. Culp to the commissioner of Indian affairs (February 17, 1934, NARA, box 4). The cemetery was arranged in six tiers. Tiers 1, 2, and 3 were on the west side. Tiers 4, 5, and 6 were on the east side, with a vacant space between tier 3 and tier 4. Spellings of patient and tribal names are per Culp's report.

Tier 1, or west row, beginning at north end					
Plot #	Name	Age	Death date	Interment date	Agency/tribe
96	Clafflin, Charles	83	2/28/14	3/3/14	Keshena WI / Menominee
95	Hall, John	34	5/25/14	5/27/14	Sacaton AZ / Pima
94	Deere, Amos	38	7/11/14	7/13/14	Shawnee OK / Abs. [Absentee] Shawnee
93	Ne-bow-o-sah	50	12/18/14	12/21/14	Mayetta KS / Potawatomi
92	Chasing Bear, Thomas	31	2/2/15	2/5/15	Ft. Yates ND / Sioux
91	Danachonginiwa	41	3/27/16	3/29/16	Keams Canyon AZ / Moqui
90	Bigmane, Joseph	30	3/27/16	Unknown	Ft. Yates ND / Sioux
89	Walkkas	79	1/21/17	Unknown	Mayetta KS / Potawatomi

88	Simons, Steve	45	10/8/17	Unknown	Muskogee OK / Cherokee
87	Two Crows, James *or* John	27	11/26/17	11/28/17	Ft. Berthold ND / Gros Ventre
86	Chargingeagle, Frederick	43	9/1/18	Unknown	Rosebud SD / Sioux
85	Dancer, Andrew	24	11/21/18	Unknown	Yankton Agcy SD / Sioux
84	Miranda, Apolonio	54	1/14/19	Unknown	Sells Agcy AZ / Papago
83	Miller, Harry	16	4/20/19	4/23/19	Walker River NV / Paiute
82	Iron, Herbert	41	5/18/19	5/19/19	Ft. Washakie WY / Arapaho
81	Collins, Fred	21	5/30/19	6/3/19	Towaoc CO / Ute Mt.
80	Coal-of-Fire, John	32	6/17/19	6/20/19	Cantonment OK / Arapaho
79	Marshall, John D.	25	11/17/19	11/20/19	Rosebud SD / Sioux
78	George, Willie	24	11/18/19	11/22/19	Walker River NV / Paiute
77	Hathorn, James	7[1]	11/26/19	11/29/19	Ft. Defiance AZ / Navajo
76	Gristeau, Ira	14	3/24/20	Unknown	Keshena WI / Menominee
75	Hedges, Edward	51	3/18/20	5/21/20	Santee NE / Sioux
74	Omudis (male)	30	6/2/20	6/5/20	White Earth MN / Chippewa
73	Crow Neck, Guy	19	7/26/20	7/29/20	Cantonment OK / Cheyenne
No #[2]	Big John	38	8/25/20	Unknown	Ft. Defiance AZ / Navajo
No #	Kennedy, Alex	64	2/15/21	2/19/21	Ft. Yates ND / Chippewa

Tier 2, second row from west side					
Plot #	Name	Age	Death date	Interment date	Agency/tribe
49	Brown Ears, Amos	31	5/1/21	Unknown	Pine Ridge SD / Sioux
50	Crow, Lightning	61	5/8/21	Unknown	Santee NE / Sioux
51	Masten, John	30	4/4/22	Unknown	Hoopa Valley CA / Klamath
52	Red Crow	84	4/8/22	4/12/22	Crow Creek SD / Sioux
53	Blackeye, James	20	5/4/22	Unknown	Redlake MN / Minn. Chippewa
54	Meacham, Abraham	62	11/7/22	Unknown	Neah Bay WA / Makah
55	Moore, Aloysius	29	5/12/23	Unknown	Rosebud SD / Sioux
56	Floodwood, Tom	62	9/26/23	9/29/23	Cass Lake MN / Minn. Chippewa
57	Black Bull, James	40	2/6/26	Unknown	Rosebud SD / Sioux
58	Juan, Benito	33	3/21/26	Unknown	Sells Agcy AZ / Papago
59	Wauketch, Seymour	71	5/27/26	5/31/26	Keshena WI / Menominee
60	Lucas, Anselmo	40	12/19/26	Unknown	Sells Agcy AZ / Papago
61	Francisco, Chico	51	4/17/27	Unknown	Sells Agcy AZ / Papago
62	Wolfe, Roy	18	3/28/28	3/30/28	Tahlequah OK / Cherokee
63	Smith, Matt	51	11/28/28	Unknown	Parker AZ / Chemehueve
64	Two Teeth	79	7/16/30	Unknown	Crow Creek SD / Sioux
65	Beel, Pugay	51	9/12/31	Unknown	Shiprock NM / No. Navajo

| 66 | Conley, Herbert | 25 | 3/17/33 | Unknown | Tuba City AZ / West. Navajo |
| 67 | Root, Jack | 82 | 10/27/33 | Unknown | Ashland WI / Chippewa |

Tier 3, third row from west side, beginning at north end, all females

Plot #	Name	Age	Death date	Interment date	Agency/tribe
49	Bah, Mary	20	8/22/30	Unknown	Tuba City AZ / West. Navajo
50	Houle, Cynthia (Cynia)	69	1/17/32	Unknown	Belcourt ND / Turtle Mt. Chippewa
51	Drag toes	72	2/24/32[3]	Unknown	Tuba City AZ / West. Navajo[4]

Tier 4, fourth row from west side, beginning at north end, all males

Plot #	Name	Age	Death date	Interment date	Agency/tribe
48	Brown, Charles	60	11/3/07	Unknown	Wisconsin / Winnebago
47	Hayes, Jacob (Satsch)	65	10/4/07	Unknown	Sacaton AZ / Pima
46	Toby *or* Koz-he-la	35	3/6/06	Unknown	Mescalero NM / Apache
45	Trucha	46	11/17/05	Unknown	Dulce NM / Jicarilla Apache
44	Hon-sah-sah-kah	23	10/23/05	Unknown	Pawhuska OK / Osage
43	Big Day	45	7/3/05	Unknown	Crow Agency (Pryor) / Mont. Crow
42	Tatsup, Fred	45	2/6/05	Unknown	Fort Hall ID / Bannock
41	Greenwood, Peter	42	9/22/03	Unknown	Rosebud SD / Brule Sioux

40	Brings Plenty, Robert	21	5/20/03	Unknown	Pine Ridge SD / Sioux
39	Nadesooda	63	2/8/08	Unknown	San Carlos AZ / Apache
38	Toistoto	32	5/17/08	Unknown	Shiprock NM / Northern Navajo
37	Chief Crow, James	28	10/28/08	Unknown	Browning MT / Piegan
36	Yells at Night	33	11/21/08	Unknown	Browning MT / Piegan
35	Woodruff, John[5]	51	5/15/09	5/17/09	Pine Ridge SD
34	Battise, George	17	5/30/09	Unknown	Wittenberg WI / Winnebago
33	Gingras, Baptiste	19	12/19/09	Unknown	Dixon MT / Flathead
32	Lone War, Thomas	53	12/24/09	Unknown	Pine Ridge SD / Sioux
31	Hawk, Silas	24	5/12/10	Unknown	Oklahoma / Sac & Fox
30	Red Cloud	58	12/7/10	Unknown	Pine Ridge SD / Sioux
29	Howling Wolf	59	3/30/11	Unknown	Ft. Berthold ND / Arickaree
28	Antone	42	4/4/12	4/6/12	Sells Agency AZ / Papago
27	Wolf, Arch	38	7/2/12	Unknown	Union Agcy OK / Cherokee
26	Starr, Frank	31	4/28/13	4/30/13	Leech Lake MN / Minn. Chippewa
25	Taylor, Joseph	24	9/18/13	Unknown	White Earth MN / Minn. Chippewa

Tier 5, fifth row from west side, beginning at north end, all females					
Plot #	Name	Age	Death date	Interment date	Agency/tribe
1	Long Time Owl Woman	34	8/25/08	Unknown	Browning MT / Blackfeet
2	Casildo, Juanita	40	6/22/08	Unknown	Laguna NM / Pueblo
3	Fairchild, Mary	58	4/29/07	Unknown	Siletz OR / Klamath
4	Reed, Lucy	22	4/19/07	Unknown	Union Agcy OK / Creek
5	LeCount or LaCount, Minnie	34	7/5/06	Unknown	Union Agcy OK / Chicka-saw
6	Ridley, Sylvia	34	6/12/05	Unknown	Union Agcy OK / Choctaw
7	Standingbear, Edith	17	5/13/05	Unknown	Pine Ridge (Allen) SD / Sioux
8	Chu-e-rah-rah-he-kah, Kittie	72	1/1/05	Unknown	Pawnee OK / Pawnee
9	House, Ollie	69	2/11/09	Unknown	Ft. Washakie WY / Shoshoni
10	Asal, Tchee	29	2/11/09	Unknown	Ft. Defi-ance AZ / So. Navajo
11	Short, Alice	34	4/7/09	Unknown	Fort Hall ID / Bannock
12	E-nas-pah[6]; E-nas-pah, Ruth	26; 2 mos.	9/30/09	10/14/09	Shiprock NM / No. Navajo
13	Sloan, Agnes	17	2/14/10	Unknown	Puyallup WA / Puyallup
14	E-we-jar	45	10/4/10	Unknown	Fort Hall ID / Bannock
15	Kay-gway-dah-se-gaik	71	10/14/10	10/15/10	Cass Lake MN / Minn. Chippewa

16	Chee	37	5/4/11	5/6/11	Ft. Defiance AZ / So. Navajo
17	Gregory, Emma	46	3/12/12	3/14/12	Union Agency OK / Creek
18	May-go-wun-e-be-quay[7]	87	3/23/12	Unknown	Leech Lake MN / Minn. Chippewa
19	Kay-zhe-ah-bow *or* Maggie Francis	95	6/22/12	6/24/12	White Earth MN / Minn. Chippewa
20	Kay-ke-gay-aush-eak *or* Martha Smith	21	3/12/13	3/14/13	Leech Lake MN / Minn. Chippewa
21	Bluesky, (Mrs. Charles)[8]	68	6/18/14	Unknown	Odanah WI / Bad River Chippewa
22	McIntosh, Louisa (Porter)	60	4/12/15	4/13/15	Union Agcy OK / Cherokee
23	Burch, Jane	35	3/1/16	Unknown	Ignacio CO / So. Ute
24	Dasia *or* Dasue (Pidajoltaha)	29	5/20/16	5/23/16	San Carlos AZ / Apache

Tier 6, row on east side beginning at north end Canton Asylum Cemetery, all females except Number 37

Plot #	Name	Age	Death date	Interment date	Agency/tribe
25	Snow, Maggie	29	7/7/16	Unknown	Wittenberg WI / Chippewa
26	Maria, Lupe	27	10/27/16	10/30/16	Laguna-Paguate NM / Pueblo
27	Pierre, Mary	76	5/16/17	Unknown	Flathead Agcy MT / Flathead
28	Vipont, Lizzie	41	4/17/17	Unknown	Walker River NV / Paiute
29	Chewie, Nancy	23	2/7/18	2/9/18	Fort Yuma AZ / Cherokee

30	Chief on Top, Ruth	25	5/11/18	5/14/18	Fort Berthold ND / Arickaree
31	Buck, Mary G.	27	12/14/18	Unknown	Ignacio CO / South. Ute
32	Comes-at-night, Cecile	25	8/9/19	Unknown	Flathead Agcy MT / Piegan
33	Magpie, Maud	41	4/22/20	4/24/20	Lamedeer MT / Northern Sheyenne
34	Poke ah doo ah	72	12/22/20	Unknown	Anadarko OK / Comanche
35	Sits in It	75	1/22/21	Unknown	Crow Creek SD / Sioux
36	Wells, Josephine	36	6/27/21	Unknown	Redlake MN / Minnesota Chippewa
37	Blair, Andrew Bray (male)	16	8/4/21	Unknown	Rosebud SD / Sioux
38	Pejihutaskana, Josephine	33	9/25/21	Unknown	Ft. Totten ND / Devils Lake Sioux
39	Caldwell, Delores	7 mos.	10/31/21	11/1/21	Keshena WI / Menominee
40	Seabolt, Sallie	46	7/9/22	Unknown	Muskogee OK / Cherokee
41	Pilon, Celina	35	10/14/22[9]	10/14/22	Rapid City School SD / Chippewa (¼).
42	Two Teeth (Mrs.)	69	1/1/25	Unknown	Crow Creek SD / Sioux
43	Kayso	59	3/23/23	Unknown	Keshena WI / Menominee
44	DeCoteau, Josephine	18	4/5/23	Unknown	Belcourt ND / Turtle Mt. Chippewa
45	Hallock, Jessie	21	6/8/23	Unknown	Oklahoma / Caddo

46	Pancho, Marie	43	10/14/23	10/17/23	Sells Agency AZ / Papago
47	Snowboy, Ebe	58	8/9/28	Unknown	Yankton Agcy SD / Sioux
48	Kiger No Walk	64	7/2/29	Unknown	Stewart NV / Paiute

[1] Hathorn's age when committed.

[2] On the first page of Culp's report, the last two plots in this tier are marked with an asterisk, with an accompanying note that reads "No Number on plot, but bodies buried there." The plot information on the following page indicates that Big John and Alex Kennedy are buried in these two unnumbered plots.

[3] Dr. Hummer's notification letter states February 21, 1932, as the date of death.

[4] Immediately under the information for plot 51, the following note appears in Culp's report, with no additional explanation: "About 40 feet east and west between Tiers three and four."

[5] Culp's report notes, "Records state above was a Negro and not an Indian."

[6] Culp's report: "The above mother and babe buried in same grave."

[7] Magwon died on March 23, 1912. A letter from Dr. Hummer to the commissioner of Indian affairs stated that she was to be buried in the asylum cemetery on March 26.

[8] Mrs. Charles Blue Sky died on June 18, 1914. A letter from Dr. Hummer to the commissioner of Indian affairs stated that she was to be buried in the asylum cemetery on June 20.

[9] Dr. Hummer's notification letter states October 11, 1922, as the date of death.

Notes on other burials: One patient, Jule Brien, died on February 5, 1918, and was buried at Canton Asylum Cemetery on February 8. The family was not notified in a timely manner and could not be present. Brien was disinterred on February 13, 1918, and taken to Nebraska. A patient named Joseph Jordan died on March 1, 1916, and a letter from Dr. Hummer to the commissioner of Indian affairs stated that Jordan was to be buried in the asylum cemetery on March 4, 1916; however, I could not ascertain whether the burial actually took place.

Patients Transferred to St. Elizabeths

These names are taken from a list requesting funds "for the board and care of Indian patients, transferred to St. Elizabeths Hospital, Washington, DC from Canton Asylum, Canton, South Dakota, 69 patients on December 22, 1933, and 2 patients on December 30, 1933, 71 patients in all." The request is dated January 3, 1934, and signed by M. Sanger, assistant to the superintendent and can be found in RG 418, entry 13, box 1, NARA, Washington DC.

Female Patients:

Augusta, Joanna
Benally, Priscilla (admitted December 28, 1933)
Black Cat, Maggie
Blanchard, Maggie
Canoe, Kate
Chavez, Lillian
Chico, Marie
Dauphinais, Madeline
Ensign, Meda
Espinoza, Frances
Espinoza, Juanita
Fast Horse, Stella
Gondosayquay
Goodbear, Frances
Gould, Gertrude
Hale, Mrs. Maggie, alias Ozowshquah
Hall, Lulu L. V.
Hurley, Nellie
Ignatio, Mary

Jim, Grace
Kalonuheskie, Edith
Moss, Amelia
Nesba
Nicholson, Maggie
Rising Fire, Bessie
Sheayounena, Minnie
Shortwoman, Sarah
Smoke, Annie
Spicer, Kittie
Spotted Elk, Nellie
Three Stars, Sophia
Tsinnijinni, Mabel
Wash, Rose
Wauketch, Mary
Williamson, Leda
Yarlott, Ollie
Yazza, Zonna

Male Patients

Bear, Frank
Blaine, Albert
Carpenter, Joseph
Catron, Kee
Charlie
Creeping, Charley
Deroin, William
Enos, John
Fairbanks, Richard
Fishtrap, James
Gray Blanket, John
Hart, Mark
Jackson, Robert
Kirk, Simon
Leve Leve, Earl
McCarter, Watt
McEwin, Joe
Marlow, George
Martin, John
Menoza, Juan
Mitchell, Willie J. S.

Montoya, Jose A. (admitted December 28, 1933)
Pappan, George
Picotte, Peter
Richards, Alfred
Stands By Him, Luke
Sweet Medicine, Jacob
Tafoya, Cleto
Thomas, Leonard
Turpin, Peter
Vigil, Fidel
Wolfe, Joe
Yazzie, Hoskee
Young Bird, Pete

NOTES

Abbreviations

NARA   National Archives and Records Administration, Washington DC
NARA KC National Archives and Records Administration, Kansas City MO

Introduction

1. Gorwitz, "Enumeration of the Mentally Ill," 184; and Geller and Harris, *Women of the Asylum*, 96, 256.

2. Kokecki and Mashburn, *Beyond the Asylum*.

3. These facilities were at Steilacoom, Washington; the Oregon State Insane Asylum in Salem; and finally at Morningside Hospital in Portland, Oregon. Congress passed the Alaska Mental Health Act on January 18, 1956, granting Alaska permission to construct its own mental health facilities.

1. Where Will the Indians Go?

1. Dr. Hummer to commissioner of Indian affairs, September 27, 1926, and report on the accident by attendant E. B. Colby, dated the same day, NARA, RG 75, box 17.

2. The early history of Canton Asylum is summarized in a thirteen-page report, *Indian Insane Asylum*, August 17, 1908, NARA, RG 75, box 1.

3. Anderson, *Creatures of Empire*, 19. This book elaborates on the role domestication issues played in the clashes between native peoples and Europeans.

4. Congress appropriated $150,000 to establish these trading houses.

5. Jackson and Galli, *History of the Bureau of Indian Affairs*, 27, 29; italics added.

6. Jackson and Galli, *History of the Bureau of Indian Affairs*, 33.

7. The United States gave $2,234.50 in goods and $1,000 a year in perpetuity for this land.

8. Tyler, *History of Indian Policy*, 48.

9. Jackson and Galli, *History of the Bureau of Indian Affairs*, 38.

10. This salary translates to approximately $81,300 today, according to MeasuringWorth's standard of living value, www.measuringworth.com.

11. *Johnson & Graham's Lessee v. McIntosh*, 21 U.S. (8 Wheat.) 543 (1823).

12. Frontier citizens tended to be considerably more hostile toward Indians than were easterners or the government itself. Men and families pushing westward bore the brunt of the outrage of Indians fighting for the land, which in many cases had been explicitly promised to them by the federal government. Both sides committed atrocities, though citizens expected no punishment for theirs and considerable help in punishing the Indians for theirs.

Battles between whites and Native Americans were costly and not always supported by the populace, and eventually the government decided to assimilate Indians into white culture. In an effort to protect them while they were being "civilized," it created a protector/ward relationship with Indians that resulted in many restrictions being placed on Indian property. Policy and practice continued to evolve over many years, and it is beyond the scope of this book to embrace all the issues involved with the complicated relationship between the U.S. government and Native Americans. Tyler, *History of Indian Policy*, describes these evolving policies and gives an especially illuminating account of early Spanish, French, Dutch, and English political thought on the status of Indians and international law.

The U.S. government is now paying for some of its past missteps. In September 2014 the Obama administration signed a $554 million settlement with the Navajo Nation for mismanagement of reservation resources and funds. Since 2009, the administration has negotiated settlements amounting to $2.61 billion with eighty tribes for accounting and trust management claims.

13. Couchman's letter, Senator Richard Pettigrew's follow-up, and other relevant correspondence can be found in U.S. Senate, *Asylum for Insane Indians*.

14. *Cherokee Nation v. Georgia*, 30 U.S. (5 Pet.) 1 (1831).

15. The act of May 5, 1832, ch. 75, 4 Stat. 514, was the first congressional appropriation specifically for Indian health care; it authorized the purchase and administration of smallpox vaccine.

16. The Snyder Act (Pub. L. No. 67-85, 25 U.S.C. § 13) is a one-page document that delineates several Bureau of Indian Affairs responsibilities and includes a one-line provision for relief of distress and conservation of health. The act also specifies that the bureau will employ "inspectors, supervisors, superintendents, clerks, field matrons, farmers, *physicians* . . ." The Bureau of Indian Affairs' obligation to provide health care to Native Americans was transferred to the Public Health Service in 1955. Responsibility today falls under the Indian Health Service, a part of the U.S. Department of Health and Human Services.

17. Even in the West, both the general public and lawmakers were well aware of the need to deal with insanity. Among the list of Lincoln County officials in 1887 were K. C. Stabeck and Dr. J. M. Lewis, respectively attorney and physician for its Board of Insanity.

18. In his earlier career as a lawyer, Pettigrew left the courtroom during an acrimonious trial in 1874. He came back with his pockets full of money. When his partner asked him what he was going to do, Pettigrew replied that he was going to pay the money out in fines for contempt of court.

19. "Wolcott Used a Lash," *Washington Post*, January 16, 1900.

20. Information about Canton and the fight to pass a bill to create Canton Asylum comes from Lincoln County Historical Committee, *History of Lincoln County*; "History," City of Canton, South Dakota, www.cantonsd.org/history; and correspondence between Pettigrew, the secretary of the interior, the commissioner and acting commissioner of Indian affairs, and Dr. W. W. Godding, in NARA, RG 48, Indian Division, LR 4658.

21. To add insult to injury, inferior reservation rations were subject to fraud. Indian agents sometimes misstated the weights of goods (averring that a four-hundred-pound cow weighed five hundred pounds) or issued corn in husks instead of shelled corn. (Two bushels of corn in husks would "shell out" to only a bushel and a half, thus cheating recipients of half a bushel of corn.) Foreman, *Five Civilized Tribes*, 159.

22. Indian landholdings shrank from 155,632,312 acres in 1881 to 77,865,373 acres in 1900. Tyler, *History of Indian Policy*, 97.

23. The Iroquois had medical societies that specialized in rituals for particular conditions, like hallucinations or nervous tremors.

24. Jewitt was captured in 1803 by the Nootka (Nuu-chah-nulth) in what is now Canada and remained with them until 1805.

25. Dodge, *Our Wild Indians*, 220.

26. Hewitt, *Notes on the Creek Indians*, 156–57.

27. Hrdlička, *Physiological and Medical Observations*, 243. Despite its indifference to many important elements of Indian life and culture, the federal government spent a great deal of time and manpower studying certain aspects of it. Hrdlička's *Physiological and Medical Observations* is an exhaustive study that went so far as to measure rates of yawning, snoring, and flatulence among Indians as compared to the white population (finding them comparable). This study looked at rates of insanity, finding that among a population of 125,000, the proportion of insane was 1 to 2,730 or 0.38 per 1,000—as against the white population's rate of 1.81 per 1,000.

28. The Night Chant was a Navajo ritual that took place at night and also incorporated sand paintings with healing symbols.

29. Explanations of Native Americans' approaches to mental illness are taken from Gamwell and Tomes, *Madness in America*; Brady, *Healing Logics*, particularly Barre Toelken's chapter, "The Hozho Factor: The Logic of Navajo Healing"; J. Murphy, "Psychiatric Labeling in Cross-Cultural Perspective", which makes a strong case for the near-universal recognition of mental illness by non-Western societies; Nielsen, *Disability History of the United States*; Hurd et al., *Institutional Care of the Insane*; and the Smithsonian Institution's Bureau of American Ethnology, Bulletin 123, a group of works compiled over a number of years by field researchers who investigated and wrote detailed reports about native peoples throughout the United States and beyond. Alvord and Van Pelt, *Scalpel and the Silver Bear*, is a fascinating, firsthand account of the many differences between traditional Navajo healing practices and modern medicine.

30. Capitol Chat, *Washington Post*, March 3, 1904.

31. Durban's ordeal was reported in "Governor Durbin Lost," *Washington Post*, September 25, 1904.

32. Bill S. 2042 (1897), for the construction of an insane asylum for Indians; referenced as an enclosure in Pettigrew to secretary of the interior, June 24, 1897, NARA, RG 48, box 227.

33. Smith to "The Honorable, The Secretary of the Interior," July 2, 1897, NARA, RG 48, box 227.

34. This assessment and copies of agent letters are in U.S. Senate, *Asylum for Insane Indians*, 1, 13.

35. An insane Indian was such a curiosity, in fact, that when a patient named Bobtail Bear died at St. Elizabeths, the *Washington Post* wrote a short item about her passing. "Death of 'Bobtail Bear," December 19, 1902.

36. Information about the Government Hospital for the Insane (St. Elizabeths) can be found in "Historic Saint Elizabeth's Hospital Building," Historic Medical Sites in the Washington, DC Area, U.S. National Library of Medicine, www.nlm.nih .gov/hmd/medtour/elizabeths.html; and "History of St. Elizabeths Hospital," http:// www.allfortheunion.com/ste/history.htm.

37. Most asylums were enthusiastically welcomed by area residents, since an asylum represented an economic boost for the town and jobs for some of its citizens. Sometimes a number of towns vied for the prize of serving as the location for a new asylum. Upon being alerted by area legislators that a selection committee was coming, residents in Weston (now West Virginia) whitewashed their homes, mended and painted fences, and repaired their streets and sidewalks to make a good impression. To top off their efforts, the townspeople sponsored a children's parade that led the committee to what they hoped would be the site for the new asylum. (They succeeded in their efforts.)

38. Lincoln County Historical Committee, *History of Lincoln County*, 36.

39. Range toilets (water closets) had several toilets that shared a common pipe. The unified system flushed at intervals, rather than individually, after use. Waste sat in the bowls, discharging odors, until the automatic flush occurred. Without proper—and powerful—ventilation, these water closets could become unpleasant quickly. The risk of contamination was high as well, considering that waste was held for a period of time and that some patients undoubtedly misused the appliance. Information about them comes from *Standard Practical Plumbing* and *Modern Plumbing Illustrated*, 1910 and 1915.

40. The description of Canton Asylum comes from annual reports made to the commissioner of Indian affairs; and James McLaughlin, inspector, "Inspection of Asylum for Insane Indians at Canton, S.D.," July 21, 1910, NARA, RG 75, box 2, FF 76237–150.

41. According to an article in *Sunshine Magazine*, Canton Asylum's first patient, Edward Hedges, was a professional ballplayer. Orbuck Olson, "The Only Indian

Asylum in the U.S.," *Sunshine Magazine*, n.d. [1924/25?], Canton Asylum folder, Canton Public Library, Canton sd.

2. Life in an Asylum

1. Stawicki, "Haunting Legacy."

2. The history of early care for the insane in America has been given in only the most general terms here, but it is a fascinating topic. For more information, readers might begin with works in the bibliography, and if particularly intrigued, find a copy of Hurd, et al., *Institutional Care of the Insane*, a four-volume work of more than a thousand pages. The study of insane asylums is a popular one, and the Internet can provide many images, firsthand accounts, and journal articles on the subject.

3. Grob, *Mad among Us*, 43.

4. Tuke, a Quaker, founded the York Retreat in England in 1796, about the same time that Pinel began his radical work in France. Tuke also rejected harsh methods of control and instead emphasized reading, quiet amusements and light labor, and conversation as of far greater assistance in curing insanity.

5. Dix took a break from these efforts during the Civil War to become superintendent of women nurses for the Union.

6. For a comprehensive look at how asylum architecture was considered a therapeutic part of patient treatment, see Yanni, *Architecture of Madness*.

7. Across the globe, extreme poverty exposes families to higher mortality rates and more psychiatric disorders. Murali and Oyebode, "Poverty, Social Inequality, and Mental Health" brings a concise discussion of these issues to readers. Native Americans certainly fit into a model of a marginalized, impoverished people ripe for mental health problems. Protective elements within their culture would have included strong kinship groups and a shared language—elements that a removal to Canton Asylum disrupted.

8. Foreman, *Five Civilized Tribes*, 62.

9. Days began early for attendants (6:00 a.m. between March 1 and October 16 and 6:30 a.m. the rest of the year) and ended around 9:00 p.m.; the cook would be up by four or five each morning.

10. Patients did not work when they first arrived, nor did epileptics, the frail, or any who could not understand and follow directions. As a protection, rules stated that patients could not be taken from the wards to work without the permission of the asylum's physician.

11. Susan Wishecoby to commissioner of Indian affairs, March 12, 1923, NARA, RG 75, box 8.

12. Information about patient routines at the Canton Asylum comes from employee affidavits, August 1907, NARA, RG 75, box 1; letters from Susan Wishecoby to the commissioner of Indian affairs, August 19?, 1921, and March 12, 1923, NARA, RG 75, box 15; and from asylum rules developed in 1903, NARA, RG 75, box 1.

13. Descriptions of McLean Asylum for the Insane come from Beam, *Gracefully Insane*; Hurd, et al., *Institutional Care of the Insane*, vol. 2; and *Massachusetts General Hospital Memorial*.

14. U.S. Indian agent (name unintelligible), Union Agency, November 19, 1907, to Honorable Commissioner of Indian Affairs; and Gifford to commissioner of Indian affairs, December 4, 1907, NARA, RG 75, box 12.

15. Information about Good Boy's case come from psychiatric and psychological examinations at the Canton Asylum, case records for Good Boy, a synopsis written by an unidentified person at St. Elizabeths, and affidavits from the District Court of the United States in *United States v. Peter Thompson Good Boy*, NARA KC, RG 75, box 9.

16. "Argued Her Sanity before Magistrate," *New York Times*, August 30, 1910, 11.

3. The Bad Start Begins

1. Information about psychiatric terminology comes primarily from Blumer, "History and Use of the Term Dementia"; and Murray, Harold, and Bosanquet, *Quain's Dictionary of Medicine*.

2. Discussions about the validity of diagnoses of insanity are fascinating. The psychiatrist Thomas S. Szasz strongly believed that the whole field of mental illness smacked of coercion and control. His books *The Myth of Mental Illness* and *The Manufacture of Madness* were informed protests written in the 1960s and 1970s. He particularly argued that mental illnesses are not real in the same way that cancer is real and that only a few brain diseases, like Alzheimer's, present any verifiable evidence of their existence. Another influential critic, Michel Foucault, considered psychiatric labeling and institutions a means of social control.

3. In addition to cited articles, information about hydrotherapy comes from articles in the *American Journal of Insanity* and from Braslow, *Mental Ills and Bodily Cures*.

4. Schools were built before churches in many areas of Lincoln County. The county's first school district was established in Canton, and classes were held there in 1869. Most of the one-room schools scattered about the county were painted white—not red.

5. Information about Gifford's life comes from Lincoln County Historical Committee, *History of Lincoln County*; the *Biographical Directory of the United States Congress*; and from *Memorial and Biographical Record of Turner, Lincoln, Union and Clay Counties, South Dakota*.

6. Dr. John Turner reported that Brings Plenty died of a "violent nocturnal convulsion," which would likely translate to the classic grand mal seizures that frightened bystanders into believing the person experiencing them was insane. This description of a seizure is taken from an article in the 1911 *Encyclopaedia Britannica*; it is reasonable to assume that only an unattended, violent seizure of this kind would cause a young man to injure himself sufficiently to result in death.

7. Potassium bromide was the first effective medication for epilepsy and acted as an anticonvulsant.

8. The first salary list for fiscal year 1903 included the following personnel: Superintendent Oscar S. Gifford; Assistant Superintendent John F. Turner, MD; financial clerk Charles Seely; attendant Roy Carley; laborer Joh Gessler; laborer Hans Lou; laborer Julia Johnson; and night watch S. D. Freeland.

9. This list of duties comes from an affidavit sworn before Inspector Reuben Perry on August 14, 1907, NARA, RG 75, box 1, and from a letter sent to the commissioner of Indian affairs, August 13, 1929, NARA, RG 75, box 20.

10. Oscar S. Gifford, "Report of Superintendent of Asylum for Insane Indians," in U.S. Office of Indian Affairs, *Annual Report of the Commissioner of Indian Affairs*, 1905, p. 334.

11. Oscar S. Gifford, "Report of Superintendent of Asylum for Insane Indians," in U.S. Office of Indian Affairs, *Annual Report of the Commissioner of Indian Affairs*, 1903, pp. 325–27.

12. Information about the Hathorn case is taken from a paper Dr. John Turner read before the South Dakota State Medical Association. He discussed the boy's case and that of several other patients in the report, which was also printed in the *New Albany Medical Herald*, August 1907, under the headline "Insane Indians." Turner did not give the name of the boy, but he is the only Navajo brought to the asylum at that age and the only patient with this particular diagnosis. Turner said in the article that the boy's mind was bright; however, there is an annotation on Hathorn's records that he had congenital imbecility. This may have been added later by someone else, because of the boy's inability to speak.

13. Information about Indian boarding schools comes from many sources, including Child, *Boarding School Seasons*; and Cash and Hoover, *To Be an Indian*, an oral history compilation.

14. This allotment was usually 160 acres per head of household and 80 acres for single people over the age of eighteen.

15. U.S. Office of Indian Affairs. *Annual Report of the Commissioner of Indian Affairs*, 1902, pp. 13–16.

16. The qualifications needed for Canton employment are taken from a civil service exam notice in the *Sioux Valley News*, September 4, 1904.

17. This situation is described in a report from Indian Office supervisor Reuben Perry, filed August 17, 1907, NARA, RG 75, box 1.

18. Soft coal is more prone to burning with black smoke and soot; it also releases sulfur dioxide and acts as an upper respiratory tract irritant.

19. Black Buffalo was discovered by the conductor, who didn't put him off for fear he would freeze in the December chill. Dr. Turner picked up the patient and returned him to the asylum after a brief two days of freedom. "A Stray Indian," *Sioux Valley News*, December 1, 1905.

20. Details about the escapes of Moxey and Lo come from items in the *Sioux Valley News*, March 16, 1906, and July 7, 1905, respectively.

21. The asylum did not have cells or strong rooms in which to hold violent patients.

22. Hysteric angina pectoris mimicked true angina (chest pain), but symptoms like rapid pulse, shortness of breath, and feelings of terror usually came on suddenly, at night, which was not typical of organic angina.

23. Bull-yards, or airing courts, were small enclosures with high wooden fences where patients could walk.

4. Helpless

1. An observer said that Tom "would commit murder at the drop of a hat, and drop the hat himself." Account of this visit taken from "Bob Visits 'Bug' House," *Sioux Valley News*, August 4, 1905.

2. The details are taken from the act, Pub. L. No. 177, April 27, 1904.

3. Rosebud superintendent James McGregor to Hummer, July 11, 1923, NARA, RG 75, box 16.

4. The incident regarding O'Keefe is taken from U.S. House, *Report of the Special Committee*.

5. Smith, "How Doctor Brigham Met the Challenge."

6. Helen Groth to the Investigation Committee of Affairs at Indian Asylum, September 20, 1933, NARA, RG 75, box 6.

7. Susan Wishecoby to Commissioner of Indian Affairs, March 12, 1923, NARA, RG 75, box 8.

8. Fifth annual sanitary report to the Department of the Interior, September 1, 1907, NARA, RG 75, box 1.

9. *Proceedings of the American Medico-Psychological Association at the Fifty-Ninth Annual Meeting*, May 12–15, 1903, 67.

10. By the 1920s, medical men thought that only 4–5 percent of patients could be cured.

11. Bethlem Royal Hospital, a priory in 1247, was converted circa 1400 for the care and confinement of the mentally ill. Also called Bedlam, the hospital could be so chaotic and noisy that today the word *bedlam* refers to any place of unusual confusion and uproar.

12. Most staff members were given room and board at the asylum as part of their wages.

13. The comedians' testimonials were for Murad cigarettes.

14. *Annual Report of the Commissioners of the District of Columbia, Year Ended June 30, 1907* (Washington DC: Government Printing Office, 1907), 1:84.

15. Working and living conditions are largely taken from descriptions in Schlereth, *Victorian America*; Freedman, *Kids at Work*; and Egan, *Worst Hard Times*.

16. The annual wages for the civil service positions mentioned in the chapter were: male attendant, $480; female attendant, $420; cook, $480; assistant cook, $360; dining room girl, $360; laundress, $480; night watchman, $480. In contrast, a schoolteacher in Hand County, South Dakota, could earn $40 a month teaching

fewer than ten students. Clerks and accountants could earn from almost $800 to $1,300 annually, depending upon experience.

17. No cause was ever found. The supposition was that either a tramp who had asked for food at the asylum earlier in the day crawled into the barn to sleep and accidentally set it on fire or that a large quantity of new hay may have spontaneously combusted.

5. A Superintendent in Trouble

1. Information about Vipont's pregnancy is taken from Turner to Charles H. Dickson, December 11, 1906, and corroborated by witnesses interviewed during a subsequent investigation, NARA, RG 75, box 1.

2. Turner to Dickson, December 11, 1906, NARA, RG 75, box 1.

3. Gifford and Seely sometimes took their wives on these "patient-fetching" trips, indicating that Turner's charge was not unfounded.

4. *Sioux Valley News*, March 16, 1906.

5. There is no information about Vipont's husband's reaction to his wife's pregnancy. The baby lived at the asylum for nearly a year but then was hastily given to the children's home at Sioux Falls, South Dakota.

6. Gifford lived about a mile and a half away and could easily be reached by telephone.

7. Information about Gifford and his staff and the various problems that arose between July 1906 and September 1908 are taken from reports written by investigating agents Reuben Perry and Edgar Allen, affidavits gathered for those reports, and letters from individuals concerned, including Corrigan to Allen, April 7, 1908, and Turner to Allen, April 10, 1908, NARA, RG 75, box 1.

8. Report of Inspector Perry, NARA, RG 75, box 1.

9. Larrabee to Superintendent, Insane Asylum, October 12, 1907, NARA, RG 75, box 6.

10. Lizzie Vipont died April 17, 1917, at Canton, owning $156.25 that she had made washing laundry and doing beadwork. Some of the money went for a headstone ($35) and a burial robe ($5), and eventually the rest of the money was given to Vipont's daughter. Lizzie Vipont was buried at Canton Asylum's cemetery. Hummer to commissioner of Indian affairs, May 14, 1919, NARA, RG 75, box 8.

11. C. Bell, *Medico-Legal Journal*.

12. Feeding tubes were forced through a nostril and down the throat of patients who refused to eat; they had a reputation for being painful.

13. One reason that St. Elizabeths had higher per capita costs was that it didn't have the extensive grounds that other institutions had and therefore couldn't raise crops or livestock to offset its expenses.

14. Table prepared by the Medico-Legal Society, in U.S. House, *Report of the Special Committee*, 916. Other insane asylums had rates of discharge from as low as 11 percent (Massachusetts Insane Hospital, Northampton) to as high as 55 percent (Illinois Asylum for Insane Criminals) for the year in question, 1904. Can-

ton Asylum would have been in operation less than two years and would have had no meaningful statistics.

15. Details of the St. Elizabeths investigation are taken from U.S. House, *Report of the Special Committee.*

16. Testimony showed that Turner's horse was occasionally used to capture runaways. Gifford said that he had been authorized to keep two private horses at government expense.

17. Christopher was quickly relieved of duty but immediately sent the commissioner of Indian affairs his own list of charges against Dr. Turner.

18. Seely had already racked up thirty days in patient fetching since January.

19. There may have been a bit of miscommunication over the question of wages. White apparently received a letter stating the position would pay $2,500 per annum, but Dr. Logie received a letter stating the salary would be $2,000. Whatever happened, Logie declined the position.

20. Charles's report, June 9, 1908, NARA, RG 75, box 1.

21. Indian Office memo, August 17, 1908, NARA, RG 75, box 1.

22. Hummer to commissioner of Indian affairs, October 29, 1908; and Commissioner to Hummer, November 3, 1908, NARA, RG 75, box 1.

6. Which Way to Canton?

1. A report entitled *Medical Education in the United States and Canada*, commonly called the Flexner Report after its author, Abraham Flexner, was published in 1910. The report documented the many glaring problems with U.S. medical education, a primary one being that far too many medical schools were diploma mills more concerned with earning money than training qualified physicians.

2. Edgar Albert Guest wrote more than ten thousand poems in his lifetime and was known as the "People's Poet." An example of his light verse is "A Toast to the Men," which begins,

> Here's to the men! Since Adam's time
> They've always been the same;
> Whenever anything goes wrong,
> The woman is to blame.

3. Perhaps it is telling that in an account of a ballgame between St. Elizabeths and Randle Heights (*Washington Post*, June 10, 1908) Hummer is listed as the umpire.

4. Though the *Sioux Valley News* certainly reported on national events, it reveled in its local news. Here is a sample of "local interest" reporting from May 22, 1914: "On Saturday Merritt Thayer having reached his ninth birthday about twenty-two kiddies of like age were invited to a party which was held on the spacious lawn surrounding the Thayer residence. Tables were spread out of doors and after games suited to their age and surroundings had been indulged in, an elegant birthday luncheon concluded the happy affair."

5. Grocers Chraft & Hansen sold the ultimate booster coffee: a line known as Chraft & Hansen Canton Coffee.

6. *Sioux Valley News*, October 2, 1908.

7. This was one of many Indian boarding schools set up by the Indian Office in an attempt to weaken children's ties to their families and culture.

8. Hummer to commissioner of Indian affairs, October 9, 1908, NARA, RG 75, box 12.

9. Replacing the kinder label of *unfortunate*, "defective" was the new term applied to institutionalized persons; it was one that Hummer frequently used.

10. Claud H. Kinnear, M.D., to Superintendent H. H. Johnson, Puyallup Indian School, October 11, 1908, and Oscar H. Keller, acting superintendent, Puyallup Consolidated Agency, to Hummer, October 27, 1908, NARA, RG 75, box 13.

11. She didn't get the seat.

12. The *Sioux Valley News* reported that temperatures had hit forty-two degrees below zero on February 3, 1905.

13. Admitted July 28, 1906, Yells-at-Night's cause of death was tuberculosis. He was buried two days later in what Hummer was already referring to as the hospital cemetery.

14. Native American population and mortality statistics in 1900 from Hacker and Haines, *Construction of Life Tables*. Statistics on tuberculosis from Rieder, "Tuberculosis among American Indians."

15. Trachoma is usually spread by contact with the discharge from the eyes or nose of an infected person. It is also transmitted by flies and gnats, which are attracted to eyes and runny noses. The disease will often strike entire communities.

16. In 1923 secretary of the interior Hubert Work asked for, and received, an increase in appropriations for Indian health care, specifically to combat trachoma. In 1925 he asked the American Medical Association to appoint a committee to advise him on trachoma, and the committee recommended public health education as a preferred means of controlling the disease. The reformer John Collier wrote in 1929 that the trachoma rate for Indians was 19.5 percent and affected about sixty thousand Indians. Measures taken to combat trachoma included isolation schools for infected children, special government trachoma hospitals and field clinics, immigrant screening, and improvements in hygiene and sanitation. See S. Allen and Semba, *Survey of Ophthalmology*; DeJong, *If You Knew the Conditions*; and Trafzer and Weiner, *Medicine Ways*.

17. According to the U.S. Centers for Disease Control and Prevention, blindness from trachoma has been eliminated in the United States today.

18. A description of a perineal douche, from Hinsdale, *Hydrotherapy*: The patient sits upon a stool with a hollow or circular seat and receives the douche upon the perineum (a small, sensitive area between the genitals and anus; in women it extends from the vagina to the anus, and in men from the anus to right below the testicles). The usual form is that of a jet, about a half inch in diameter, but it may take the form of a spray. The temperatures employed are usually comparatively

low, sixty to eighty degrees Fahrenheit, in order to overcome weakness of the bladder, chronic proctitis, sexual depression, and psychic impotence.

19. W. White, *Outlines of Psychiatry*, 28–33.

20. In 1900 dementia praecox also implied an irrevocable mental decline.

7. Hummer's Reign Begins

1. Hummer finally received an elderly man named John Fowles as a financial clerk, but Fowles didn't know how to perform his duties or even use a typewriter.

2. Onion sets are tiny onion bulbs grown from seed the previous year. Farmers plant onion sets as soon as the ground can be worked in the spring and harvest the first shoots as green onions or let the planted sets mature into large bulbs. In that rural community, such knowledge was so basic that young children would be expected to know it. Hay is harvested, baled, and fed to cattle, while straw consists of dead, dried stalks and is used for bedding material or mulch.

3. It was also a dry year, which hurt all farmers.

4. The duties of the asylum matron included:

> 1. She shall supervise all the domestic departments of the asylum, under the direction of the superintendent. She shall enforce discipline, sign all requisitions for supplies needed for their work.
>
> 2. She shall be responsible generally for the condition of the clothing, bedding and linen in all parts of the asylum.
>
> 3. She shall . . . be accountable for the careful keeping and economical use of all furniture, stores, and other articles provided for the asylum.
>
> 4. She shall visit all portions of the asylum, at least once daily, in order that she might ascertain the needs and requirements of the patients for their comfort, and supervise generally the work of all employees, except the attendants. ("Rules and Regulations for Asylum for Insane Indians, Canton, S.D.," 1903, NARA, RG 75, box 1)

5. Hummer used more than eight government towels each week in his private quarters.

6. Patients allowed liberty often congregated in the basement area, where the water closet was locked for some reason. Many patients, having no convenient place to answer the call of nature, defecated in the coal bins and urinated in the halls and recreation rooms if they weren't watched closely.

7. Apparently Hardin was the victim of a politically motivated investigation.

8. Information about the conditions at Canton Asylum during Dr. Hummer's first year comes from affidavits from employees, correspondence from Hardin, and inspection reports submitted by Charles L. Davis, supervisor of Indian schools, and Dr. Joseph A. Murphy, medical supervisor, NARA, RG 75, box 2.

9. The Hummers were finally mentioned in the paper when this trip was reported. They came back to an unexpected snowstorm.

10. The Indian Office's opinion was that Hardin should accept the quarters Hummer had offered him.

11. Smith apparently resisted any attempts to get her out of bed and fought her attendants ferociously at times. In an affidavit, the attendant who helped Hardin said that she couldn't handle Smith by herself, and Hummer wouldn't give her the assistance she needed. Hardin himself said that he had to take Smith to the bathroom "with some force" in order to clean her up.

12. Most of the charges had additional elements to them, but this list captures the vital complaints.

13. Information about Hummer's early background comes from census records and information from St. Elizabeths' congressional investigation, NARA, RG 418, box 1.

14. Hardin came from an Indian school, where this was not the practice. He did not allow staff to clean his quarters.

15. Davis did not find confirmation for the nineteenth charge, that Hummer had called the asylum "the joke of the Indian Service." It may have been, at most, an idle remark and possibly had not been made at all or was made in a different context.

16. Tyler, *History of Indian Policy*, 107.

17. Mrs. Hummer continued to work occasionally; she went to North Carolina to pick up three insane patients for the asylum in 1922.

18. Valentine to Hummer, March 5, 1910, NARA, RG 75, box 2.

19. Hardin to Indian Rights Association, NARA, RG 75, box 2; and Hardin to *Argus-Leader*, April [?], 1910, NARA, RG 75, box 5.

8. Reforms and Canton Asylum

1. Beers, *A Mind That Found Itself*, 107. Clifford Beers, who probably suffered from bipolar disorder, was institutionalized for varying periods of time in three different hospitals from 1900 to 1903. He spent the greater part of his confinement at the facility he described in his book (where the grounds, he mentioned, were lovely). In 1908 he published *A Mind That Found Itself*, which he hoped would become an *Uncle Tom's Cabin* for the mentally ill. In 1909 he and several others formed the National Committee for Mental Hygiene, which was renamed the National Mental Health Association in 1950. As a result of his untiring efforts, he helped change the country's attitudes toward, and treatment for, the mentally ill.

2. Beers was not the first person to divulge the details of the hidden—and often horrendous—life within insane asylums. Twenty years earlier, in 1887, the *New York World*'s editor, John A. Cockerill, had received an idea for a sensational story from his newly hired female reporter Nellie Bly (the pen name of Elizabeth Jane Cochrane Seaman): she would get herself committed to a notorious insane asylum so she could write about conditions there. He agreed, and the twenty-three-year-old Bly fooled alienists completely when she faked catatonic amnesia. She was committed to the Women's Lunatic Asylum on Blackwell's Island in New York.

There, Bly's first supper consisted of a piece of bread and five prunes; subsequent meals did not improve, as she also received spoiled beef, hard bread (once with a spider in her slice), and dirty water for drinking. Later she saw patients sitting in the cold for hours at a time, while rats ran loose around them.

When Bly was first examined, one doctor said she was "positively demented," and another decided that she was a "hopeless case." Once she made it inside the asylum as planned, Bly stopped her acting and reverted to her normal, sane self. Surprisingly, doctors still considered her insane and would not let her go until a "family friend" (the newspaper's attorney) took her out under his guardianship.

Embarrassed doctors had a hard time explaining themselves to the public and the grand jury that eventually convened to investigate Bly's account of her stay. It was evident, however, that just like Hummer's and Superintendent White's opposition to releasing patients from St. Elizabeths, alienists anywhere resisted changing their diagnoses or admitting error once they had committed a patient to their institutions.

The *New York World* serialized Bly's account of her ordeal, and each installment sold out to an enthralled public. Her exposé and subsequent book, *Ten Days in a Mad-House*, prodded New York officials into investigating and cleaning up some of the worst abuses at Blackwell's Island.

3. Perhaps not coincidentally, Beers's book came out about the time (1908) that Luepp decided upon his "common sense" approach at Canton Asylum and replaced Gifford.

4. Information about these two scandals comes from the *New York Times*, August 27, 1908, and April 30, 1911.

5. The federal Pure Food and Drug Act of 1906 was a direct response to Upton Sinclair's graphic description of the meat industry in his novel *The Jungle*. On December 1, 1911, the *Sioux Valley News* published a list of adulterated food that South Dakota's food and drug commissioner had found during inspection and analysis. Among the fifty-eight items were artificial ice containing putrid animal or vegetable matter, hamburger sausage adulterated with borax, and tomato catsup composed of spoiled material.

6. Teddy Roosevelt's administration (1901–9) set aside forty-two million acres of public land for national forests, wildlife refuges, and other protected areas, like the Grand Canyon.

7. Upon his arrival in New York at the age of twenty, Collier was naive enough to mistake a three-dollar-per-week room in New York's red-light district as a bargain in boarding. Later he tried to organize railroads and southern chambers of commerce into a distribution system to help unemployed immigrants in the North find work in the South.

8. *Winters v. United States*, 207 U.S. 564 (1908).

9. Cahill, *Federal Fathers and Mothers*, 222; and Tyler, *History of Indian Policy*, 107–8.

10. House Reports (Private), vol. B, 62nd Cong., 3d sess., December 2, 1912–March 4, 1913. In 1913 Valentine was appointed chairman of the First Massachusetts Minimum Wage Board. Later he became an industrial counselor (settling labor disputes). He died quite suddenly, on November 14, 1916, after falling ill at Delmonico's in New York.

11. The *Sioux Valley News* reported on the asylum's masquerade and Christmas parties on November 4, 1910, and December 27, 1912, respectively.

12. For example, a patient who was discharged and later relapsed would represent two cured patients if he or she were discharged once again.

13. This was an illegal expense unless appropriations had been specifically set aside for these items.

14. Hummer's beef with South Dakota's medical board is taken from a sworn statement by Dr. John Turner, November 20, 1909, NARA, RG 75, box 2.

15. The smell had been described by some inspectors as "almost unbearable."

16. Pringle to commissioner of Indian affairs, August 10, 1912, NARA, RG 75, box 2.

17. Report from Breid to commissioner of Indian affairs, January 31, 1912, NARA, RG 75, box 2.

18. Canton Asylum often had to send escorts with discharged patients to make sure they made it home safely. Hummer asked for authority to provide an escort for Oche-chago-oke-zhig-oke, a recovered patient, to Red Lake, Minnesota, because she spoke no English and would have to change trains on her way home. Hummer to Commissioner of Indian Affairs, March 9, 1910, NARA, RG 75, box 13.

19. Wallin, *Experimental Studies of Mental Defectives.*

20. John Carpenter to F. G. Colett (or Collett), November 18, 1925, NARA, RG 75, box 17.

21. Kentuck had been arrested after a fight in a poolroom. Two white men began to tease and roughhouse with him, and Peter stuck the blade of a pocketknife into the thigh of one of them. His family wasn't told when the trial would be held and learned about his fate as he was on his way to Canton Asylum.

22. Answers to these questions might have been hard to get at because of language difficulties or lack of knowledge on the part of the reservation superintendent requesting the commitment. If used, however, they would have been bona fide attempts to understand what might be going on with an Indian patient.

23. W. White, *Outlines of Psychiatry*, chap. 7, "Examination of the Insane."

24. The American eugenics movement may not be particularly well known to modern readers, yet it was a popular social program that began in the mid-1800s and peaked in the 1920s. The movement drove legislation in many states and foreshadowed the ideology of Nazi Germany. With its emphasis on pedigree charts, breeding, and laws against interracial marriages, American eugenics focused on keeping whites pure-blooded. For a wealth of fascinating information about this topic, see Cold Spring Harbor Laboratory, Image Archive on the American Eugenics Movement, www.eugenicsarchive.org.

25. Born in Birmingham, England, Galton (February 16, 1822–January 17, 1911) was a first cousin to the naturalist Charles Darwin.

26. Hummer to commissioner of Indian affairs, December 30, 1918, NARA, RG 75, box 14.

27. Hummer to commissioner of Indian affairs, July 25, 1925, NARA, RG 75, box 17.

28. Parole privileges allowed patients unrestricted movement outdoors.

29. Information about Isabella Porter is taken from correspondence between Hummer, Josephine Grasshopper, and the commissioner of Indian affairs, March–June 1910, NARA, RG 75, box 13.

30. Both are buried in Canton Asylum's cemetery.

9. Let the Investigations Begin

1. Information about Deere as well as the following accounts of Omudis, Papa, and other incidents of misconduct come from a ten-page letter headed "Treatment of Patients as seen by James Herman," written by James Herman, a patient at the time, no date given but stamped as received by the Office of Indian Affairs on June 17, 1915, and from an investigation on June 8, 1915, led by Dr. L. F. Michael, NARA, RG 75, box 5.

2. James Two Crows did not have an easy life at the asylum himself. Night watchman Albert H. Chappell was dismissed from the asylum for beating him up in December 1909.

3. Patients were sleeping in the hallway where the game was being played, because their rooms were being painted.

4. Putney, "Canton Asylum for Insane Indians," 12.

5. *Sioux Valley News*, September 19, 1913.

6. Leahy, "Canton Asylum," 78.

7. *Cedar Falls Daily News*, October 21, 1912; *Sumner (IA) Gazette*, August 29, 1929.

8. *Sioux Valley News*, August 29, 1913.

9. Isabella Smith left in September 1913 and Joe Emerson in February 1914.

10. In May 1914, probably for smallpox.

11. Examples of Hummer's detail-oriented chores are taken from correspondence to and from the commissioner of Indian affairs, NARA, RG 75, boxes 7, 9, and 10.

12. Raymond Smoots to a friend, January 22, 1914, NARA, RG 75, box 5.

13. Knox was known for her irritability and quarrelsomeness.

14. Landis called it a "rubber article."

15. Ewing was an Indian who also went by the name Flying Iron.

16. Hummer may have been referring to Landis, as he further stated that Ewing wanted to "square" matters when the woman was dismissed.

17. Norman Ewing was transferred to Fort Peck Agency.

18. Information about Hummer's sexual misconduct is taken from a report by Dr. L. F. Michael and an unsigned twelve-page statement and summation that included the text of Landis's May 29, 1915, affidavit concerning her automobile ride with Hummer and its aftermath, NARA, RG 75, box 5. The statement was written

by someone (perhaps Assistant Commissioner of Indian Affairs E. B. Meritt) who had the authority to recommend a course of action beyond Michael's. This writer accused Michael of not making a recommendation on the Landis case because he and Hummer were both physicians.

Though their profession may have given them common ground, Michael also made his investigation without knowledge of Hummer's prior conduct. Only after he had listened to Hummer's ranting when faced with Landis's charges did Michael understand that this was not the first time Hummer had been in a similar predicament. Like so many others before him, Michael added, "It is quite evident that those who have, in any way, said anything not complimentary to the institution or the Doctor have fallen in his estimation."

Landis's failure to immediately report Hummer's attempted seduction is not unusual; most young ladies of that era would have been mortified to have their names associated with anything sordid. Because she had plainly bested him, she may have felt safe enough at the asylum, surrounded by patients and other employees.

Landis wanted to save money to educate herself for a better position, and Hummer actually helped her to apply for the position of cook. He had no desire for publicity, either, and this may have originally been a way to assure Landis's silence. When his wife began goading her, along with Hummer's incessant criticism (there is no knowing what passed between him and his wife concerning Landis), the truce no longer held. Once she was fired, Landis probably still struggled with the idea of making her situation public, and it took her four months to come to the conclusion that Hummer deserved to be exposed.

19. Sells to Hummer, May 15, 1916, NARA, RG 75, box 5.

20. Report from special supervisor Dr. R. E. L. Newberne to the commissioner of Indian affairs, January 20, 1916, NARA, RG 75, box 2.

10. Life among the Indians

1. Agnes Caldwell to Commissioner of Indian Affairs Cato Sells, January 1, 1920, NARA, RG 75, box 14. Caldwell's husband later remarried and had four more children while she was still in the asylum.

2. Hummer to commissioner of Indian affairs, November 8, 1920, NARA, RG 75, box 14. Information about Caldwell's work for Hummer is found in a memorandum from medical officer William G. Cushard to Dr. H. C. Woolley, January 9, 1934, NARA, RG 418, entry 13.

3. E. White, *Service on the Indian Reservations*, 334–35; and Cahill, *Federal Fathers and Mothers*, 50.

4. The asylum was designed to house twenty-four male and twenty-four female patients, though the ratio always skewed toward a greater proportion of males. The Indian Office's supervisor of construction John Charles wrote that the asylum had been built to accommodate fifty-six patients, either a misstatement on his part or a worse-case scenario.

5. Hardin (writing on behalf of Hummer during his absence) to commissioner of Indian affairs, September 22, 1909, NARA, RG 75, box 2.

6. Hummer to commissioner of Indian affairs, January 15, 1916, NARA, RG 75, box 14.

7. Hummer to commissioner of Indian affairs, September 21, 1926, and commissioner to Hummer, September 18, 1926, NARA, RG 75, box 10.

8. Per capita costs at Canton derive from Edgar B. Meritt to Fred G. Coldren, April 21, 1915, NARA, RG 75, box 18. National figures are quoted from the *Eighty-Ninth Annual Report of the South Carolina State Hospital for the Insane for the Year 1912* (Columbia SC: Gonzales and Bryan, State Printers, 1913).

9. St. Elizabeths' per capita costs ran $220 in 1909; the figure comes from the District of Columbia appropriation bill for 1909. Other reports show that this cost remained remarkably stable for a number of years.

10. Though economy may have been one consideration, the real outcome of that decision was that Hummer remained the only medical man at the facility. No one could argue with his diagnoses, challenge him on any medical issue, or swear out charges against him based on competent, comparable knowledge about how patients ought to be treated.

11. Meritt's questions about per capita costs and Hummer's reply with his plans for expansion and projected savings are contained in correspondence between the two: January 15, February 24, March 3, and March 6, 1916, NARA, RG 75, box 14.

12. Hummer was still dealing with the minutia of administering a large facility. In August 1917 he tartly informed the Herbert Boiler Company in Chicago that a casting on the hot water heater it had sold him was defective, leaving the asylum without hot water. He added, "We have notified you at two different times to ship a boiler to us at once . . . and if this is not done very soon I shall be compelled to take other means to secure it from you."

In this exchange with his supplier, Hummer came away the definite loser. The president of the company told Hummer that *he* had written back telling the superintendent that he wouldn't ship another heater until he received the one the asylum already had. Then he snapped,

As far as your threatening language . . . you can take such steps as you see fit, as your bluffs don't go here for a cent.

You had the use of this heater for pretty near over a year, and there must be some cause for its cracking.

If you desire to ship the body of this heater back, send it here, and if it is defective we will make it good. If it is not our fault, we will do nothing, except to sell you another heater. (W. E. Herbert, Pres., Herbert Boiler Company, to Hr. R. Hummer, MD, August 6, 1917, NARA, RG 75, box 11)

13. Act of March 2, 1917, 39 Stat. 988, in C. F. Hauke, chief clerk, Office of Indian Affairs, to T. E. Bancroft, March 15, 1929, NARA, RG 75, box 1.

14. Correspondence between the National Committee for Mental Hygiene, White, Hummer, and the commissioner of Indian affairs, June 4, 6, 20, 1917, NARA, RG 75, box 14.

15. As always, the Indian Office had denied Hummer's proposal for an epileptic cottage. This time, however, Assistant Commissioner Meritt cited the tremendous building program going on and the subsequent scarcity of labor and high cost of materials to support the war effort as the basis for its decision.

16. These numbers were up from thirteen new patients in 1916 and only four in 1915.

17. On Mary Walking Day, see Hummer to commissioner of Indian Affairs, May 17, 1918, NARA, RG 75, box 14; on Fisher, see Hummer to commissioner of Indian Affairs, July 18, 1918, and E. B. Meritt to Charles D. Munro, superintendent, Winnebago Agency, December 12, 1918, NARA, RG 75, box 14; Meritt quotes from a letter he had received from Hummer dated December 3, 1918.

18. An American Medical Association–sponsored study estimated that 21 million people worldwide died in the 1918 flu pandemic. Out of a population of 105 million, the U.S. death toll was around 675,000. Barry, *Great Influenza*, 396–97.

19. Hummer to commissioner of Indian affairs, July 4, 1918, NARA, RG 75, box 1.

20. Francis was pictured with his cup in the *Washington Post*'s retrospective picture press section, August 31, 1919.

21. Cahill, *Federal Fathers and Mothers*, 243.

22. Hummer to the commissioner of Indian affairs, August 16, 1918, NARA, RG 75, box 7. During World War I, most Indian males were not subject to the draft because they weren't citizens. Despite this, approximately fifteen thousand voluntarily enlisted once the United States joined the combat; hundreds of men from northern tribes crossed the border to join the Canadian army even before the United States entered the war. Tyler, *History of Indian Policy*, 109. Though they have been somewhat overshadowed by the famed Navajo code talkers of World War II, Choctaw Indians used their language to create an unbreakable code in World War I.

23. Hummer to commissioner of Indian affairs, December 30, 1918, NARA, RG 75, box 14. As Hummer pleaded for his favored new construction, he pushed aside Dr. Newberne's recommendation (probably made following another routine inspection) for separate cottages for the tidy and untidy and separate sitting rooms for the quiet and disturbed cases: "It would produce a weird looking institution if we erected a small building here and one there to meet all the varying needs of such a mixture of cases as we have here." He reserved the privilege of asking for these buildings and such others as might be needed at a later time.

24. Agnes Caldwell to Cato Sells, February 24, 1920, NARA, RG 75, box 15. Perhaps one reason letters like these exist is due to Elizabeth Packard. Besides lobbying for fairer commitment laws, she lobbied for laws to prevent the censorship of patient mail; due to her efforts, most states gave the power to screen mail to a supervisory committee rather than the superintendent of an insane asylum. This

law provided that the names and addresses of the committee members be posted in every inmate's room. Though this procedure may not have been in place at Canton, patients did seem to know that they could write to the commissioner of Indian affairs without interference.

11. Another Sort of Prison

1. Blood quantum is a way of measuring ethnicity based on bloodline; for Indians, it looks at the number of marriages outside the group against a baseline of pure-bloodedness in a person's family tree, usually from the early 1800s, when some of the first record keeping was initiated. Blood quantum is important today, as it is the basis by which the federal government acknowledges Indian entitlements. The government issues a CDIB, or Certificate of Degree of Indian Blood, to Native Americans who can prove their bloodlines. A recipient of benefits must be enrolled in a tribe as well, and blood quantum is often used by tribes (along with other requirements) to decide who can enroll. Each tribe decides how much blood is needed to be a member, usually no less than one-sixteenth.

2. Jackson and Galli, *History of the Bureau of Indian Affairs*, 69.

3. Jackson and Galli, *History of the Bureau of Indian Affairs*, 75.

4. Keller and Ruether, *Encyclopedia of Women and Religion*, 99; and Cahill, *Federal Fathers and Mothers*, 30–31.

5. U.S. Office of Indian Affairs, *Annual Report of the Commissioner of Indian Affairs*, 1886.

6. It is perhaps unsurprising that the Indian Office created a new holiday in boarding schools—Indian Citizenship Day—which was celebrated on the anniversary of the Dawes Act. Its irony is manifest after reading the many firsthand accounts of life in Indian boarding schools that can be found on the Internet and in books. Cahill, *Federal Fathers and Mothers*, gives a clear history of Indian policy and the role it played in boarding schools and assimilation. Child, *Boarding School Seasons*, is also an illuminating work that will give readers a good idea of daily life at boarding schools.

7. Keller and Ruether, *Encyclopedia of Women and Religion*, 99–100; and Philp, *John Collier's Crusade for Indian Reform*, 98–99.

8. Child, *Boarding School Seasons*, 98.

9. Meritt's bulletin concerning the Indian Bureau is relentlessly laudatory until the section "Indian Bureau Critics." In it, he accuses selfish interests of promoting propaganda against the Indian Bureau "for the purpose of releasing all Indians from Government supervision. The billion and a half dollar Indian estate looks mighty tempting to the Indian land grafters."

10. There were several groups that advocated for Indians, such as the Indian Rights Association (IRA), formed in 1882 by men who wanted to "bring about the complete civilization of the Indians and their admission to citizenship." Members were genuinely shocked by the mistreatment of Indians; unfortunately, they felt that any reform had to be based on education and assimilation. Their efforts

to help Indians included petitioning for day schools rather than off-reservation boarding schools and supporting Indians' legal rights. For the most part, however, the IRA and similar organizations supported the Dawes Act.

11. Herman's testimony about Amos Deere's death and other maltreatment at the asylum was influential in getting attendant Van Winkle dismissed.

12. These were mainly expenses for the escort who came to get him and bring him back.

13. Newberne's report on James Herman contains an odd element. Besides giving background on his subject and an assessment of his current status, Newberne weighed in on the state of affairs between Herman and his wife. "It is she who *demands* and *deserves* the best of the bargain in the property settlement which she and her husband are trying to effect. She has borne alone the family burdens since her husband was sent to the asylum upon her initiative."

Why Newberne felt that Mrs. Herman deserved so much is unclear, especially when he explains that she "has been able to do this because she has been the beneficiary of the proceeds from the rented lands—something like $1800 per annum." NARA, RG 75, box 13.

14. That is, the acreage released to him by the Department of the Interior.

15. Information about James Herman's case comes from NARA, RG 75, box 13.

12. The World Outside

1. Information about Johnson is taken from correspondence between the concerned parties, dated June 7, 1920, to August 4, 1920, NARA, RG 75, box 15.

One issue that Hummer raised earlier in Rowley Johnson's case was the drain on the asylum's finances to accept Johnson, care for him, and then let him go. Hummer went on record as opposing the admission of "these cases" on the grounds of economics, because the expenditures on Johnson were a "total loss." Since he continued to accept epileptics, one possible interpretation of his words is that he didn't want to accept patients who might get well and cost him money to send home.

Johnson's mother wrote to Hummer in 1920, saying that she had a reliable Indian cure for epilepsy that she had seen work in others: mix a healthy woman's menstrual blood with a little lukewarm water, pour it over the patient's head, neck, and shoulders, and rub it in with vigor while he is in a convulsion. After the patient gained consciousness, he was to drink half a cup of the mixture.

In a somewhat similar case to Johnson's, Hummer released a woman he described as a constitutional psychopath, a pathological liar, and a nymphomaniac. During outbreaks, he said, "she is very troublesome." Hummer to commissioner of Indian affairs, June 30, 1919, NARA, RG 75, box 14.

2. Wishecoby to Cato Sells, July 22, 1920, NARA, RG 75, box 15.

3. Hauke to Walter G. West, superintendent, Klamath Agency, May 21, 1920, NARA, RG 75, box 15.

4. Hummer apparently did not learn his lesson. When James Blackeye's mother requested his return home, Hummer told the commissioner that the nineteen-year-

old had suffered 313 recorded epileptic convulsions in less than two years, two of which nearly killed him. However, he would let the boy go if his mother understood his condition and would accept full responsibility for him. Blackeye died at the asylum in 1922 and was buried there.

5. Owl promised to "obey the public & government laws from now on," which implied that he may have been taken to Canton because he was difficult on the reservation.

6. Owl to the commissioner of Indian affairs, December 16, 1919, and Hummer's reply, December 17, 1919, NARA, RG 75, box 14.

7. Indian Office Circular 1571, "Admission of Patients," October 14, 1919, NARA, RG 75, box 14. The intent was for Indians who were citizens or could pay their own way to receive treatment in state or private hospitals. Citizenship did not preclude admission to Canton, but preference was given to noncitizen wards. Citizens committed to Canton had to go through due process of law, unless they were violent or had to be restrained; in that case the nearest relative or guardian could consent to commitment.

Milas Lasater of District 9 in Wichita, Kansas, wrote to Commissioner of Indian Affairs Charles H. Burke in October 1921 concerning Emily Waite, a girl who was not a federal ward. Lasater had apparently spoken to Burke about her and was granted permission to keep the girl at Canton, provided it was at no cost to the government. Lasater expressed his gratitude for the decision and added, "I came back by Canton on my return and told Dr. Hummer of my conference with you. . . . I am convinced that in Dr. Hummer we have a most humane and competent Superintendent who takes a personal interest in his patients, giving them every consideration possible and necessary for their well being under his care, and turning them out if and when he has been able to restore them to normal." NARA, RG 75, box 15.

8. Lane took eighteen bath towels, a white blanket, an electric lamp with a green shade, and a silver toilet set (hand mirror, comb, and brush) belonging to one of the patients, Josephine Wells.

9. The baby girl, Delores, died six months later.

10. Christine Amour, Caldwell's roommate, also received their visits.

11. Information about the employee problems (Lane, Juel, and Lewis) Hummer suffered can be found in correspondence between Hummer to the commissioner of Indian affairs and employee statements concerning the incidents, dated March 26 to April 5, 1920, and July 26, 1920, NARA, RG 75, box 7 and box 5.

12. Indian school authorities anxious to thwart students' healthy hormones sometimes nailed windows shut and locked fire escapes in the girls' dormitories so boys couldn't visit.

13. Hardin deposition, November 19, 1909, NARA, RG 75, box 2.

14. Hummer's older son, Francis, would eventually also act as an escort for new patients being fetched to the asylum.

15. When Hummer brought his parents to live with him is unclear; his mother died at the asylum in 1921.

16. Hurd et al., *Institutional Care of the Insane*, 2:269.

17. Chlorpromazine was said to induce a "medical lobotomy."

18. The American Neurological Association formed in 1875.

19. Pellagra was a true scourge that baffled doctors, who for years had believed there was a dietary link. In 1909 the superintendent of Peoria State Hospital hosted a Public Health Service study during which two physicians from its Medical Corps examined two hundred cases (one hundred of whom had died) for a month. Hurd et al.'s monumental *Institutional Care of the Insane* discusses an experiment the staff conducted to test the theory that pellagra was caused by corn: for a year, fifty patients ate an exclusive corn diet and fifty others ate a diet heavy in corn and corn products. They did not develop pellagra.

20. Grob, *Mad among Us*, 142. This concentration on a spectrum of behavior was called "dynamic psychiatry."

21. Prandoni and Gold, "St. Elizabeths Hospital Celebrates 150 Years"; and "St. Elizabeths West Campus, Washington, DC," www.stelizabethsdevelopment.com/docs /Full_History_of_St_Elizabeths.pdf, 12.

22. Hurd et al., *Institutional Care of the Insane*, 2:269, 414–15, 752.

23. He called these episodes "psycholeptic," a term associated with fits brought on by painful emotional memories.

24. Information is taken from letters and charts in Lucy Gladstone's file, NARA KC, RG 75, box 9.

25. The Burke Act had an additional stipulation that made it unlawful for Indians under wardship to obtain liquor—they could buy it legally as citizens, but not as wards.

26. Hummer to Commissioner Burke, May 12, 1921, NARA, RG 75, box 10.

27. Burke to Hummer, May 23, 1921, NARA, RG 75, box 10.

28. Hummer's tally usually fluctuated by a body or two during the year; in July 1922 he had ninety patients, with three under the age of ten and another nine patients between ten and nineteen.

29. In a letter sent April 9, 1921, NARA, RG 75, box 8, Meritt told Hummer firmly that the government did not want the money returned and that Hummer should spend it on necessary improvements and future needs.

30. Statistics are taken from *Mental Hygiene*, January 1919.

31. U.S. Office of Indian Affairs, *Report of the Commissioner of Indian Affairs*, 1920, 64. "Figures compiled from reports of Indian School superintendents, supplemented by information from 1910 census for localities in which no Indian Office representative is located."

32. Hummer to superintendents of Indian schools and agencies, June 21, 1921, NARA, RG 75, box 15.

33. Report dated June 27, 1921, and Southern Pueblos Indian Agency report, July 21, 1921, NARA, RG 75, box 15.

34. Philp, *John Collier's Crusade for Indian Reform*, 4–8.

35. Philp, *John Collier's Crusade for Indian Reform*, 32.

36. The superintendent was later forced out of office.

37. Downes, "Crusade for Indian Reform," 343–44.

38. The assistant commissioner of Indian affairs, Edgar Meritt, later drove the agent out of office.

39. Information about the fight over the Bursum Bill is taken from Collier, *From Every Zenith*; Philp, *John Collier's Crusade for Indian Reform*; and Downes, "Crusade for Indian Reform," among other sources.

Albert Fall also proved himself no protector of Indians when he ruled in 1922 that prospectors could lease public lands to drill for oil and mine coal and phosphates. In a report to the House Indian Affairs Committee, Fall included Indian reservations among those public lands since they were created through executive order. Philp explains that Indians would get no royalties for the leases on their reservations, which would instead go into the general reclamation fund, to the state where the reservation was located, and to the federal government.

Burke did not agree with his superior's assessment of reservation accessibility, though he did not challenge it. When Hubert Work succeeded Fall, Burke wrote to him and asked that the Interior Department's solicitor reevaluate Fall's decision. In rare and transitory agreement, both Burke and Collier opposed Fall's ruling that reservations were ordinary public lands. However, Burke eventually supported an alternative piece of legislation called the Indian Oil Bill, which gave Indian land more protection and Indians a share in oil royalties. The protections did not go far enough in Collier's opinion. He believed that the royalties were insufficient and that the provisions of the bill ended up treating Indians as though they were guests on public land and could be asked to leave.

Collier drummed up congressional support from Representative James A. Frear and Senators Burton Wheeler and Robert La Follette. He and his colleagues also held public meetings to attack the oil bill. Eventually, President Coolidge signed a bill in 1926 that allowed prospectors to lease land but gave Indians 100 percent of their royalties. The bill also protected reservation land by prohibiting any changes in boundaries except by act of Congress. It was a satisfactory win for Collier, who felt that Indians gained much that they had lost under Fall.

Indian policy and the many acts and bills consequent to it are complicated subjects, and I have of necessity merely skimmed over the ones I mention. Philp, *John Collier's Crusade for Indian Reform*, has several examples of the type of legislation that enraged reformers and gives a clear idea of the energy and determination that many people dedicated to changing old mind-sets and bringing federal policy to a new footing.

40. Abraham Meachem, released June 6, 1922, had been "entirely restored to his normal mental state." Hummer to commissioner of Indian Affairs, June 18, 1922, NARA, RG 75, box 16.

41. McGregor to Hummer, July 11, 1923, NARA, RG 75, box 16.

42. Correspondence between Gensler and Hummer, October 8, 1924, and between Fitzgerald and Meritt, November 16 and 24, 1924, NARA, RG 75, box 17.

43. This woman is almost certainly a patient on record as Edith Schroder, a spelling I have used throughout this book. Her name also appears with the spellings "Shroader" and Shroder."

44. Figures are taken from U.S. Senate, *Hearings before the Subcommittee of the Committee on Appropriations on H.R. 15130*, 66th Cong., 3d sess., 1921. Testimony is from Wednesday, January 12, 1921.

45. The subcommittee met to determine the Interior Department appropriation bill for 1924.

46. Film rentals for the treasured moving pictures came to $200 each year. Medical supplies came to $123.52.

47. During these hearings Meritt stated, "It may be interesting to the committee to know that there are fewer insane Indians per capita than there are among the white people."

48. "Report on Canton Asylum for Insane Indians (July 15–17, 1922)," to commissioner of Indian affairs, cover dated July 17, 1922, NARA, RG 75, box 10.

49. Correspondence between Espinoza, Manby, Hummer, and Burke, January–March 1924, NARA, RG 75, box 17.

50. "Hiawatha Asylum Is Only One in World," *Sioux Valley News*, October 28, 1926.

51. Vaux's comments about Canton Asylum come from his report to the Board of Indian Commissioners, June 30, 1923, NARA, RG 75, box 2.

13. Hummer Can't Keep Up

1. Hummer to commissioner of Indian affairs, March 5, 1923, NARA KC, RG 75, box 1. Though the Peyote Road was eventually recognized by the Indian Bureau, it had not been a traditional practice; instead, it had become popular with young men returning from government schools. Waters, *Masked Gods*, 135–37.

2. Also, Turner wrote that Dr. Corrigan operated on two of Turner's patients, for which Turner paid him cash. This would indicate that Turner couldn't perform operations at the asylum himself. Statement to Reuben Perry, August 18, 1907, NARA, RG 75, box 1.

3. These items sometimes show up on eBay.

4. Anderson, "World's Only Indian Insane Asylum," *Canton Farm News*, March 23, 1923.

5. Wishecoby to commissioner of Indian affairs, August 19, 1921, NARA, RG 75, box 15. Since she was not a Canton employee, Mrs. Marbles probably was someone in authority at Wishecoby's home reservation. Wishecoby's records don't show any particular diagnosis, but she mentions having "fits" at home, and in other correspondence, Hummer mentions epilepsy as a problem for her.

6. Hummer to commissioner of Indian affairs, September 19, 1921, NARA, RG 75, box 15.

7. Kraepelin's work eventually led to the *Diagnostic and Statistical Manual of Mental Disorders*, published and used by the American Psychiatric Association today.

8. Tertian malaria is malaria in which the febrile paroxysms (feverish convulsions) occur every forty-two to forty-seven hours, or every third day, counting the day of occurrence as the first day of the cycle.

9. Wagner-Jauregg was an Austrian physician. Among other achievements, he was appointed Extraordinary Professor at the Medical Faculty of the University of Graz and Extraordinary Professor of Psychiatry and Nervous Diseases, and director of the Clinic for Psychiatry and Nervous Diseases in Vienna.

10. Information about the state of psychiatric thought in the 1920s comes from articles in the *American Journal of Insanity* and *American Journal of Psychiatry*, 1920–24.

11. Silk, *Asylum for Insane Indians*, September 1933, 6, and cover letter addressed to commissioner of Indian affairs, October 3, 1933.

12. Amos Red Owl to commissioner of Indian affairs, November 18, 1929, NARA, RG 75, box 18.

13. After a congressional investigation, Fall was convicted of bribery in 1929 and sentenced to prison—the first cabinet official in U.S. history to be convicted of a felony.

14. Statement by Ava Dunn, August 1923, NARA, RG 75, box 16.

15. Patient Philip Carson echoed this complaint, saying in 1918 that "your place is unfitted for treatment. no medicine to take the treatment with." NARA, RG 75, box 14.

16. Information about this episode is found in letters from the principals, NARA, RG 75, box 16; and NARA KC, RG 75, box 1. Court's explanatory letters are headed "Trouble with a girl" and "The breaking out of the asylum" and dated September 6 and September 7, 1923, respectively. Hummer stated in a letter to the commissioner of Indian affairs, November 6, 1923, that Court had been chained in his room since September 4, 1923.

14. Ripples in the Waters

1. Al Capone died of paresis in 1947.

2. Diefendorf, *Clinical Psychiatry*, 318.

3. Olmsted and Blaxill, *Age of Autism*, 9.

4. Olmsted and Blaxill, *Age of Autism*, 7.

5. Wassermann tests are diagnostic for syphilis.

6. Hutchinson teeth is a deformity in the incisors that is indicative of congenital syphilis.

7. Information about Kraepelin's visit can be found in Kraepelin to White, Munich, February 16, 1925; Burke to White, March 5, 1925; Department of the Interior, circular 2119, June 12, 1925; and Felix Plaut and Emil Kraepelin to Burke, Munich, December 9, 1925, all in NARA, RG 75, box 17; Kraepelin and Plaut, *Paralysestudien Bei Negern Und Indianern*; and "General Paralysis in Primitive Races," a summary.

8. Hummer told Burke that his staff had made an outfit that tied up the back so the patient couldn't remove it. Even if Hummer *had* purposely left the patient

naked to make his point, it seems that the specialized garment had never been in use before.

9. Under his predecessor, Gifford, restraints had been used for violent patients or repeat escapees. Dr. Turner did not allow restraints for merely troublesome patients, a policy made clear in one attendant's bitter remarks in a deposition (August 14, 1907) about not being allowed to restrain patients who fought with her.

10. Burke to Hummer, October 20, 1925; and Hummer to Burke, October 24, 1924, NARA, RG 75, box 6.

11. Stevens, "Medical Report on Canton Asylum" to commissioner of Indian affairs, September 1925, cover dated October 12, 1925, NARA, RG 75, box 10.

12. Kentuck appears to have been railroaded into committal after a skirmish with some white men. Kentuck's relatives were especially concerned about his release in 1925 because the superintendent of the Hoopa reservation wanted to sell Kentuck's allotment (four acres) to the highest bidder.

13. This incident is taken from a series of letters: John Carpenter to attorney Frederick G. Collett, November 18, 1925; Collett to commissioner of Indian affairs, December 5, 1925; Hummer to John Carpenter and Emma Frank, December 20, 1925; and Hummer to Burke, December 21, 1925, NARA, RG 75, box 17.

14. Canton's population stood at three thousand in 1920, but many of its citizens would have already been employed.

15. Information about the employee situation comes from a report by special inspector T. B. Roberts Sr., September 23, 1926, NARA, RG 75, box 5.

16. Information about this visit comes from Meritt to Hummer, August 4, September 18, 1926; Krulish's report dated August 5, 1926; and Hummer to commissioner of Indian affairs, September 21, 1926, NARA, RG 75, box 10.

17. Report of Supervisor Elinor D. Gregg, November 1925, and Hummer's reply, December 15, 1925, NARA, RG 75, box 3.

18. Grob, *Mad among Us*, 67–68.

19. Susan [Wishecoby] to Hummer, June 14, 1925, NARA, RG 75, box 17.

20. Archibald to Hummer, May 11, 1926, NARA, RG 75, box 11.

21. Faribault had a girl, Winona, who remained at Canton Asylum for four years. The baby's father was thought to be another patient, Willie Dayea.

22. In the same manner, Hummer conveniently overlooked Agnes Caldwell's deficiencies so she could keep house for him. Faribault's situation as caretaker to Hummer's parents is detailed in Burch, "Dislocated Histories."

23. Herman Van Winkle boarded at the Canton facility in a two-room apartment with his wife and five children. Mrs. Van Winkle worked there as a seamstress and was included in the personnel brouhaha but received little of Hummer's vindictiveness because she was willing to resign. Hummer's complaint against her was that she couldn't do her work properly because of child care duties; no one disputed him on this.

Van Winkle, in his letter to Commissioner Burke, stated that in the summers of 1923 and 1924, swill from the institution was taken to Hummer's own farm and fed to his hogs, while the government's hogs were fed corn. He further stated that Hummer instructed him to bring Hummer's cattle and hogs to the institution and care for them there.

Along with other details, Van Winkle quoted Hummer as saying, "We will let the government office by [sic] corn for the government hogs and maybe they will buy more land." (If Van Winkle's statement was true, apparently Hummer felt that if he withheld free swill and let the government pick up the tab for all the extra corn, he could justify asking for more farmland for the institution.) Van Winkle further stated that he had to take forty hogs of Hummer's to market to sell them, receiving a check for them in Hummer's name.

Special inspector Roberts reported that Hummer, in a signed statement, admitted the truth of all that was charged except "that he says he paid Van Winkle $20 to do the work and that no government grain was fed." Roberts explained that Hummer had apparently made an unwise investment a few years earlier, "when the land boom was on," purchasing land mortgaged at $300 an acre. He had been hard-pressed to raise the interest and taxes and had tried "by outside ventures, such as buying and feeding hogs, to keep his head above the water."

Roberts added that Hummer's explanation was probably true, since land as good as Hummer's was being purchased by the government for $150 an acre at the time he made his statement. Hummer suffered no reprisals for this moral slip. All of this information comes from NARA, RG 75, box 5.

24. This reconstruction of events comes from Hummer's letters to the commissioner of Indian affairs and the commissioner's replies; Hummer's letters stating and defending his accusations; Herman Van Winkle's explanatory letter to the commissioner, August 20, 1926; Mrs. Lena Wilson's (Jobin's niece) letter to commissioner of Indian affairs, October 16, 1926; special investigator T. B. Roberts Sr.'s report to the commissioner, September 23, 1926; and Dr. Emil Krulish's subsequent report on January 15, 1927, all in NARA, RG 75, box 5. Within this body of reports and letter writing is a rather extraordinary missive from Hummer to Commissioner Burke, in which Hummer practically froths at the mouth over old grievances, continually refers to himself as "your superintendent," and launches a minute and convoluted account of his every action in the matter of Van Winkle's dismissal.

25. Burke to Krulish, December 15, 1926, NARA, RG 75, box 5.

26. See Hummer's report for Jobin, April 24, 1923, NARA KC, RG 75, box 6; and Dr. Emil Krulish, efficiency reports for Mary Coleman, Mabel Van Winkle, and Lucie Jobin, November 1, 1926, included in Krulish's report on the personnel situation, January 15, 1927, NARA, RG 75, box 5. Jobin was terminated from Canton Asylum on February 28, 1927, and assigned to the Chin Lee School at Fort Defiance, Arizona. Hummer apparently wanted Jobin out of the Indian Service (where she had served since 1901) entirely. That she was transferred instead was probably because of Krulish's recommendation.

1. An extremely influential publication was Gertrude Bonnin's *Oklahoma's Poor Rich Indians: An Orgy of Graft and Exploitation of the Five Civilized Tribes—Legalized Robbery*, an Indian Rights Association pamphlet.

2. For an excellent overview of the mid-1920s reform efforts, see Downes, "Crusade for Indian Reform."

3. The Board of Indian Commissioners had been authorized by executive order in 1869, partially as an oversight committee over the disbursement of Indian appropriations.

4. Quoted from Parman, "Lewis Meriam's Letters," 280.

5. Deloria and Lytle, *Nations Within*, 43–45.

6. Hummer to commissioner of Indian affairs, April 21, 1927, NARA KC, RG 75, box 2.

7. Hummer to commissioner of Indian affairs, May 9, 1927, NARA, RG 75, box 5.

8. Dawson to Hummer, April 16, 1927; Hummer to commissioner of Indian affairs, April 19, May 5, 1927, NARA, RG 75, box 17.

9. In 1925 Assistant Commissioner Meritt required reservation superintendents to reimburse Canton Asylum for the expense of patient care when patients had sufficient funds to make that possible. Caldwell's expenses were partially reimbursed by her agency, which helped Hummer's bottom line.

10. Information about Agnes Caldwell's situation comes from Caldwell to commissioner of Indian affairs, April 30, 1927, NARA, RG 75, box 17; Josephine Johnson to Burke, October 18, 1928, NARA, RG 75, box 18; A. E. Schaal to Hummer, December 4, 1929, NARA KC, RG 75, box 3; memorandum from medical officer William G. Cushard to Dr. H. C. Woolley, January 9, 1934, NARA, RG 418, box 1.

11. Superintendent William A. Light to Hummer, May 25, 1927, NARA KC, RG 75, box 1.

12. The details of what Edwards found on his visit to Canton Asylum can be found in Meriam, *Problem of Indian Administration*, 304–14 (the Meriam Report).

13. Only a month later, Hummer submitted his 1930 "Estimate of Needs." Interestingly, out of a $129,770 budget (of which $76,000 would go for new construction and equipment), Hummer allotted only $300 for medical and surgical expenses.

14. He said that it had the highest average use of available beds of any hospital in the Indian Service.

15. Hummer to commissioner of Indian affairs, October 19, 1928, NARA KC, RG 75, box 2.

16. Hummer to commissioner of Indian affairs, February 23, 1928, NARA KC, RG 75, box 2.

17. B. G. Courtright to commissioner of Indian affairs, February 15, 1920 [1929], NARA, RG 75, box 4.

18. Hummer to commissioner of Indian affairs, February 16, 1929, NARA, RG 75, box 5.

19. Sioux Falls Committee, Report to the Indian Affairs Committee, March 5, 1929, NARA, RG 75, box 4.

20. Pettigrew to Burke, March 6, 1929, NARA, RG 75, box 5.

21. Gilland to commissioner of Indian affairs, March 11, 1929, NARA, RG 75, box 5.

22. Undated memorandum from Dr. Krulish during the course of his investigation, NARA, RG 75, box 5.

23. Krulish report, March 23, 1929, NARA, RG 75, box 5.

24. Krulish report, April 9, 1929, NARA, RG 75, box 5. Hummer appeared able to manipulate the Sioux Falls committee to his advantage, but he was obviously aware that he had made several vocal enemies in Canton.

25. The jackasses opposed higher tariffs.

26. Hummer to commissioner of Indian affairs, March 2, 1928, NARA, RG 75, box 17.

27. Patients received no dental care at all, and Silk had to recommend that the staff pass out toothbrushes.

28. The asylum had camisoles (strait jackets), ten pairs of metal wristlets with locking devices, and a pair of shackles borrowed from a sheriff six months earlier.

29. The Silk Report (Silk, *Asylum for Insane Indians*, April 18, 1929) is an outstanding snapshot of life at Canton Asylum, particularly considering that Hummer knew about the proposed visit and had just been investigated by Krulish. Like the Meriam Report, Silk's language was measured and fair, though his dismay is evident in the details he presents. His survey was conducted March 20–26, 1929.

30. Burke to Dr. William A. White, May 8, 1929, NARA, RG 418, box 1.

31. Putney, "Canton Asylum for Insane Indians," 21.

32. Cramton to Rhoads, January 20, 1930, NARA, RG 75, box 3.

16. The Gale Blows

1. Hummer to commissioner of Indian affairs, November 4, 22, 1930, NARA, RG 75, box 18. The letter dated November 22 indicates that he expected Schroder (he spelled the name "Shroder") to lose all the fingers on her right hand, as well as her thumb.

2. Hummer had never mentioned these restraints to Burke or other Indian Office personnel who sought to push more staff on him, and of course, he had never had the authority to make such a promise to Cramton in the first place.

3. Hummer's financial decisions come from Hummer's letter to Rhoads, November 30, 1930, and Statement of Superintendent, November 30, 1930, NARA, RG 75, box 11.

4. When questioned, Chico said she was not afraid of pregnancy because she had menstruated since being with Ball, implying a sexual liaison of some sort.

5. Information about Ball and Chico come from statements by Marie Chico, Emma Henke, Anna Tjelstad, Frances Caldwell RN, and nurse Lorena L. Sinning, as well as one unsigned statement, NARA KC, RG 75, box 6. Though not nearly so disturbing in character, even the asylum's professional staff were sometimes less

than ideal; nurse Elsie Behrman slacked off on her duties enough to be reported by the other nurses. She left sometime before the end of 1932.

6. Report from Holst to commissioner of Indian affairs, August 16, 1932, NARA, RG 75, box 4.

7. Report from Lowndes to the commissioner of Indian affairs, December 15, 1932, NARA, RG 75, box 4. Lowndes, like many other inspectors, confined most of his commentary to the buildings. Like Holst, he deplored the *situation* of the patients without being able to appreciate specific problems with Hummer's treatment. Lowndes did include a menu in his report and termed the food good but not well-balanced. Breakfast almost always included bacon and gravy, along with a starch of some kind, and coffee. The midday meals for a typical Friday through Wednesday featured beef and gravy; pork and gravy; fish and gravy; pork and gravy; beef and gravy; and pork and gravy, along with potatoes and a vegetable each day. Suppers were more problematic. Friday's supper consisted of stewed peas, hot rolls, peaches and prunes, and hot tea; two other meals that week were beans, bread, stewed apples, and hot tea. Meat, in the form of stew, was featured only once that week for supper.

8. Moley was a powerful New Dealer who had supported Governor Roosevelt before the election, recruiting some of his fellow professors at Columbia University to form FDR's Brain Trust. The trust advised FDR during his campaign and then followed him to Washington to advise him on the New Deal.

9. Dementia praecox being the old term for schizophrenia.

10. Evidence that Tafoya was involved in protests against the Maisel Company comes from the fact that a letter from T. F. McCormick, superintendent of the Northern Pueblos, to Tafoya was cited in the Federal Trade Commission's case against Maisel; see Jacobs, *Engendered Encounters*, 243. Information about the Maisel case comes from Jacobs's book and from Hoerig, *Under the Palace Portal*, 60–61.

11. Information about Collier's visit to Santa Clara Pueblo and Cleto Tafoya is found in Memorandum to Secretary Ickes, August 4, 1933, NARA, RG 75, box 3; admission note, case no. 39257, NARA, RG 418, box 1; in Philp, *John Collier's Crusade for Indian Reform*.

12. The details of Charles Fahy's legal opinion come from his memorandum for the secretary, April 21, 1933, and two additional memoranda dated August 24 and August 28, 1933, NARA, RG 75, box 4.

13. Silk, *Asylum for Insane Indians*, September 1933.

14. Details of the maneuvering to keep Canton Asylum open are found in telegrams from Bennett, Hildebrandt, Howes, Bulow, and Norbeck, all dated September 8, 1933; Bennett to Ickes, September 8, 1933; Collier to Hummer, September 12, 1933; Norbeck to Collier, telegram, September 13, 1933, all in NARA, RG 75, box 3; Collier to Silk, September 9, 1933, NARA, RG 418, box 1; and Ickes to Norbeck, September 9, 1933; Silk to White, September 11, 1933, NARA, RG 75, box 4.

15. Silk to White, September 23, 24, 1933, NARA, RG 418, box 1.

16. Collier to Moen, September 26, 1933; and memorandum for Secretary Ickes, February 1, 1934, NARA, RG 75, box 4.

17. "The Village Speakeasy," *Sioux Valley News*, September 28, 1933.

18. Groth to Investigation Committee of Affairs at Indian Asylum at Canton, S.Dak., September 20, 1933, NARA, RG 75, box 6. Hoover sent Groth's letter to Commissioner Collier.

19. Karlson to Silk, October 21, 1933, NARA, RG 75, box 3.

20. Hummer to Mr. Martin, agent, September 29, 1933, NARA, RG 75, box 4; and Collier to Hon. Henrik Shipstead, October 6, 1933, NARA, RG 75, box 3.

21. Collier to Hummer, October 5, 1933, NARA, RG 75, box 3.

22. The headlines quoted are from the *Spokane Spokesman-Review* and the *Sioux Falls Argus Leader*, respectively, both October 15, 1933. Details about Hummer's dismissal come from a Department of the Interior "Memorandum for the Press," October 16, 1933, NARA, RG 75, box 4. The release quoted Secretary Ickes's telegram to Hummer: "Your answer October nine to charges not satisfactory. You are hereby dismissed effective when Superintendent Balmer, Pipestone, receipts to you for funds and property in your charge. Have wired him proceed immediately to Canton and receipt."

23. "30,000 Indians to Petition to Retain Asylum," *Sioux Valley News*, October 26, 1933.

24. Clement Valandra, "Indian Committee," *Sioux-Falls Argus-Leader*, October or November 1933. Valandra's letter appeared in the paper's Reader's Letters section, and Valandra apparently sent the clipping to John Collier on November 1, 1933.

25. Ickes to Hon. Fred H. Hildebrandt, September 20, 1933, NARA, RG 75, box 4.

26. Executive Order, n.d. [1933], NARA, RG 75, box 4.

27. "Dr. Hummer Opens Office in S. Falls for Mental Disease," November 2, 1933, *Sioux Valley News*.

28. Two other patients made the trip a few days later, and eight others remained in the asylum waiting on arrangements to return home.

Epilogue

1. Cleto Tafoya, the initiating cause of Canton Asylum's closure, was one of those admitted.

2. L. L. Culp to commissioner of Indian affairs, February 17, 1934, NARA, RG 75, box 4.

3. Wilkens and Stark, *American Indian Politics*, 260. The constitution itself, showing Tafoya as a signer, can be found at the Native American Constitution and Law Digitization Project, coordinated by the University of Oklahoma Law Library and the National Indian Law Library, http://thorpe.ou.edu/IRA/nmsccons.html.

4. Trujillo, *Española*, 105; Rothman, *On Rims and Ridges*, 239.

5. Powers, *Navajo Trading*, 77.

BIBLIOGRAPHY

Files at the National Archives and Records Administration (NARA) in Washington DC (Record Groups 75 and 418) and Kansas City, Missouri (Record Group 75), hold thousands of documents pertaining to the Canton Asylum for Insane Indians. These files provided the core information within this book and allowed for detailed glimpses into the administration of the asylum.

Adams, G. S., and Leo Kanner. "General Paralysis among the North American Indians: A Contribution to Racial Psychiatry." *American Journal of Psychiatry* 6, no. 1 (July 1926): 125–33.

Allen, John R. "On the Treatment of Insanity." *American Journal of Insanity* 6, no. 3 (January 1850): 263–83.

Allen, Shannen K., and Richard D. Semba. *Survey of Ophthalmology* 47, no. 5 (September 2002): 500–509.

Alvord, Lori Arviso, and Elizabeth Cohen Van Pelt. *The Scalpel and the Silver Bear: The First Navajo Woman Surgeon Combines Western Medicine and Traditional Healing.* New York: Bantam, 1999.

Anderson, Virginia DeJohn. *Creatures of Empire: How Domestic Animals Transformed Early America.* New York: Oxford University Press, 2004.

"Asylum for the Insane of the Army and Navy and the District of Columbia." *American Journal of Insanity* 9, no. 4 (April 1853): 384–96.

Barkley, Frederick R., R. G. List, Robert S. Maxwell, and Ray Tucker. *Sons of the Wild Jackasses.* Reprint, Seattle: University of Washington Press, 1970. Questia Online Library, http://www.questia.com/PM.qst?a=o&d=59646162.

Barry, John M. *The Great Influenza: The Epic Story of the Deadliest Plague in History.* New York: Viking, 2004.

Barsh, Russel Lawrence. "American Indians in the Great War." *Ethnohistory* 38, no. 3 (Summer 1991): 276–303.

Bates, James. "Report on the Medical Treatment of Insanity, and the Diseases Most Frequently Accompanying It." *American Journal of Insanity* 7, no. 2 (October 1850): 97–111.

Beam, Alex. *Gracefully Insane: The Rise and Fall of America's Premier Mental Hospital.* Cambridge: Perseus, 2001.

Bear, Charla. "American Indian Boarding Schools Haunt Many." *Morning Edition* (National Public Radio). May 12, 2008. Transcript. http://www.npr.org/templates /story/story.php?storyId=16516865.

Beers, Clifford Whittingham. *A Mind That Found Itself.* Reprint, Pittsburgh: University of Pittsburgh Press, 1981.

Bell, Clark, ed. *Medico-Legal Journal* 9 (1891). Google e-book.

Bell, Luther V. "On the Coercive Administration of Food to the Insane." *American Journal of Insanity* 6, no. 3 (January 1850): 223–35.

B. L. R. "Reports of Hospitals for Insane." *American Journal of the Medical Sciences* 143 (July 1876): 254–58.

Blumer, G. Alder. "The History and Use of the Term Dementia." *American Journal of Insanity* 63, no. 3 (January 1907): 337–47.

Bly, Nellie. *Ten Days in a Mad-House.* New York: Ian L. Munro, 1887. http://digital .library.upenn.edu/women/bly/madhouse/madhouse.html.

Brady, Erika, ed. *Healing Logics: Culture and Medicine in Modern Health Belief Systems.* Logan: Utah State University Press, 2001.

Braslow, Joel. *Mental Ills and Bodily Cures: Psychiatric Treatment in the First Half of the Twentieth Century.* Berkeley: University of California Press, 1997.

Bucknill, John Charles. "Modes of Death Prevalent among Insane." *American Journal of Insanity* 19, no. 3 (January 1863): 354–62.

———. "Notes on Asylums for the Insane in America." *American Journal of Insanity* 33, no. 1 (July 1876): 21–41; 33, no. 2 (October 1876): 137–60.

Burch, Susan. "Dislocated Histories: The Canton Asylum for Insane Indians." *Women, Gender, and Families of Color* 2, no. 2 (Fall 2014): 141–62.

Butler, Ray. "Etherization in the Treatment of Insanity." *American Journal of Insanity* 11, no. 2 (October 1854): 164–69.

Cahill, Cathleen D. *Federal Fathers and Mothers: A Social History of the United States Indian Service, 1869–1933.* Chapel Hill: University of North Carolina Press, 2011.

Cash, Joseph H., and Herbert T. Hoover, eds. *To Be an Indian: An Oral History.* St. Paul: Minnesota Historical Society Press, 1971.

Chesler, Phyllis. *Women and Madness.* Garden City NY: Doubleday, 1972.

Child, Brenda J. *Boarding School Seasons: American Indian Families, 1900–1940.* Lincoln: University of Nebraska Press, 1998.

Churchill, Fleetwood. "On the Mental Disorders of Pregnancy and Childbed." *American Journal of Insanity* 7, no. 3 (January 1851): 259–66.

Collier, John. "Amerindians." *Pacific Affairs* 2, no. 3 (March 1929): 116–22.

———. *From Every Zenith: A Memoir.* Denver: Sage Books, 1963.

Collins, James P. "Native Americans in the Census, 1860–1890." *Prologue* (quarterly magazine of the National Archives) 38, no. 2 (Summer 2006).

Courtwright, David T. "The Hidden Epidemic: Opiate Addiction and Cocaine Use in the South, 1860–1920." *Journal of Southern History* 49, no. 1 (February 1983): 57–72.

Dain, Norman. *Concepts of Insanity in the United States, 1789–1865*. New Brunswick NJ: Rutgers University Press, 1964.

Davenport, Charles B. *Heredity in Relation to Eugenics*. New York: Henry Holt, 1911.

DeJong, David H. *If You Knew the Conditions: A Chronicle of the Indian Medical Service and American Indian Health Care, 1908–1955*. Lanham MD: Lexington Books, 2008.

———. "Unless They Are Kept Alive: Federal Indian Schools and Student Health, 1878–1918." *American Indian Quarterly* 31, no. 2 (Spring 2007): 256–82.

Deloria, Vine, and Clifford M. Lytle. *The Nations Within: The Past and Future of American Indian Sovereignty*. New York: Pantheon Books, 1984.

Dent, Emmet C. "Hydriatric Procedures as an Adjunct in the Treatment of Insanity." *American Journal of Insanity* 59, no. 1 (July 1902): 91–101.

Dick, Everett. *The Sod-House Frontier, 1854–1890: A Social History of the Northern Plains from the Creation of Kansas and Nebraska to the Admission of the Dakotas*. Lincoln NE: Johnsen Publishing, 1954.

Diefendorf, Allen Ross. *Clinical Psychiatry: A Text Book for Students and Physicians, Abstracted and Adapted from the Seventh German Edition of Kraepelin's "Lehrbuch Der Psychiatrie."* New York: Macmillan, 1915.

Dilenschneider, Anne. "An Invitation to Restorative Justice: The Canton Asylum for Insane Indians." *Northern Plains Ethics Journal*, 2013, 105–28.

Dodge, Colonel Richard Irving. *Our Wild Indians: Thirty-Three Years' Personal Experience among the Red Men of the Great West*. Reprint, Freeport NY: Books for Libraries Press, 1970.

Downes, Randolph C. "A Crusade for Indian Reform, 1922–1934." *Mississippi Valley Historical Review* 32, no. 3 (December 1945): 331–54.

Drucker, Philip. *Cultures of the North Pacific Coast*. San Francisco: Chandler, 1965.

Duran, Eduardo, and Bonnie Duran. *Native American Postcolonial Psychology*. Albany: State University of New York Press, 1995.

Dwyer, Ellen. *Homes for the Mad: Life Inside Two Nineteenth-Century Asylums*. New Brunswick NJ: Rutgers University Press, 1987.

Egan, Timothy. *The Worst Hard Time: The Untold Story of Those Who Survived the Great American Dust Bowl*. New York: Houghton Mifflin, 2006.

Elsner, Henry L. *Monographic Medicine*. Vol. 6, *The Prognosis of Internal Diseases*. New York: D. Appleton, 1916. Google Books.

Field, James A. "The Progress of Eugenics." *Quarterly Journal of Economics* 26, no. 1 (November 1911): 1–67. JSTOR.

Foreman, Grant. *The Five Civilized Tribes*. The Civilization of the American Indians Series, vol. 8. Norman: University of Oklahoma Press, 1934.

Freedman, Russell. *Kids at Work: Lewis Hine and the Crusade against Child Labor.* New York: Clarion, 1998.

Gamwell, Lynn, and Nancy Tomes. *Madness in America: Cultural and Medical Perceptions of Mental Illness before 1914.* Ithaca NY: Cornell University Press, 1995.

Geller, Jeffrey L., and Maxine Harris. *Women of the Asylum: Voices from Behind the Walls, 1840–1945.* New York: Doubleday, 1994.

"General Paralysis in Primitive Races." *British Medical Journal,* December 4, 1926, 1064.

Gilchrist-Stalnaker, Joy. *A Short History of Weston Hospital (Trans-Allegheny Asylum for the Insane).* Horner wv: Hacker's Creek Pioneer Descendants, 2001.

Gorwitz, Kurt. "Enumeration of the Mentally Ill and the Mentally Retarded in the Nineteenth Century." *Health Service Reports* 89, no. 2 (March–April 1974): 180–87.

Gould, Lewis L. *The Most Exclusive Club: A History of the Modern United States Senate.* Cambridge: Basic Books, 2005. Google Books.

Grimes, G., an inmate of the Lunatic Asylum of Tennessee. *A Secret Worth Knowing: A Treatise on the Most Important Subject in the World, Simply to Say, Insanity.* Nashville, 1846.

Grob, Gerald N. *The Mad among Us: A History of the Care of America's Mentally Ill.* New York: Free Press, 1994.

———, ed. *Mental Illness and Social Policy: The American Experience.* New York: Arno Press, 1973.

———. *Mental Institutions in American: Social Policy to 1875.* New York: Free Press, 1973.

Hacker, J. David, and Michael R. Haines. *The Construction of Life Tables for the American Indian Population at the Turn of the Twentieth Century.* Working Paper 16134. Cambridge MA: National Bureau of Economic Research, June 2010.

Hagan, William T. "Tribalism Rejuvenated: The Native American since the Era of Termination." *Western Historical Quarterly* 12, no. 1 (January 1981): 4–16.

Hamilton, William. "On Forced Alimentation." *American Journal of Insanity* 13, no. 3 (January 1857): 278–80.

Heckewelder, Rev. John. *An Account of the History, Manners, and Customs of the Indian Nations Who Once Inhabited Pennsylvania and the Neighboring States.* Philadelphia: Abraham Small, 1819. Reprinted as *The First American Frontier.* New York: Arno Press, 1971.

Hewitt, J. N. B. *Notes on the Creek Indians.* Edited by John R. Swanton. Smithsonian Institution, Bureau of American Ethnology, Bulletin 123; Anthropological Papers, No. 10. Washington DC: Government Printing Office, 1939.

Hinsdale, Guy. *Hydrotherapy.* Philadelphia: W. B. Saunders, 1910. Google Books.

Hodge, Frederick Webb, ed. *Handbook of American Indians North of Mexico.* Smithsonian Institution, Bureau of American Ethnology, Bulletin 30. Washington DC: Government Printing Office, 1907.

Hoerig, Karl A. *Under the Palace Portal: Native American Artists in Santa Fe*. Albuquerque: University of New Mexico Press, 2003.

Hrdlička, Aleš. *Physiological and Medical Observations among the Indians of Southwestern United States and Mexico*. Smithsonian Institution, Bureau of American Ethnology, Bulletin 34. Washington DC: Government Printing Office, 1908.

Hummer, H. R. "Insanity among the Indians." *Proceedings of the American Medico-Psychological Association at the Sixty-Eighth Annual Meeting*, May 28–31, 1912.

Hunt, Isaac H. *Three Years in a Madhouse!* N.p.: Published by Isaac H. Hunt, 1851. Disability History Museum, http://www.disabilitymuseum.org/lib/docs/736 .htm.

Hurd, Henry M., William F. Drewry, Richard Dewey, Charles W. G Pilgrim, G. Alder Blumer, and T. J. W. Burgess. *The Institutional Care of the Insane in the United States and Canada*. Vols. 1–4. Edited by Henry M. Hurd. Reprint, New York: Arno Press, 1973.

Jackson, Curtis E., and Marcia J. Galli. *A History of the Bureau of Indian Affairs and Its Activities among Indians*. San Francisco: R & E Research Associates, 1977.

Jacobs, Margaret D. *Engendered Encounters: Feminism and Pueblo Cultures, 1879–1934*. Lincoln: University of Nebraska Press, 1999.

Jewitt, John R. *A Narrative of the Adventures and Sufferings of John R. Jewitt, Only Survivor of the Crew of the Ship Boston, during a Captivity of Nearly Three Years among the Savages of Nootka Sound*. Ithaca NY: Andrus, Gauntlett, 1851.

Jones, Robert. "The Evolution of Insanity." *Lancet* 2 (September 8, 1906): 635–38. Google Books.

Kappler, Charles J., ed. *Indian Affairs: Laws and Treaties*. Vols. 1, 3, 4, 5. Washington DC: Government Printing Office, 1904, 1941.

Keller, Rosemary Skinner, and Rosemary Radford Ruether, eds. *The Encyclopedia of Women and Religion in North America*. Bloomington: Indiana University Press, 2006.

Kelly, Lawrence C. *The Assault on Assimilation: John Collier and the Origins of Indian Policy Reform*. Albuquerque: University of New Mexico Press, 1983.

Kirkbride, Thomas S. *On the Construction, Organization and General Arrangements of Hospitals for the Insane*. Philadelphia, 1854. Google Books.

Kokecki, Paul R., and Janice D. Mashburn. *Beyond the Asylum: The History of Mental Handicap Policy in Tennessee, 1796–1984*. Nashville TN: Department of Mental Health and Mental Retardation, 1984.

Kraepelin, Emil, and Felix Plaut. *Paralysestudien Bei Negern Und Indianern*. Berlin: Verlag Von Julius, 1926.

Kunitz, Stephen J., and John Collier. "The Social Philosophy of John Collier." *Ethnohistory* 18, no. 3 (Summer 1971): 213–29.

Landis, Barbara. "Carlisle Indian Industrial School History." 1996. http://home.epix .net/~landis/histry.html.

Leahy, Todd E. "The Canton Asylum: Indians, Psychiatrists, and Government Policy, 1899–1934." PhD diss., Oklahoma State University, 2004.

Lerner, Paul. *Hysterical Men: War, Psychiatry, and the Politics of Trauma in Germany, 1890–1930*. Ithaca NY: Cornell University Press, 2003.

Lincoln County Historical Committee. *The History of Lincoln County South Dakota*. Freeman SD: Pine Hill Press, 1985.

MacBride, Henry J., and W. L. Templeton. "The Treatment of General Paralysis of the Insane by Malaria." *Journal of Neurology and Psychopathology* 5 no. 17 (May 1924): 13–27.

MacDonald, Arthur. *Statistics of Crime, Suicide, Insanity, and Other Forms of Abnormality, and Criminological Studies, with a Bibliography, in Connection with Bills to Establish a Laboratory for the Study of the Criminal, Pauper, and Defective Classes*. 58th Cong., March 13, 1903. S. Doc. 12.

Marr, Carolyn J. "Assimilation through Education: Indian Boarding Schools in the Pacific Northwest." American Indians of the Pacific Northwest Collection, University of Washington Digital Collections. http://content.lib.washington.edu/aipnw/marr.html.

Massachusetts General Hospital Memorial & Historical Volume. Boston: Griffith-Stillings Press, 1921.

McCandless, Peter. *Moonlight, Magnolias and Madness: Insanity in South Carolina from the Colonial Period to the Progressive Era*. Chapel Hill: University of North Carolina Press, 1996.

McGovern, Constance M. *Masters of Madness: Social Origins of the American Psychiatric Profession*. Hanover NH: University Press of New England, for University of Vermont, 1985.

Medico-Legal Society of the District of Columbia. *Report of the Special Committee on Care and Treatment of the Insane in the District of Columbia and Elsewhere*. Records Relating to the Investigation of 1906, 1903–6, Record Group 418, box 3, folder 1, no. 46, NARA, Washington DC.

Memorial and Biographical Record of Turner, Lincoln, Union and Clay Counties, South Dakota. Chicago: Geo. A. Ogle, 1897.

Meriam, Lewis, et. al. *The Problem of Indian Administration*. Baltimore: Johns Hopkins Press, 1928. ERIC (Education Resources Information Center), http://www.eric.ed.gov/PDFS/ED087573.pdf.

Meritt, Edgar B. *The American Indian and Government Indian Administration*. Office of Indian Affairs, Bulletin 12. Chilocco, Oklahoma: Indian Agricultural School, Indian Print Shop, 1926. Indian Office Publications, 1926–1930, Record Group 75, box 3, folder 005-110, NARA, Kansas City.

Mintz, Steven. *Native American Voices: A History and Anthology*. St. James NY: Brandywine Press, 1995.

Morton, Thomas G. "Removal of the Ovaries as a Cure for Insanity." *American Journal of Insanity* 49, no. 3 (January 1893): 397–401.

Munro, John C. "Report of Cases of Trephining for Epilepsy." *Boston Medical and Surgical Journal* 150, no. 5 (February 4, 1904): 109–15. http://www.nejm.org/doi/full/10.1056/NEJM190402041500501.

Murali, Vijaya, and Femi Oyebode. "Poverty, Social Inequality and Mental Health." *Advances in Psychiatric Treatment* 10 (2004): 216–24.

Murphy, Jane M. "Psychiatric Labeling in Cross-Cultural Perspective." *Science*, n.s. 191, no. 4231 (March 12, 1976): 1019–28.

Murphy, P. L. "Colony Treatment of the Insane and Other Defectives." *Transactions of the Medical Society of the State of North Carolina, Fifty-Third Annual Meeting*, May 29–31, 1906.

Murray, Montague, John Harold, and W. Cecil Bosanquet. *Quain's Dictionary of Medicine*. 3rd ed. London: Longmans Green, 1902.

Nathan Kline Institute. NKI Center of Excellence in Culturally Competent Mental Health. Native Americans. http:ssrdqst.rfmh.org/cecc/index.php?q=node/22. Accessed January 1, 2014.

Nielsen, Kim E. *A Disability History of the United States*. Boston: Beacon Press, 2012.

Niles, H. R. "Static Electricity in the Treatment of Nervous and Mental Diseases." *American Journal of Insanity* 53, no. 3 (January 1897): 390–95.

Notes and Comments. *American Journal of Psychiatry* 79, no. 4 (April 1923): 721–23.

Olmsted, Dan, and Mark Blaxill. *The Age of Autism: Mercury, Medicine, and a Man-Made Epidemic*. New York: Thomas Dunne Books, 2010.

Packard, Elizabeth P. W. *Modern Persecution; or, Insane Asylums Unveiled*. Hartford CT: Case, Lockwood, and Brainard, 1874. Disability Museum, http://www.disabilitymuseum.org/lib/docs/1663card.htm.

Paine, Harlan L. "Psychotic Symptoms of Epilepsy." *American Journal of Psychiatry* 79, no. 4 (April 1923): 713–19.

Parman, Donald L. "Lewis Meriam's Letters during the Survey of Indian Affairs, 1926–1927." Pt. 1. *Arizona and the West* 24, no. 3 (Autumn 1982): 253–80.

Philp, Kenneth R. "Albert B. Fall and the Protest from the Pueblos, 1921–23." *Arizona and the West* 12, no. 3 (Fall 1970): 237–54.

———. *John Collier's Crusade for Indian Reform, 1920–1954*. Tucson: University of Arizona Press, 1977.

Powel, T. O. "A Sketch of Psychiatry in the Southern States." *American Journal of Insanity* 54, no. 1. (July 1897): 21–36.

Powers, Willow Roberts. *Navajo Trading: The End of an Era*. Albuquerque: University of New Mexico Press, 2001.

Prandoni, Jogues R., and Liza H. Gold. "St. Elizabeths Hospital Celebrates 150 Years." *Psychiatric Services* 56, no. 3 (March 2005): 370.

Pratt, Richard H. "Kill the Indian and Save the Man." History Matters: The U.S. Survey Course on the Web. http://historymatters.gmu.edu/d/4929. Originally published in *Official Report of the Nineteenth Annual Conference of Charities and Correction*, 1892, 46–59.

Putney, Diane T. "The Canton Asylum for Insane Indians, 1902–1934." *South Dakota History* 14, no. 1 (Spring 1984): 1–29.

Ray, Isaac. "The Insanity of Women Produced by Desertion or Seduction." *American Journal of Insanity* 23, no. 2 (October 1866): 263–74.

Reiss, Benjamin. *Theaters of Madness: Insane Asylums and Nineteenth-Century American Culture.* Chicago: University of Chicago Press, 2008.

"Restraint in British and American Insane Asylums." *American Journal of Insanity* 34, no. 4 (April 1878): 512–30.

Rhein, John W. W. "Insanity in Children." *American Journal of Insanity* 71, no. 3 (January 1915): 471–87.

Rieder, Hans L. "Tuberculosis among American Indians of the Contiguous United States." *Public Heath Report* 104, no. 6 (November–December 1989): 653–57.

Riney, Scott. "People and Powerlessness: The People of the Canton Asylum for Insane Indians." *South Dakota History* 27, nos. 1 & 2 (Spring/Summer 1997): 41–64.

Robertson, Paul. *The Power of the Land: Identity, Ethnicity, and Class among the Oglala Lakota.* New York: Routledge, 2002.

Robinson, Doane. *History of South Dakota.* Vol. 1. Indianapolis: B. F. Bowen, 1904.

Rothman, Hal K. *On Rims and Ridges: The Los Alamos Area since 1880.* Lincoln: University of Nebraska Press, 1992.

Rusco, Elmer R. *A Fateful Time: The Background and Legislative History of the Indian Reorganization Act.* Reno: University of Nevada Press, 2000.

Schlereth, Thomas J. *Victorian America: Transformations in Everyday Life, 1876–1915.* New York: Harper Perennial, 1991.

Schlup, Leonard. "Charles Henry Burke and the Department of Indian Affairs in the Harding and Coolidge Administrations." *International Review of History and Political Science* 17 (1980): 1–14.

Scull, Andrew, ed. *Madhouses, Mad-Doctors, and Madmen: The Social History of Psychiatry in the Victorian Era.* Philadelphia: University of Pennsylvania Press, 1981.

Shelton, Brett Lee. *Legal and Historical Roots of Health Care for American Indians and Alaska Natives in the United States.* Issue brief. Menlo Park CA: Henry J. Kaiser Family Foundation, 2004.

Silk, Samuel A. *Asylum for Insane Indians Canton, S.D.* Initial report. April 18, 1929. South Dakota State Historical Society Archives, Pierre.

———. *Asylum for Insane Indians Canton, S.D.* Second report. September 1933. South Dakota State Historical Society Archives, Pierre.

Smith, Stephen. "How Doctor Brigham Met the Challenge to Diagnose Insanity at Sight." *Proceedings of the American Medico-Psychological Association at the Fifty-Ninth Annual Meeting*, May 12–15, 1903.

Spaulding, John M. "The Canton Asylum for Insane Indians: An Example of Institutional Neglect." *Hospital and Community Psychiatry* 57, no. 10 (October 1986): 1007–11.

Stacey, Michelle. *The Fasting Girl: A True Victorian Medical Mystery.* New York: Putnam, 2002.

Stawicki, Elizabeth. "A Haunting Legacy: Canton Asylum for Insane Indians." Minnesota Public Radio. December 9, 1997. Transcript. http://www.rootsweb.com/~sdlincol/hiawatha.htm.

Stowe, Steven M. *Doctoring in the South.* Chapel Hill: University of North Carolina Press, 2004.

Swain, Donald C. "Harold Ickes, Horace Albright, and the Hundred Days: A Study in Conservation Administration." *Pacific Historical Review* 34, no. 4 (November 1965): 455–65.

Sweet, Kelli. "Controversial Care: The Canton Indian Insane Asylum: 1902–1934." MA thesis, University of Nebraska at Omaha, 2000.

Szasz, Thomas S. *The Age of Madness.* Garden City NY: Anchor Books, 1973.

"Thoughts on the Causation of Insanity." *American Journal of Insanity* 29, no. 2 (October 1872): 264–83.

Tighe, Janet A. "'What's in a Name?': A Brief Foray into the History of Insanity in England and the United States." *Journal of the American Academy of Psychiatry and the Law Online* 33, no. 2 (2005): 252–58.

Trafzer, Clifford E., and Diane Weiner, eds. *Medicine Ways: Disease, Health and Survival among Native Americans.* Walnut Creek CA: AltaMira Press, 2001.

Trennert, Robert A. "Corporal Punishment and the Politics of Indian Reform." *History of Education Quarterly* 29, no. 4 (Winter 1989): 595–617.

Trujillo, Camilla. *Española.* Images of America series. Charleston SC: Arcadia, 2011.

Tyler, S. Lyman. *A History of Indian Policy.* Washington DC: Department of the Interior, 1973.

Tucker, Ray. "Those Sons of Wild Jackasses." *North American Review* 229, no. 2 (1930): 225–33.

U.S. Commission on Civil Rights. *Broken Promises: Evaluating the Native American Health Care System.* Washington DC: Government Printing Office, 2004. www.usccr.gov/pubs/nahealth/nabroken.pdf.

U.S. Congress. House. *Report of the Special Committee on Investigation of the Government Hospital for the Insane.* 2 vols. 59th Cong., 2d sess., 1907. H. Rep. 7644. Records Relating to the Investigation of 1906, Record Group 418, box 1, no. 46, NARA, Washington DC.

U.S. Congress. Senate. *Asylum for Insane Indians.* 55th Cong., 2d sess., February 11, 1898. S. Rep. 567.

U.S. Department of Commerce. Bureau of the Census. *Patients in Hospitals for Mental Disease, 1923.* Washington DC: Government Printing Office, 1923.

U.S. Office of Indian Affairs. *Annual Report of the Commissioner of Indian Affairs.* Washington DC: Government Printing Office, 1886, 1903, 1904, 1905, 1906, 1907, 1910, 1920.

Wallin, J. E. Wallace. *Experimental Studies of Mental Defectives: A Critique of the Binet-Simon Tests and a Contribution to the Psychology of Epilepsy.* Baltimore: Warwick & York, 1902.

Walling, William H., ed. *Sexology.* Family Medical Edition. Philadelphia: Puritan, 1904.

Waters, Frank. *Masked Gods: Navaho and Pueblo Ceremonialism.* Reprint, Athens: Swallow Press/Ohio University Press, 1984.

White, E. E. *Service on the Indian Reservations: Being the Experiences of a Special Indian Agent While Inspecting Agencies and Serving as Agent for Various Tribes*. Little Rock AR: Diploma Press, 1893.

White, William A. *Outlines of Psychiatry*. New York: Journal of Nervous and Mental Disease Publishing Company, 1907.

Wilkens, David E., and Heidi Kiiwetinepinesiik Stark. *American Indian Politics and the American Political System*. Lanham MD: Rowman & Littlefield, 2011.

Willis, Frank N., Larry M. Dean, and Larry Larsen. "The First Mental Hospital for American Indians, 1900–1934." *Bulletin of the Menninger Clinic* 45, no. 2 (1981): 149–54.

Winslow, Kenelm. *The Home Medical Library*. New York: Review of Reviews, 1909.

Woodward, Grace Steele. *The Cherokee*. The Civilization of the American Indians, vol. 65. Norman: University of Oklahoma Press, 1963.

Woodward, Samuel B. "Observations on the Medical Treatment of Insanity." *American Journal of Insanity* 7, no. 1 (July 1850): 1–34.

Yanni, Carla. *The Architecture of Madness: Insane Asylums in the United States*. Minneapolis: University of Minnesota Press, 2007.

Yellow Bird, Pemina. "Wild Indians: Native Perspectives on the Hiawatha Asylum for Insane Indians." MindFreedom. http://www.mindfreedom.org/kb/mental

-health-abuse/Racism.

Index

Page numbers in italics refer to illustrations.

acreage, 12, 13, 69, 201; as allotment, 161, 171, 355n14; at Canton Asylum, 24, 184, 191, 193, 231, 232, 246; on reservations, 51, 161, 187, 351n22

act, Congressional, 22, 161, 246, 259, 264, 349n3, 350n15, 350n16, 366n13, 372n39. *See also* Burke Act; Dawes Act

Alaska, 4, 185, 241, 277, 349n3

alcohol abuse, alcoholism, 42, 65, 131, 165, 168, 212

alienist(s), 29–30, 41–42, 44, 57, 60, 62–63, 66, 125, 128–30, 149, 175, 178–79, 277, 361–62

Allen, Edgar A., 82–84

allotments (land), 17, 51, 161, 164, 170–71, 184, 186, 355n14, 375n12

Alvord, Lori Arviso, 28, 276

American Indian Defense Association, 190, 228, 254

American Journal of Insanity, 15, 42, 44, 45, 63, 175, 179

American Medical Association, 89, 205, 359n16, 367n18

American Medico-Psychological Association, 90, 124, 129, 179, 216

Amyotte, Emma, 257, 269

Anglo culture and norms, 17, 28–29, 129, 161–62, 188, 277, 281

assimilation, 6, 28, 51, 162, 164, 275, 368n10

asylum architecture, 31, 201

asylum medicine, 29, 41–42, 49, 50–51, 99, 179, 203, 277, 280

Ball, Vernon E., 250–51, 378n4

Balmer, James W., 267, 380n22

basket-making, 66, 194

bedbugs, 105, 108, 110

beadwork, beading, 37, 66, 200, 357n10

Bear, Frank, 9, 222

Beers, Clifford, 119, 157, 203, 361n2

Bennet, Claude A., 259–60

Beyer, W. R., 207–8

Big Sioux River, 24, 127

bills, legislative, 16–17, 21, 23, 47, 246, 372n39. *See also* Bursum Bill

blood quantum, 161, 368n1

Bly, Nellie, 361–62n2

Board of Indian Commissioners, 164, 193, 227, 240, 377n3

booster, boosterism, 20, 54, 92, 140, 359n5

brain, 50, 167, 179, 197, 101–2, 241, 354n2

Breid, Jacob, 127–28, 142

Brings Plenty, Robert, 47–48, 53, 354n6

bromides, 42, 48, 57, 355n7

Brown, Charles, 81, 82, 83, 84

Brown, John, 100, 194, 203–4

bull-yards, 356n23

Bureau of Indian Affairs, 11–15, 21, 33, 121, 164, 188–89, 350n16; medical personnel, 114, 235; resignations from, 106, 116; transfers within, 245, 261, 376. *See also* Indian Office

Burke, Charles, 184, 190–91, 196, 205, 214, 224, 227–28, 236–37, 249; and asylum patients, 184, 186, 190, 207–8, 217, 230;

Burke, Charles (*continued*)
as congressman, 108–9, 116; reaction to
asylum inspections and visits, 215–16,
223, 238, 240–41, 245; and reformers,
184, 189, 247, 372n39. *See also* Burke Act;
Bursum Bill
Burke Act, 183, 371n25
Bursum Bill, 187–90, 196, 205, 241

Caldwell, Agnes, 133, 151–52, 155, 160, 176,
178, 230, 264, 269, 375n22, 377n9; and
daughter Delores, 370n9
Calhoun, John C., 13–14
Canton, South Dakota, 23–24, 46–47, 68,
92–93
Canton Asylum: battles concerning,190,
222, 236, 259, 261–62; commitment
process, 5, 31–33, 35–37, 64, 130–31, 174,
191, 203, 254–55, 261, 269, 370n7; court
orders for commitment, 5, 261, 269;
descriptions of, 24–25, 53, 55–56, 57–59,
67, 70, 97, 105–7, 143, 154, 198–99, 200,
214, 233, 235; distance issues, 27–28, 54,
73, 155, 196, 220, 266; economies at, 112,
155, 214, 250, 360n4, 366n10, 369n11; food
at, 5, 50, 56, 57, 82, 103–4, 112–13, 122, 154,
159, 224, 244, 285; hospital, 86, 141, 153,
217, 242; medical care, 48, 49–52, 57, 158,
203, 373n2; patient processing at, 33–34;
quarters at, 48, 86, 91, 104, 106–7, 112–13,
229, 237, 239, 285, 360n5, 361n14; sane
patients at, 234, 264, 265, 269, 285; stench
from poor housekeeping, 138, 154, 217,
244, 352n39; stench from sewer, 82, 86,
127, 363n15; visitors to, 31–32, 59, 67, 70,
141–42, 194, 199, 212. *See also* epilepsy
Canton Asylum cemetery, 53, 269, 270,
357n10, 359n13, 364n30
Canton Asylum employees: abuses by, 137–
39, 221, 242–43, 249, 250–51, 258, 284, 285,
364n2; affidavits of, 83, 114–15, 144, 148–
49, 361n11, 364n18; duties of, 34, 48–49,
76, 154, 215, 284, 360n4; shortages of, 48,
146, 160, 175, 229, 232, 239, 243, 250, 251,
252. *See also* Canton Asylum matron
Canton Asylum matron, 39, 350n16, 360n4;
under Gifford, 54, 83; under Hummer,

95, 104–5, 108, 137, 144, 146, 149, 219–21,
224–25
Canton Asylum patients, 71, 94, 105–6;
accidents and injuries, 9, 222, 249;
babies born to, 74, 134, 175–76, 222, 243,
269, 357n5, 370n9, 375n21; children as, 1,
50–51, 71, 81, 94, 95, 175, 178, 233, 241–42,
281, 285, 370n7; clothing of, 59, 105, 199,
242; daily occupations of, 34, 49–50, 59,
65; entertainments for, 56, 65, 66, 67, 141,
150, 155, 184, 193–94; escapes by, 56–57, 59,
74, 102, 129–30, 168, 169, 206–8, 222, 231,
235, 250, 375n9; deaths of, 5, 48, 51, 53, 65,
80, 86, 96, 102, 115, 134, 138, 232, 242, 243,
258, 269, 357n10, 369n11, 369n4, 370n9;
deaths of, causes, 47–48, 81–82, 96, 134,
158, 229, 242, 354n6, 359n13; fighting
among, 154, 177, 193, 217, 256, 284; first
patient at, 25, 352–53n41; funds belonging
to, 230, 231–32, 251, 357n10, 377n9; illness
among, 56, 57, 85–86, 97, 102, 158, 213;
interaction among, 34, 73–74, 138, 176,
193; letters from, 151, 160, 173, 192, 200,
221, 230; numbers of, 48, 59, 65, 86, 152,
158, 184; tribes represented among, 53,
177; work done by, 34, 65, 152, 174, 182–83,
200, 237, 257. *See also* Brown, Charles;
Smith, Martha
Canton Chamber of Commerce, 198, 252,
261, 263
Carlisle Indian School, 29, 161
Carpenter, John, 130–31
ceremonies, 18, 20, 32, 270, 276–77, 279
Charles, John, 85–87, 97, 127, 365n4
Chico, Mary, 250–51, 378n4
children, 67–68, 70, 98, 120, 132–33, 142,
151–52, 155, 160, 165, 176, 199, 276, 360n2;
of Canton staff, 67–68, 83, 106, 229,
375n23; in insane asylums, 4; insanity
among, 44, 175. *See also* Canton Asylum
patients: children; Gifford, Oscar S.;
Hummer, Harry R.; schools
chlorpromazine, 179, 371n17
Chraft & Hanson, 68, 359n5
Christmas, 122, 140, 166, 231, 251
Christopher, Berney, 82–83, 93, 358n17
Christopher, Clara, 27, 224, 231, 244

churches, 29, 46, 66, 126, 140, 153, 354n4

citizens: of Canton, 77, 92, 93, 127, 128, 139, 140; U.S., 4, 23, 59, 60, 142, 166, 167, 195, 240, 350n12; and Native Americans, 168, 184, 186, 256, 367n22, 370n7

citizenship, 368n6, 368n10, 370n7, 371n25

civilization, 15, 52, 162, 368n10

civil service, 75, 152, 232, 278, 356; exams, 53, 89

Civil War, 3, 23, 29, 93, 179, 353n5

Clapp, W. H., 22

coal, 56, 70, 84, 105, 112, 143, 186, 206, 242, 355n18, 360n6, 372n39

Coleman, Elizabeth, 219, 222, 224

Coleman, Mary, 224, 225

Collier, John, 120, 186–87, 254–55; as Indian rights advocate, 190, 227–28, 247, 253; efforts to close Canton Asylum, 255–56, 262, 264, 265, 267. *See also* Bursum Bill

commissioner of Indian Affairs, 13; assistant commissioner, 75, 85, 223; correspondence from, 88, 143, 149–50, 156, 264–65; and patients, 134, 151, 184, 208. *See also* Burke, Charles; Collier, John; Jones, William A.; Meritt, Edgar B.; Valentine, Robert G.

Committee on Indian Affairs, 13, 15, 22, 189, 227, 240

competent, incompetent (mental condition), 56, 170, 186, 227, 240

concepts of insanity, 17–20, 30, 42–44, 61, 66

Congress, 11, 13, 23, 61, 78, 121, 157, 161, 167, 184, 189–90, 227, 241, 247, 253, 264, 276, 349n4

Coombs, Josiah, 169–72

corn, 65, 238, 249, 351n21, 371n19, 375–76n23

Corrigan, John W., 77, 81–83, 373n2

cottages, 35, 70, 201, 229, 367n23

Couchman, Peter, 14–15

Court, Jerome, 206–8

Cramton, Louis C., 163, 191, 246–47, 250, 276, 378n2

crops, 249, 357n13

Culp, L. L., 267, 269

culture, 18, 43, 64, 103, 128, 130, 132, 164–65, 170, 190, 227, 273, 281, 351n27, 353n7; clashes between, 10–11, 33, 51, 129; disre-

gard for Native American, 17, 29, 32, 33, 53, 161–62, 177, 220, 275, 277, 350n12

custodial care, 30, 128, 245

Dakota Territory, 24, 46–47, 140

Davenport, Charles, 132

Davis, Charles L., 109–16, 126, 148, 155, 166, 259, 275, 361n15

Dawes Act, 51, 161, 170, 183, 368n6, 368n10

Deere, Amos, 137–38, 144, 369n11

defectives, 42–43, 66, 95, 132–33, 153, 155, 176, 246, 278, 280, 285, 359n9

Department of the Interior, 2, 4–5, 15, 89, 95, 170, 188, 195–96, 205, 214–15, 227–28, 246, 254, 256, 265, 285, 372n39

Deroin, William, 257–58

Diagnostic and Statistical Manual of Mental Disorders, 43, 373n7

Dickson, Charles, 74–75

discharges (not Canton patients), 79; furloughs, 201; rates of, 79, 357n14; readmission, 363n12

Dix, Dorothea, 23, 31, 353n5

domesticated animals, 10–11

Donohue, P. J., 167–68

Dorrington (inspector), 144, 148, 149

Dunn, Ava, 206–7

Durbin, Winfield, 21

East, the (U.S.), 20–21, 46, 69, 87, 107, 123, 139, 221, 266, 279

easterners, 90, 92, 96, 350n12

editors, 15, 60, 67, 85, 91, 102, 115, 142, 189, 190, 361n2

Edwards, Herbert R., 231–35, 242, 252

Elliot, James D., 260, 267

epilepsy, 5, 42, 47, 65, 94, 202–3, 233–34, 244, 373n5; cottages for, 153, 156, 158, 160, 192, 194, 229, 244, 280; treatments for, 48, 57, 197–98, 203, 355n7, 369n1

escorts, patient, 36, 102, 183, 261, 363n18, 369n12, 370n14

Espinoza, Frances, 192–93

eugenics, 132, 176, 281, 363n24

Europeans, 9–11, 18, 29, 41, 157

Evans, Richard P., 79, 85

Ewing, Norman, 147, 364n15, 364n16, 364n17

farms and farming, 34, 51–52, 69, 72, 104, 110, 189, 191, 193, 217, 222, 231, 233, 237, 250, 257

Fall, Albert B., 187–89, 195, 205, 372n39, 374n13

Faribault, Elizabeth, 222, 243; and daughter Winona, 249, 375n21

feces, 101, 108, 115, 154, 235, 285

feeblemindedness, 43, 132–33, 151, 186, 191, 203, 260, 281

fever, 43, 175, 258, 374n8

fever therapy, 202

Fillius, Grace O., 232, 235–40, 245

filthy patients, challenges of, 50, 101, 107, 110, 154, 244

fire extinguishers, 82, 86, 112

Flandreau, South Dakota, 47, 93, 94, 116

food: at Canton Asylum, 5, 50, 56, 57, 82, 103–4, 112–13, 122, 154, 159, 224, 244, 285; on reservations, 17, 51–52, 162

Fowles, Jacob A., 107, 148, 360n1

Freud, Sigmund, 42, 124, 180

funds, 25, 98, 102, 121, 124, 142, 155, 194, 214, 231–32, 251–52, 255, 264, 267, 380n22; belonging to patients, 230, 231–32, 251, 357n10, 377n9; for construction, 70, 229

Gandy, Harry L., 167–71

gardens, 34, 56, 57, 65, 103, 104, 159

General Federation of Women's Clubs, 187, 189

ghost, 18, 20

Gifford, Oscar S., 23, 45–47, 67, 80, 93, 140; conflict with Turner, 70, 74–75, 80, 81; death of, 140–41; employee favoritism by, 54, 76–77; family members of, 45–46, 72, 76, 139, 140; honors and achievements of, 46–47, 93, 140–41; performance of, at asylum, 53, 65, 71–72, 77, 83–84. *See also* Brown, Charles

Giles, Leon, 230–31

Gilland, Dewey, 237–38, 240, 244

Gladstone, Lucy, 181–83

Godding, W. W., 22–23, 49, 180, 245

Good Boy, Peter Thompson, 37

Government Hospital for the Insane. *See* St. Elizabeths (Government Hospital for the Insane)

grand mal seizure, 354n6

Grasshopper, Josephine, 133–34

grave markers, 88, 194, 269

Great Depression, 247, 250–51

Gregory County, 165, 167

Groth, Helen, 63–64, 262, 263

guardhouse, 15, 32, 53

guardianship, 11, 240; over Native Americans, 14, 195, 227, 245; of patients, 173, 370n7

Guest, Edgar, 90, 358n2

habeas corpus, writ of, 62

hallucinations, 18, 37, 131, 179, 200, 211, 213, 222, 264, 351n23

Hardin, L. M., 106–13, 115–17, 127, 139, 153, 177–78, 240, 360n7, 361n10, 361n11, 361n14

Harding, Warren G., 187, 188, 195, 205

Hathorn, James, 50–51, 65, 355n12

Hauke, C. F., 174, 223

Hawk, Charles, 231–32, 242

health care, 14, 114, 276, 350n15, 350n16, 359n16

Hedges, Edward, 25, 65, 352n41

Hendricks, Randy (matron), 137, 144

Herman, Blanch, 165, 167, 169–71, 369n13

Herman, James, 147, 164–72, 369n13

Hiawatha, 55

Holst, John H., 251–52, 259

Hoopa reservation, 375n12

Hot Springs, South Dakota, 165–66, 204

House Appropriations Committee, 163, 215, 276

House Committee on Indian Affairs, 189, 240, 372n39

Hummer, Harry R.: accusations against employees, 147, 206, 219, 221, 224, 235–39; background of, 89–90, 111, 274, 279; children of, 90, 101, 102, 104, 113, 143, 159, 178, 221–22, 370n14; concerning patients, 94, 133–34, 151–52, 158, 174, 193, 200, 216; corresponding with Indian Office, 88, 95–96, 147–48, 160, 185, 237; post–Canton Asylum, 270–71; at St. Elizabeths, 61–62, 79, 89–90, 102, 358n3; temper of, 102–3, 107, 111, 113–15, 127, 139, 144, 147–48, 364–65n18,

376n24; with vendors, 222. *See also* Court, Jerome; Hendricks, Randy (matron); Herman, James; investigations into abuses; Landis, Ione; sterilization of patients

Hummer, Levi, 111, 178

Hummer, Norena (wife of Harry), 90, 96, 104–5, 106, 108, 109, 115, 141, 142, 143, 146, 258, 271, 361n17

hydrotherapy, 35, 44, 49, 98–99, 180, 359–60n18; at Canton Asylum, 97, 98–99, 178, 194, 196, 242

Ickes, Harold, 190, 253–55, 259–60, 265–67, 270, 275, 380n22

immigrants, 69, 120, 128, 186–87, 359n16, 362n7

Indian agent, 14, 21, 32, 36, 37, 51, 63, 102, 351n21

Indian boarding schools, 29, 39, 51, 80, 82, 141, 161–63, 266, 282, 359n16, 368n6, 368–69n10; cruelty in, 163, 266; runaways from, 163

Indian Office, 15, 52, 108, 148–49, 240–41, 264; challenges to Hummer's authority by, 95, 174; coercion by, 52–53, 164; insensitivity of, toward Native Americans, 33, 51, 52–53, 162–63, 275. *See also* Bureau of Indian Affairs

Indian Oil Bill, 372n9

Indian Rights Association, 116, 253, 368n10

Indian soldiers, 367n22

Indian Territory, 14, 21, 72, 256

influenza (grippe), 97, 140, 158–59, 367n18

injunction, 127, 260–62, 263, 265, 267

insane asylums, 29–31, 34–35, 49, 68, 119, 179, 181, 201; commitment procedures, 4, 38–39, 59–61; decline of, 66, 125, 181; overcrowding at, 23, 34–35, 66, 85–86, 97, 113, 124, 127–28, 153; oversight of, 39, 60, 67, 88, 196; patient labor in, 35, 64–65; patients in, 41–42, 70–71, 78, 120; as tourist destinations, 67; visits to patients at, 220, 266; wards in, 1–2, 24, 34, 49, 70, 73–74, 104–5, 137–38, 175–76, 200, 234, 237, 242–44, 256, 258. *See also* Canton Asylum; McLean Asylum

insanity: acute, 18, 42, 95, 125, 181, 258, 277;

causes, 17, 19, 29, 42, 66, 175, 179, 201, 277; chronic, 3, 42, 47, 125, 128, 179–80, 258, 277, 280; cure rates, 30–31, 60, 125–26; diagnosing, 43, 63, 129, 131–32; in general population, 3, 29, 128, 185, 351n27; in Native American population, 19, 22, 29, 141, 185, 351n27; treatments for, 18–20, 29–31, 32, 35, 44, 67, 99, 124, 176–77, 179–80. *See also* fever therapy; hydrotherapy; moral treatment; phototherapy

insanity board, 4, 62, 263

insanity commission, 37, 38, 63, 165, 167

interpreters, 12, 39, 183, 275, 282

investigations into abuses, 9, 22, 56, 121, 168, 197, 227, 240–41, 374n13; at Canton Asylum under Gifford, 75, 77, 80, 83–84, 93; at Canton Asylum under Hummer, 9, 109, 111–13, 139, 147–48, 150, 216–18, 224, 232, 236–37, 250–51, 275–76, 364n18. *See also* Silk, Samuel

jail, 4, 29–31, 32, 35, 36, 37, 64, 206–7, 208

Jobin, Lucie, 219–25, 227

Johnson, Rowley, 173–74, 369n1

Jones, William A., 21–22, 52

journals, professional, 15, 78, 124, 197, 202, 214, 219. See also *American Journal of Insanity*

Kanner, Leo, 212–14, 216

Karlson, G. W., 263

Kentuck, Peter, 130–31, 217–18, 269, 363n21, 375n12

Kirkbride, Thomas, 60

kiva, 276

Knights Templar, 213, 256

Knox, Katherine (Katy), 145, 364n13

Koepp, Doretta L., 236, 238–39, 240

Kraepelin, Emil, 201, 212–14, 373n7

Krulish, Emil, 219–20, 223–26, 229, 235–36, 238–40, 259, 276, 376n26

Landis, Ione, 145–49, 218, 259, 276, 364n14, 364n16, 364–65n18

language, 7, 12, 17, 28, 32, 51, 53, 66, 94, 103, 108, 109, 113, 162–63, 183, 190, 256, 353n7, 367n22; as barrier, 73, 128, 212; as barrier

language (*continued*)
for patients, 4, 33, 71, 129, 177, 180, 213, 220, 234, 237, 275, 282
Larrabee, C. F., 75, 76–77, 84, 85
Lasater, Miles, 370n7
laundry, 48, 176, 182–83, 200, 357n10
laundry (facility), 34, 105, 108, 110–11, 153, 160, 206, 249
Liberty Loan, 159, 232
Lincoln County, 23, 46, 159, 206, 263, 350n17, 354n4
livestock, 10, 55, 65, 189, 193–94, 219, 285; cattle, 64, 160, 164, 171, 217, 360n2
Logie, B. R., 85, 87, 358n19
Lowndes, Charles T., 252, 255, 259, 379n7
loyalty, 11, 46, 127, 140; in employees, 72, 75, 143, 178, 218, 280; disloyal employees, 224
Luepp, Francis, 84–85, 94, 250, 275, 362n3
Luhan, Antonio, 187, 188

magazines, 155, 189, 190, 352–53n41
malaria, 202, 374n8
McLean Asylum, 35, 123, 181
medicine man, 19, 59, 276
Medico-Legal Society, 78–79
mental classifications, 21, 201, 252
mental disorders: alcoholic insanity, 165, 167; amentia, 129–30; constitutional inferiority, 37, 234; dementia, 42, 47, 57, 124, 222, 234; dementia praecox, 100, 201, 233, 255, 360n20, 379n9; depression, 17, 132, 179, 211, 359n18; idiocy, 19, 21–22, 76, 94, 95, 130, 152, 234; imbecility, 21, 74, 129, 130, 133, 138, 153, 186, 229; mania, 37, 43, 176, 179, 254, 369n1; mania, acute, 18, 45, 99; melancholia, 73, 95, 201; moronic, 21–22, 129–31, 217, 230; nymphomania, 176, 369n1; paranoia, 17, 100, 192, 234; schizophrenia, 100, 201, 379n9. *See also* insanity
mental health, 3, 17, 29, 32, 41, 77, 203, 353n7
mental health care, 9, 67, 68, 70, 120, 281; in Alaska, 4, 277, 349n3; as a family matter, 29; organizations for, 157, 203, 276; reformers, 22–23, 119, 361–62n2
mental retardation, 21–22, 129
Meriam, Lewis, 227–28, 241, 253, 254;

Meriam Report by, 232, 241, 247
Meritt, Edgar B., 143, 205, 228, 253–54, 368n9; and asylum investigations, 148–49, 236–37, 276, 364–65n18; interest of, in asylum finances, 156, 191–92, 232, 367n15; 371n29, 377n9; intervention by, with patients, 156, 165–66, 168–71, 191
Michael, L. F., 147–49, 276, 364–65n18
Moen, G. J., 261–62, 267
moral treatment, 30
moth sickness, 19–20
movies, 174, 184, 230, 373n46
muckrakers, 120, 186, 189–90, 227
Murphy, Joseph A., 114–17, 259, 275

Nash, George, 91–93, 102, 115
National Committee for Mental Hygiene, 157, 203, 361n1
Native Americans: contact with Europeans, 9–11; cultural behaviors, 60, 129; as federal wards, 4, 14, 15, 64–65, 114, 168, 172, 184, 186, 187–88, 195, 245, 285; healing practices, 18, 19, 20, 27, 32, 270, 276–77, 279; illness among, 52, 97, 121; land holdings of, 52, 161, 172, 187–88; poverty among, 17, 98, 220, 353n7; on reservations, 32, 52. *See also* acreage; trachoma; tuberculosis
Navajos, 19–20, 28, 351n28
Newberne, R. E. L., 150, 156, 170, 172, 192–93, 367n23, 369n13
New Deal, 69–70, 253, 379n8
New Mexico, 74, 185, 187–89, 270
newspapers, 59, 85, 102, 115, 123, 125–26, 141, 142, 147, 198–99, 260, 283, 361–62n2; *Chicago Daily*, 67; *Daily Argus Leader*, 109, 116; *Detroit Free Press*, 90; *Hudsonite*, 67; *New York Sun*, 54; *Sioux Falls Daily Press*, 116–17; *Washington Post*, 21, 64, 69, 358n3, 367n20; *Washington Herald*, 78; *Washington Times*, 78. See also *Sioux Valley News*
New York (city), 38, 46, 120, 186, 187, 362n7
New York (state), 97, 120, 132, 156, 163, 191, 212
Night Chant, 351n20
Norbeck, Peter, 259–60, 265

nurses, 102, 180–81, 353n5; at Canton
Asylum, 86, 137, 192, 196, 203–4, 219–20,
223, 225–26, 228–29, 230–32, 233, 235, 249,
250–51, 258, 274; Hummer's clashes with,
235–40, 244; lack of, 39, 282, 283

occupational therapy, 42, 179, 196, 277
O'Keefe, Daniel, 61–62, 79, 85
Oklahoma, 121, 163, 227, 231, 240, 247
Omudis, Spot, 138, 139
operation, surgical, 81–82, 97, 98, 204,
373n2
Outlines of Psychiatry, 91, 99, 131
Owl, Allen, 174, 176, 370n5

Packard, Elizabeth, 38, 367n24; and Packard Laws, 38
paresis, 202, 211–12, 374n1
parole, parole privileges, 133, 168–69, 174,
175, 176–77, 194, 204, 364n28
patent (deed), 170, 171, 172
paternalism, 6, 65, 164, 183, 278
patients, Canton Asylum. *See* Canton
Asylum patients
pellagra, 179, 371n19
per capita costs, 78, 156, 191, 357n13, 366n9; at
Canton Asylum, 155, 156, 157, 185, 245, 259
Perry, Reuben, 75–78, 80, 84, 253
petitions, 108, 121, 133, 168, 170, 263, 266,
284–85, 368–69n10
Pettigrew, Richard F., 15–17, 20, 21–24, 50,
350–51n18
phototherapy, 178–79
physicians, 14, 39, 43, 80, 84, 89, 93, 107,
120, 148, 179, 198, 214, 223, 282, 353n10,
358n1, 364–65n18; inspecting Canton
Asylum, 238, 364–65n18; in the Interior
Department, 124, 159, 246, 267, 350n16; of
mental illness, 5, 38, 42–43, 45, 67, 90, 99,
114, 131, 149, 156–57, 180–81, 275. *See also*
Hardin, L. M., Hummer, Harry R.; Krulish, Emil; Michael, L. F.; Turner, John F.
Pinel, Philippe, 30
Poe, Charles, 61–62, 79, 85
policy, 187, 196, 225, 250, 273; mental health,
3, 257, 375n9; toward Native Americans,
2, 6, 13–14, 39, 183, 190, 274–75, 278,

350n12. *See also* assimilation
Porter, Isabella, 133–34
poverty, 17, 70, 98, 182, 220, 353n7
Pratt, Richard H., 28–29, 161–62
Preston-Engle Report, 228, 241
Pringle, R. M., 127
prison, 164, 221, 234, 243, 245, 374n13
prisoners, 31, 177
psychiatry, 44, 66, 124, 180, 183, 196–97,
201, 203, 219, 226; psychiatric assessment,
36, 60, 180, 212, 213, 354n2; psychiatric care, 28, 39, 57, 123, 201–2, 274, 281;
psychiatric exams and records, 4, 100,
181–82, 233, 242
psychoanalysis, 42, 180, 277
Public Works Administration, 253, 255, 263
pueblo (place), 187–88, 254, 270
Pueblos (people), 185, 187–88, 189, 196, 253,
254, 255, 270, 279n10

race, 15, 16, 17, 28, 91, 95, 132, 163–64, 195
racial theories, 15, 16–17, 176, 363n24
radiators, 25, 154, 232
range toilets, 25, 70, 87, 105, 138, 352n39
rations, 17, 52–53, 108, 109, 155, 164–65,
351n21
records, record keeping, 172, 233, 263, 269,
274, 282; at Canton Asylum, 37, 74, 93,
204, 213, 234, 235, 281, 373n5; Hummer's
failure at, 181, 183, 233, 242, 244, 256; at
other asylums, 79, 181, 197, 214, 224
Red Owl, Lizzie, 204, 213, 245
reform: of commitment laws, 38; of Indian
policy, 368n10; of mental health care, 119,
203; of societal ills, 120
reformers, 22–23, 120, 163, 227–28, 240–41,
265, 273, 275, 359n16. *See also* muckrakers
relatives of patients, 3, 27, 39, 61, 64, 125, 131,
220, 370n7; at Canton Asylum, 5, 27–28,
36, 130–31, 158, 166, 174, 182–83, 204, 213,
220, 222, 260, 363n21, 375n12; letters
from, 130–31, 133–44, 204, 230; at other
asylums, 31, 79, 80, 220
religion: religious garb, 121; religious
organization–sponsored schooling, 162;
religious practices, 254
reporters, 39, 120, 193, 361n2

reservation superintendent, 21, 95, 102, 141, 174, 183, 203, 217, 377n9
restraints, physical, 30, 41, 49, 57, 73, 99, 216, 280, 285, 375n9
Rhoads, Charles, 246, 249–52, 253
Rice Boarding School, 163
Ritter, Robert, 221, 224
rituals, healing, 18, 19, 32
Roberts, T. B., 218, 222–24, 225, 376n23
Roosevelt, Franklin (FDR), 253, 254, 260, 263, 379n8
Roosevelt, Teddy, 68, 91, 362n6
Rosebud Reservation, 265–66

salaries, 13, 243; of Canton Asylum medical staff, 108, 116, 214, 223, 245, 358n19; of other asylum employees, 54, 122, 153–54, 160, 216, 231, 244–45, 250
Santa Clara Pueblo, 254, 270
schools, 47, 74, 89, 109, 121, 162, 163–64, 180, 199, 225, 227–28, 354n4, 358n1; day schools, 33, 47, 152, 162, 368–69n10; proprietary, 89. See also Indian boarding schools
Schroder, Edith, 191, 249, 269
secretary of the interior, 21–22, 48, 52, 85, 121, 162, 184, 205, 245, 253, 256. See also Fall, Albert B.; Ickes, Harold; Wilbur, Ray L.; Work, Hubert
Seely, Charles, 54, 57, 67–68, 71–72, 74, 75, 82–85, 92, 93, 96, 106, 122
seizures, 19, 138–39, 183, 280; epileptic, 47–48, 57, 173, 354n6; "fits," 207, 213, 229, 371n23, 373n5; "spells," 73, 182, 185, 204, 254
servants, 35, 102, 104, 111, 113
Seventh District Medical Society, 150, 271
sewer system, 25, 55, 82, 127
Sells, Cato, 149, 160, 167, 169–72, 173
Shanahan, Frank, 73–75, 80
Shawano, Annie, 229–30; and brother James, 229
Short, Alice, 57
short-hair order, 52–53
Silk, Samuel, 1, 241, 246, 260–61, 263, 276; 1929 report by, 241–45, 247, 255; 1933 report by, 256–58, 264
Sioux Falls, South Dakota, 123, 127, 145, 206, 235, 237
Sioux Falls committee, 236, 237, 239, 240, 260–61, 267, 270–71, 357n5
Sioux Valley News, 71, 91, 92, 93, 122, 126, 139–40, 142, 193, 262, 359n12, 352n5, 363n11
Smith, Alice Stanton, 38–39
Smith, Martha (Kay-ge-gay-aush-oak), 101, 107–8, 109, 110, 113, 361n11
Smith, Mary J., 48–49, 71
Smithsonian Institution, 103, 121, 351n9
Smoots, Raymond, 137, 144
sod homes, 24, 69
"sons of the wild jackasses," 241
South Dakota, 17, 23, 46, 54, 64, 102, 126, 226, 238, 270; climate, 20, 55, 96–97, 127, 266; physical characteristics of, 21, 24, 27, 69, 73, 159; residents of, 20, 21, 37–38, 87, 102, 109, 157, 260, 269; Territory of, 23–24, 47; towns in, 41, 47, 85, 93–94, 116, 231, 356n16. See also Canton, South Dakota; Sioux Falls, South Dakota
souvenirs, 194, 198
spectrums of behavior, 180
spirits, 10–11, 17–18, 33, 145, 163
Stands By Him, Luke, 199, 235
St. Elizabeths (Government Hospital for the Insane), 22, 23, 31, 37, 49, 128, 157, 191, 197, 267; commitment to, 61; employees of, 79–80; Indian patients at, 22, 37, 246, 252, 260, 269, 352n35; investigation into, 78–80, 90, 95; leadership in mental health care, 180, 198, 246, 278
sterilization of patients, 132–33, 258, 280
Stevens, Walter S., 216–17
straitjacket, 1, 41, 80, 85, 119, 241
superstitions, 19, 32, 103, 129
Supreme Court, 13–14, 161, 187
surveys: medical, 98, 121; of mental institutions, 196, 237, 256; of government policy, 205, 227–28
syphilis, 42, 65, 202, 211, 212, 213–14, 257, 374n6

Tafoya, Cleto, 254–55, 270, 379n10, 380n3
Tafoya, Severa, 254–55
Teapot Dome, 205

telegrams, 84–85, 137, 259–60, 380n22

telegraphs, 85, 169, 206, 260

telephones, 41, 46, 57, 62, 68, 81, 96, 102, 145, 261, 357n6; Hummer's spat over, 110, 112, 113

Todd, Ida, 94

toilets, 33–34, 35, 49, 110, 138, 146, 154, 235, 243. *See also* range toilets

tonics, 49, 50–51, 179

tourists, 198–99, 255, 283

trachoma, 97–98, 121, 163, 359n15, 359n17

trade, 10–11, 13, 24

trading houses, 11–12, 349n4

training, 45, 53, 95, 114; of Canton staff, 39, 102, 154, 196; medical, 36, 89, 94, 150, 180–81, 198, 225, 226, 276, 358n1

trauma: head injuries, 179, 197; mental, 29, 33

treaties, 12–13, 14, 64, 161, 187; Fort Laramie Treaty, 14; Treaty of Guadalupe, 187; Yakama Treaty, 14

trephination, 197–98

tribes, 12, 14, 17–19, 51, 53, 161, 177, 227, 350n12, 367n22, 368n1

tubercular, 56, 96–97, 208, 244, 258

tuberculosis, 102, 121, 163, 174, 233, 258, 266, 269; deaths from, 96–97, 134, 158, 229, 242, 359n13

Tuke, William, 30, 353n4

Turner, John F., 48, 51, 53, 57, 74, 83–84, 87, 122–23, 155; conflict with Gifford, 74–76, 80; conflict with Hummer, 103, 106, 109, 114–15, 127; reports and correspondence of, 48, 56; trips by, 71–72, 74, 102. *See also* Brown, Charles

Two Crows, James, 138, 364n2

"unfortunates," 29, 76, 141, 150, 197, 359n9

United States, 11–16, 41, 42, 98, 128, 132, 156, 157, 161–62, 164, 180, 185, 188, 211–12, 232, 349n7; army, 15, 23, 91, 159, 180, 205, 208, 235, 367n22; navy, 23, 180, 205; public health service, 98, 179, 350n16, 371n19

Utica State Lunatic Asylum, Utica Asylum for the Insane, 63, 221

vaccines, 14–15, 101, 142, 350n15

Valentine, Robert G., 114–16, 121–22, 123, 126

Van Winkle, Herman, 219, 222–23, 224, 229, 375–76n23

Van Winkle, Martin, 137–39, 149, 166

Vaux, George, Jr., 193–94

Vipont, Lizzie, 73–76, 357n5, 357n10

Wagner-Jauregg, Julius, 202

Walker River Agency School, 163

Walking Day, Mary, 158

warehouses, 3, 183, 277

warehousing, 181

Washington, George, 11–12, 199

Washington DC, 20, 23, 25, 36, 45, 61, 66, 69, 89, 96, 111, 241, 279–80, 366n9; as seat of government, 74, 109, 116, 117, 142–43, 171, 188–89, 249, 254–55, 262–63; transferring patients to, 256, 260, 262, 266–67. *See also* St. Elizabeths (Government Hospital for the Insane)

Wassermann tests, 212–13, 374n5

well water, 56, 200

West, the (U.S.), 2, 14, 21, 41, 46, 62, 66, 69, 90, 97, 102, 221, 254, 256, 273, 280

westerners, 16, 128, 129, 241

Wheeler, Burton, 241, 253, 372n39

White, William A., 61–62, 85, 91, 99, 131–32, 176, 212, 245

Wilbur, Ray L., 245–46, 259, 276

Willoughby, W. F., 227–28

Wilson, Edith A., 230–31, 232–33, 234–35

Wishecoby, Susan, 159, 173, 194, 200–201, 221, 373n5

Work, Hubert, 205, 215, 359n16, 372n39

work as therapy, 34–35, 64–65, 200

World War I, 98, 159, 179, 180, 191, 205, 235, 367n22

Yankton State Hospital, 64, 165, 167, 168–69, 212–13, 214, 216, 263

Yells-at-Night, 96, 359n13

Yezza, Nakai, 129–30

CPSIA information can be obtained
at www.ICGtesting.com
Printed in the USA
LVHW091953011020
667694LV00002B/2/J

9 780803 280984